GLOBAL PERSPECTIVES ON BRONCHOSCOPY

Edited by **Sai Praveen Haranath**
and **Samiya Razvi**

Global Perspectives on Bronchoscopy
Edited by Sai Praveen Haranath and Samiya Razvi

Published by InTech
Janeza Trdine 9, 51000 Rijeka, Croatia

Publishing Process Manager Jana Sertic

Technical Editor Teodora Smiljanic

Cover Designer InTech Design Team

Additional hard copies can be obtained from orders@intechopen.com

Global Perspectives on Bronchoscopy, Edited by Sai Praveen Haranath and Samiya Razvi
p. cm.
ISBN 978-953-51-0642-5

Meet the editors

Dr Sai Praveen Haranath is a physician working at Apollo Hospitals, Hyderabad, India and is also part of one of the first Tele ICU programs in India. He did his MBBS at Madras Medical College and then went to the USA. Over 15 years in America he specialized Internal Medicine, Pulmonary and Critical Care Medicine and is American Board Certified in these fields. His training and employment included the University of Connecticut, Loyola University, Oregon Health and Science University and numerous other hospitals. He also obtained a Masters in Public Health degree. He is a Fellow of the American College of Chest Physicians and is on the steering committee of the Disaster Response Network, the Occupational and Environmental Diseases Network, and also part of the Marketing Committee of this global organization. He returned to India in 2011 to pursue his lifelong desire to raise the standard of Indian and global healthcare through the ethical practice of excellent medicine. He has expertise in fiberoptic bronchoscopy and advanced bronchoscopic procedures. His prior experience in rural, community and academic settings in the USA and most recent engagement at The Permanente Medical Group/ Kaiser Permanente in the San Francisco area and his current position at Apollo Hospitals in Hyderabad have given him experience in pulmonary medicine and bronchoscopic procedures.

Dr Samiya Razvi obtained her medical degree and Diploma in Child Health from Christian Medical College and Hospital, Vellore, India. She has experience in clinical research at the All India Institute of Medical Sciences New Delhi and in basic science research at the Department of Clinical Immunology, Mount Sinai Medical Center, New York. Dr Razvi trained in Pediatrics at Long Island College Hospital and Beth Israel Medical Center, New York. Following residency, she completed a 3-year fellowship in Pediatric Pulmonology at the Morgan Stanley Children's Hospital of New York Presbyterian, Columbia University, New York. She obtained Board Certification in Pediatrics from the American Board of Pediatrics and subspecialty board certification in Pediatric Pulmonology, American Board of Pediatrics. Her keen interest in clinical research led her to pursue and obtain a Master's degree in Biostatistics, Patient Oriented Research Track in 2007, from the Mailman School of Public Health, Columbia University, New York. Dr Razvi worked as Staff Pediatric Pulmonologist at Children's Hospital at Cleveland Clinic, Ohio, where in addition to clinical responsibilities, she actively participated in resident and trainee teaching and as a mentor in research. She was awarded the Teacher of the Year, 2008 at the Pediatric Institute, Children's Hospital at Cleveland Clinic. Currently, she is Consultant Pediatric Pulmonologist at Apollo Hospitals, Jubilee Hills,Hyderabad, India. She continues to be involved in teaching and mentoring post-graduate trainees and is the Chairman of the Thesis Committee for post-graduateresearch. Dr Razvi's areas of clinical interest are pediatric asthma, lung disease of prematurity, cystic fibrosis and pediatric flexible bronchoscopy.

Contents

Preface

Bronchoscopy has become an essential part of modern medicine. Recent advances in technology have allowed integration of ultrasound with this tool. The use of lasers along with bronchoscopes has increased the therapeutic utility of this device. Globally an increasing number of pulmonary specialists, anaesthesiologists and thoracic surgeons are using the bronchoscope to expedite diagnosis and treatment. The current volume on bronchoscopy adds to the vast body of knowledge on this topic. The contributions from around the world cover the breadth of this field and include cutting edge uses as well as a section on pediatric bronchoscopy.

This was a tough job for me as an editor of the book, since the authors wrote vast and extensive chapters . It was a great experience. I would request readers to review the book and suggest areas for modification or further topic additions for future versions. Every care has been taken to ensure the accuracy of information and authors are aware of the strict rules against plagiarism. The book is divided in various sections in order to make it easier for the beginner, as well as the advanced reader to have a rapid overview of this topic. The section on pediatric bronchoscopy highlights issues specific to children that are recognizably different from adults, including airway anatomy, anesthesia considerations and the emerging field of diagnostic and therapeutic procedures in this age group. A major indication for bronchoscopy in infants and young children continues to be evaluation for congenital airway malformations, and both common and uncommon disorders are reviewed with illustrations in this text.

As a pulmonary and critical care physician it has been fulfilling to see the chapters on special areas like bronchoscopy in bronchiectasis as well as in the intensive care unit. Practical uses like managing and monitoring the airway during percutaneous tracheostomy performance has an entire chapter devoted to this evolving topic . In summary, this book is a great testament to the power of collaboration and is a superb resource for doctors in training, ancillary team members as well as practicing healthcare providers who have to perform or arrange bronchoscopy or the similar procedures. I would like to sincerely thank my associate editor Dr Samiya Razvi for ensuring the pediatric section to integrate well into this comprehensive book. I am grateful to InTech as well as Jana Sertic, my coordinator, for her patient yet firm requests for expediting this book. I hope the readers will find this book enjoyable for reading and that they will recignize a contemporary source of knowledge in our book.

Dr. Sai Praveen Haranath
Consultant Pulmonologist and Critical Care Medicine Specialist,
Axon Anesthesia Associates, Hyderabad,
Apollo Hospitals, Jubilee Hills, Hyderabad,
India

Dr. Samiya Razvi
Consultant Pediatric Pulmonologist,
Apollo Hospitals, Jubilee Hills, Hyderabad,
India

Section 1

Basics of Bronchoscopy

1

Role of Flexible-Bronchoscopy in Pulmonary and Critical Care Practice

Gilda Diaz-Fuentes and Sindhaghatta K. Venkatram
*Division of Pulmonary and Critical Care Medicine,
Bronx Lebanon Hospital Center, Bronx, New York
USA*

1. Introduction

The introduction of the flexible bronchoscope by Dr. Ikeda in 1968 revolutionized bronchoscopy around the world. Initially, bronchoscopy was performed by surgical specialists with a rigid scope only in highly specialized centers, and the main indication was for therapeutic purposes. In the 1970s, flexible fiberoptic bronchoscopy (FFB) was learned by pulmonologists and surgical specialists and proved itself as a safe and useful technique for diagnostic and therapeutic purposes. The results have been a rapid proliferation of FFB inside and outside of the academic institutions.

In the armamentarium of the pulmonary physician, FFB assumes a central position that is somewhere between the noninvasive diagnostic maneuvers such as physical examination, laboratory study, pulmonary function testing and radiologic diagnostics on one side and invasive surgical procedures such as mediastinoscopy and diagnostic thoracotomy on the other side.

A recent trend has been the emergence of "interventional bronchoscopy" and the "interventional bronchoscopist". These phrases denote a two-tier system in which one group of bronchoscopists perform "routine bronchoscopy" and the other performs special bronchoscopic procedures. Disease processes encompassed within this discipline include complex airway management problems, benign and malignant central airway obstruction, pleural diseases, and pulmonary vascular procedures. Diagnostic and therapeutic procedures pertaining to these areas include, but are not limited to, rigid bronchoscopy, transbronchial needle aspiration (TBNA), auto fluorescence bronchoscopy, endobronchial ultrasound (EBUS), transthoracic needle aspiration (TTNA) and biopsy, laser bronchoscopy, endobronchial electrosurgery, argon-plasma coagulation, cryotherapy, airway stent insertion, balloon bronchoplasty and dilatation techniques, endobronchial radiation, photodynamic therapy, percutaneous dilatational tracheotomy, transtracheal oxygen catheter insertion, medical thoracoscopy, and imaging-guided thoracic interventions. (Anders et al. 1988)

Considering the prominence of FFB in the procedural armamentarium of pulmonary physicians (among other specialties) and the new developments of interventional bronchoscopy, it is important for the non-interventional pulmonologist and physician in pulmonary training to have a clear understanding of the role of FFB.

The objective of this review is to describe the place of non-interventional FFB in the practice of modern pulmonary and critical care medicine, to review the indications, contraindications and limitations of the procedure and to discuss the role of FFB in modern intensive care units (ICUs). The versatility of the flexible bronchoscope, combined with its portability, allows one to perform the technique at the bedside, and this is of major importance in the unstable patient, who is often unable to be transported safely to the bronchoscopy suite.

2. Facilities, personnel, pre-procedure investigation and monitoring

In order to perform a FFB, a well-equipped facility, trained personnel, pre-procedure evaluation, and monitoring is highly recommended. Bronchoscopies can be performed in a bronchoscopy suite, operating room, at the bedside and in the outpatient setting. The planned bronchoscopic procedures, the availability of equipment and ancillary personnel and resources will dictate the best and safe place for the FFB.

Prior to the procedure, the patient's history must be taken and a thorough physical examination must be given. The physician must obtain information on previous therapies and current performance status. Laboratory tests (e.g. complete blood count, coagulation profile and renal function) are usually obtained despite routine preoperative coagulation screening not being recommended in patients with no risk factors for complications. (Kozak & Brath, 1994)

A minimum requirement is the availability of cardiorespiratory monitoring and oxygen and resuscitation equipment. The bronchoscopist and nursing staff should have appropriate training for the procedure to be performed. Conscious sedation can be administered by a skilled bronchoscopist or anesthesiologist. If procedures are performed under general anesthesia, the presence of an anesthesiologist and specialist nurse should be added. (European Respiratory Society/American Thoracic Society [ERS/ATS], 2002; Becker at al. 1991)

3. Fiberoptic bronchoscopic techniques

Flexible bronchoscopy is preferably performed via the transnasal approach by many bronchoscopists after appropriate topical anesthesia and conscious sedation. A complete inspection of all segments of both lungs is carried out to exclude significant endobronchial abnormalities. The following section will describe the most common bronchoscopic techniques used by the non-interventional pulmonologist.

Bronchial washings

Bronchial washings are the secretions aspirated back through the bronchoscope channel after instillation of saline into a major airway. Secretions obtained by this method do not represent material from the bronchiolar or alveolar level and in non-intubated patients they may be contaminated by secretions from the upper airway.

The main use of bronchial washings is for diagnosing pneumonia caused by strictly pathogenic organisms, such as Mycobacterium tuberculosis and endemic systemic fungi. In addition, bronchial washing can be used to collect specimens for cytology in suspected malignancy.

Protected-specimen brushing (PSB)

Protected-specimen brushing is a telescoping plugged catheter passed through the suction channel of the bronchoscope. Once beyond the tip of the scope, the internal sheet is extended, its gelatin plug expelled, and the sterile brush is dipped into either the visible airway secretions or passed more distally into the involved pulmonary segment. The brush is retrieved by reversal of the process, and then cut into a sterile container with 1mL of buffer or broth. In the microbiology laboratory, the sample is quantitatively cultured. Most investigators use the cutoff of 10^3 cfu/ml for differentiation of infection from contamination. The main value of PSB is for the diagnosis of bacterial pneumonia; therefore, only quantitative culture and possibly Gram stain of the secretions obtained by the brushing justify its use.

Bronchial brushings

The bronchial brush catheter is inserted in a similar way as the PSB. The cytology brush is stiffer than the PSB, so it makes it easier to obtain cellular material from the airway wall. The main indication for bronchial brushes is for the cytologic diagnosis of malignancies or viral inclusion bodies in airway cells. There is a slight increase in mucosal bleeding.

Bronchoalveolar lavage (BAL)

In comparison to bronchial washing, BAL samples a much larger airway and alveolar area. It is estimated that approximately 1 million alveoli (1% of the lung surface) are sampled, with approximately 1 ml of actual lung secretions returned in the total lavage fluid. Bronchoalveolar lavage requires careful wedging of the tip of the bronchoscope into the desired airway lumen, isolating that airway from the rest of the central airways. Wedging is defined as the position where the scope cannot be advanced while the distal lumen is still visible. Then, normal saline in 30 to 60 ml aliquots are instilled two or three times and after 2 respiratory cycles the fluid is intermittently suctioned out to a trap with low suction. The first 20 ml which are secretions found in the subsegmental bronchus is usually discarded as this is not representative of alveolar lavage The returned volume varies with the amount instilled but is generally 10 to 100 ml. The number of lavages needed is based on return and the number of tests ordered. In our institution the bronchoscopy nurse informs us of the adequacy of the sample.

Bronchoalveolar lavage has been proven to be very safe and can be done without fluoroscopy. The diagnostic threshold for BAL fluid has been reported to be 10^4 cfu/ml for quantitative and 10^5 for non-quantitative cultures. Bronchoalveolar lavage is the mainstay of bronchoscopic diagnosis in the immunosuppressed patient when looking for an infectious process. In addition, BAL has diagnostic utility in eosinophilic pneumonias, pulmonary alveolar proteinosis, and pulmonary malignancies especially lymphangitic carcinomatosis. (Baughman, 2007)

Transbronchial biopsy (TBBx)

This technique is performed wedging the scope in the segmental bronchus of interest, and then passing the biopsy forceps through the working channel of the scope. Fluoroscopy can assist to visualize the forceps entering the pulmonary sub segment. The biopsy forceps is advanced to the periphery of the diseased region until resistance is met. Placement of the biopsy forceps near, but not at the lung surface minimizes the risk of pneumothorax. Subsequently, the forceps is withdrawn approximately 1 cm, and the jaws are opened and advanced slightly to obtain the sample of the lung. The forceps is then advanced close to the area where resistance was encountered, and the jaws are closed. In case the patient reports pain at this point, the forceps is opened and withdrawn; only the visceral pleura is pain-sensitive.

The biopsy forceps is firmly retracted to obtain the sample which is placed in formalin and sent for histopathologic evaluation.

Ideally, 4 to 6 transbronchial biopsy specimens should be obtained, with at least 1 sample containing full-thickness bronchial mucosa and some alveolar parenchyma. The number of biopsy specimens required for optimal diagnostic yield has been reported to be 4 to 10; BTS guidelines recommend 4–6 samples in diffuse lung disease and 7–8 samples in focal lung disease. (British Thoracic Society Bronchoscopy [BTS], 2001)

We routinely disconnect the patient from the respirator for a couple of seconds during the initial part of forceps withdrawal. If there is any bleeding the scope is wedged to allow for clot formation. Other options include instillation of cold saline or topical epinephrine.

Transbronchial biopsy specimens are examined by histological techniques to exclude infections, malignancies or other disorders. Specimens can also be placed in sterile saline and cultured. TBBx have been shown to increase the diagnosis of PCP in AIDS patients by 15 %. The most important role for TBBx is probably the documentation of noninfectious etiologies. (Prakash at al., 1991; American Thoracic Society [ATS], 1987)

A comparison of the yield of transbronchial biopsy specimen between standard-sized forceps and large forceps found no significant differences in the size of the biopsies or in the amount of alveolar tissue collected. (Wang et al., 1980; Loube et al., 1993)

The tissue samples obtained by means of TBBx forceps are small, approximately 3 mm in size. Therefore, this procedure is not useful in diagnosing heterogeneous lung diseases such as idiopathic lung diseases.

Transbronchial needle aspiration (TBNA)

Transbronchial needle aspiration through the flexible bronchoscope was developed in the early 1980s for the diagnosis and staging of lung cancer. The most important indication for transbronchial needle aspiration is the mediastinal staging of lung cancer. The lymph node stations as defined by the TNM system are easily accessible with TBNA, which is cost-effective and reduces the need for exploratory surgery. TBNA have been incorporated in the training of basic bronchoscopic skills. For a detailed review, the reader is directed to some excellent reviews on the topic. (ERS/ATS, 2002; Dasgupta & Mehta, 1999)

To obtain a specimen, the needle assembly is introduced through the working channel of the bronchoscope with the needle retracted within the metal hub of the catheter. The scope is kept as straight as possible, with its distal tip in the neutral position. These precautions are necessary to prevent damaging the working channel of the scope. Once the metal hub is visible at the distal end of the scope, the needle is advanced and locked in place. The catheter is retracted until only the tip of the needle is visible at the end of the scope. The scope is advanced to the target, and the tip of the needle is anchored into the intercartilaginous space. At this stage, the goal is to penetrate the tracheobronchial wall at an angle as close to perpendicular as possible.

For peripheral lesions, TBNA should be performed with fluoroscopic guidance.

The diagnostic yield of transbronchial needle aspiration for staging of lung cancer varies between 15- 83%, with a positive predictive values of 90-100%. In evaluating peripheral lung nodules, TBNA increases the diagnostic yield of bronchoscopy by 20-25% by facilitating the sampling of lesions that are inaccessible with the forceps or brush. Transbronchial needle aspiration has also been shown to improve the yield in the evaluation of submucosal disease, sarcoidosis, and mediastinal lymphadenopathy in acquired immune deficiency syndrome (AIDS) patients. (ERS/ATS, 2002; Dasgupta &Mehta, 1999; Wang et al., 1983; Ceron et al., 2007)

In the last decades we have seen the introduction of several bronchoscopic diagnostic techniques which include, among others, endobronchial ultrasound, auto fluorescence bronchoscopy and electromagnetic navigation. The aim of these modalities is to increase the diagnostic yield of bronchoscopy and minimize the need for more invasive procedures.

However, such specialized innovations are limited to specialized centers and in general do not reflect the application of this technique in routine clinical practice. In recent years, TBNA has been incorporated as a routine in the bronchoscopy suite and is part of the routine training of pulmonary fellows.

The use of endobronchial ultrasound -transbronchial needle aspiration (EBUS-TBNA) is a relatively new, minimally invasive and an emerging diagnostic modality that has proven utility in the evaluation of patients with lung cancer for the assessment of mediastinal and hilar lymph nodes, and diagnosis of lung and mediastinal tumors. (Herth et al., 2006)

4. Indications for flexible bronchoscopy

The traditional and newer indications for diagnostic and therapeutic bronchoscopies permit greater latitude in the application of the procedure. Several reports including the North American survey on bronchoscopy reveals that the most common indications for bronchoscopy are the evaluation of suspicious lesions (nodules and masses), hemoptysis, pneumonia and infections, diffuse pulmonary process, and therapeutic. (Prakash at al., 1991; ATS,1987; Alamoudi et al., 2000) A study looking at 124 consecutive bronchoscopies, showed that suspicion of pulmonary tuberculosis (31%), lung mass (19%) and hemoptysis (18%) were the most common indications for the procedure. (Alamoudi et al., 2000) Although the availability of flexible bronchoscopy has been a major advance in adult pulmonary medicine, its role in pediatrics has remained less well defined. The most common indications for the procedure in the pediatric literature included stridor, abnormal chest roentgenogram and airway evaluation. (Brown et al., 1983; Nicolai, 2001)

It is not uncommon to perform diagnostic and therapeutic bronchoscopies simultaneously. In one study of 198 bronchoscopies performed in critical care units, 47% were done for therapeutic reasons, 44% for diagnostic reasons, and 9% for both. (Bellomo et al., 1992)

The major indications for diagnostic bronchoscopy are listed in Table 1. The overall yield of diagnostic bronchoscopy depends on the indication and the techniques used during the procedure and vary from 45% to 80%. The most common indication for diagnostic FFB is suspected malignancy, infection or tuberculosis. (Prakash at al., 1991; Joos et al., 2006)

Mass/nodule/ suspicious lesion/cancer
Hemoptysis
Pneumonia/infection
Diffuse/interstitial disease in a non-immunocompromised patient
Diffuse infiltrative pulmonary disorders in immunocompromised patients
Unexplained cough or wheezing
Persistent purulent sputum of unknown etiology
Trachea/ stridor/ vocal cord paralysis/hoarseness
Superior vena cava syndrome
Extrapulmonary symptoms with frequent pulmonary and bronchial involvement
Thermal/chemical injury
Suspected tracheo-esophageal fistula
Abnormal radiographic findings
Evaluation of abnormal pulmonary function testing like central airway stenosis
To evaluate complications of artificial airway
Tracheobronchial obstruction
Progressive or non- resolving pneumonias.
Complications in lung transplant recipients
Specific Indication in the ICU
Ventilator associated Pneumonia
Endotracheal tube placement confirmation
Airway trauma, Bronchial stump dehiscence
Smoke and Inhalational injury
Double lumen intubation for independent lung ventilation

Table 1. Indications for Diagnostic Bronchoscopy

Indications for therapeutic bronchoscopy are listed in Table 2. Often, bronchoscopy is done for diagnostic and therapeutic purposes- for example patients with airway obstruction with placement of stent, or hemoptysis. No indication is absolutely restricted to a specific location; with the current portability of the bronchoscope and the advances in monitoring and bedside care, many hospitals provide ventilator care or advanced care to patients in areas other than the intensive care unit.

Difficult intubation of airway and assessment of tube placement
Retained secretions and atelectasis
Foreign body in the tracheobronchial tree
Atelectasis/lobar collapse
Debridement of necrotic tracheobronchial mucosa
Dilatation of strictures and stenosis
Pneumothorax (fibrin glue therapy)
Delivery of brachytherapy
Percutaneous tracheostomy
Drainage of lung abscess/bronchogenic cysts
Thoracic trauma
Laser bronchoscopy
Photodynamic therapy
Electrocautery / Cryotherapy

Table 2. Indications for Therapeutic Bronchoscopy

4.1 Most common indications for bronchoscopy

4.1.1 Lung cancer

The flexible bronchoscope has become the main diagnostic tool in the evaluation of patients suspected of lung cancer, with more than 70% of lung carcinomas being approachable via bronchoscopy. Additionally, bronchoscopy plays an important role in the disease staging and an extended role in delivering therapeutic modalities. Regarding staging of the malignancy, bronchoscopy may help to determine the extension of the tumor. Bronchoscopic findings of vocal cord paralysis, tumor to the level of the right tracheobronchial junction or within 2 cm of the left tracheobronchial junction, and carinal or tracheal involvement are evidence of advanced stages of the malignancy.

An advantage of flexible bronchoscopy is that it is safe, well tolerated and readily available in most places. The flexibility of the bronchoscope allows the inspection of most of the fourth order and often up to sixth order bronchi and the direct assessment of the color and vascularity of the mucosa.

Routine bronchoscopic techniques include bronchial washings and lavage, brushings, and transbronchial biopsies. These may be augmented by the use of needle aspiration with or without the use of endobronchial ultrasound. It is still unclear if the combination of cytologic and histologic procedures provides the best diagnostic yield for lung cancer, but probably depends on the local expertise. (Alamoudi et al., 2000; Garg et al., 2007)

The diagnostic yield of bronchoscopy for malignancy depends on the location and the size of the lesion as well as the experience of the bronchoscopist.

Central endobronchial lesions carry the highest diagnostic yield of more than >90%, whereas small peripheral lesions have lower yield and usually require additional time and techniques. In visible, but intramural rather than endobronchial tumors, the diagnostic yield decreases to around 55% and is reduced further when the tumor lies beyond the bronchoscopist's vision. (Mazzone et al., 2002; El-Bayoumi & Silvestri, 2008; Gasparini et al., 1995)

The presentation of central tumors varies from an exophytic lesion, with partial or total occlusion of the bronchial lumen, to peribronchial tumors with extrinsic compression of the airway, or with submucosal infiltration of tumor. Peribronchial tumors or lesions with submucosal infiltration produce subtle changes in the mucosa that includes changes in mucosal color and vascularity, loss of bronchial markings, and nodularity of the mucosal surface. The yield of endobronchial biopsies is highest for exophytic lesions, with a diagnostic yield of approximately 90%. Central lesions are best approached with a combination of bronchial washes and brushings, and at least three to five endobronchial biopsies.

The addition of transbronchial needle aspiration may improve the yield and should be considered in submucosal lesions and peribronchial disease and extrinsic compression. The TBNA needle should be inserted into the submucosal plane at an oblique angle, and in patients with peribronchial disease and extrinsic compression, the needle should be passed through the bronchial wall into the lesion. Occasionally, the presence of crush artifact or surface necrosis will give a low yield of endobronchial biopsies for this kind of lesion. (Schreiber & McCrery, 2003; Dasgupta & Mehta, 1999) In general, the diagnostic yield is increased with the use of multiple bronchoscopic techniques.

Peripheral lesions are usually approached with a combination of bronchoscopic techniques like bronchial wash, brushes, biopsies and needle aspiration. The main determinants for the bronchoscopic diagnostic yield for peripheral lesions include:

- the size of the lesion: the diagnostic yield of bronchoscopy for lesions smaller than 3 cm varies from 14% to 50% compared with a yield of 46% to 80% for lesions larger than 3 cm.
- the distance of the lesion from the hilum and the relationship between the lesion and bronchus; a chest computed tomogram showing the presence of a bronchus sign predicts a higher yield of bronchoscopy for peripheral lung lesions.

The use of fluoroscopy increases the diagnostic yield from bronchoscopy in focal lung lesions. Fluoroscopy carries the limitation of being time consuming, requires some experience, and is not readily available in all centers. A lesion that is too small and not visible by fluoroscopy during the bronchoscopy poses a diagnostic challenge and often times require further surgical biopsy procedures. Endobronchial ultrasound and electromagnetic navigation are exciting new technologies that could help to increase the diagnostic yield in those cases. (Gasparini, 1997; Cortese & McDougall 1979; Yung, 2003; Liam et al., 2007)

The diagnostic yield of the TBBx can be significantly increased up to 73% by combining bronchoscopy with computed tomogram (CT) guidance in a dedicated low-dose protocol. The sensitivity of transbronchial biopsy for a solitary pulmonary nodule with multislice CT guidance has been reported to be 62.2% compared with 52.6% with fluoroscopic guidance. (Tsushima et al., 2006; Hautmann et al., 2010) The diagnostic yield of bronchoalveolar lavage alone for primary lung cancer is in the lower 30% for peripheral lung lesions. (De Gracia et al. 1993; Fabin et al., 1975; Fedullo & Ettensohn, 1985; Semenzato et al., 1990)

In a study of 162 patients with malignant lung infiltrates the BAL showed increased sensitivity in cases of bronchoalveolar cell carcinoma (93%) and lymphangitic carcinomatosis (83%). (Rennard, 1990)

The objective of staging for non-small cell lung cancer in the absence of distant metastases is the evaluation of mediastinal lymph node involvement. This is decisive to determine the prognosis and treatment plan for the patient. Nonsurgical staging includes minimally invasive needle biopsy techniques such as transbronchial or transthoracic needle aspiration and esophageal or endobronchial endoscopic ultrasound-guided fine-needle aspiration.

The reported diagnostic yield for EBUS-TBNA of lymph nodes is as high as 93% with a sensitivity, specificity, and accuracy of 94%, 100%, and 94%, respectively; positive predictive value of 100% and negative predictive value of 11%.(Herth et al.,2006)

A detailed discussion of EBUS if beyond the scope of this review, but the bronchoscopist must be aware that for those patients with known or suspected lung cancer, EBUS alone or in combination with EUS-FNA could likely replace more invasive and expensive surgical techniques. (Spiro & Porter, 2002; Gomez & Silvestri, 2009)

The use of Rapid On-site Evaluation (ROSE) has been shown to reduce the incidence of inadequate specimens which is an important cause of non-diagnostic TBNA aspirates. Several studies showed an increase of 15 to 25% in the diagnostic yield for malignancy and a decrease in the number of inadequate specimens. The overall reported diagnostic yield when ROSE is used is up to 80% when compared with a 50% yield when specimens are processed in the usual manner. The concordance between the preliminary diagnosis made in the bronchoscopy suite and the final diagnosis after subsequent review of material in the cytopathology laboratory was 87%, suggesting that ROSE of needle aspirate is fairly accurate but not perfect. Disadvantage of ROSE is the requirement of an expert and readily available cytopathologist in the bronchoscopy suite which involves extra time and effort. (Baram et al., 2005; Davenport, 1990; Uchida et al., 2006)

4.1.2 Pulmonary infections

The clinical-radiological and routine laboratory features of pulmonary infections often offer clues to the microbial cause of the infection, but the specific etiologic diagnosis usually requires the assistance of the microbiology laboratory.

Fiberoptic bronchoscopy is frequently used as part of the diagnostic investigation of suspected pulmonary infections in those cases where noninvasive tests have been non-diagnostic. The various methods used are bronchoscopic lavage, brushing, biopsies and occasionally TBNA which frequently are performed together to identify potential pathogens. Quantitative cultures of the specimen collected are performed to differentiate colonization from real pathogens. Rapid diagnosis is important, especially in immunocompromised patients.

In the past, bronchoscopy has been used to obtain specimens for the identification of pathogenic organisms, such as tuberculosis, in otherwise smear-negative cases, but its role in the diagnosis of lung infections in general has been limited. As a consequence of the rapid increase in the population of immunocompromised patients due to organ transplantation, human immunodeficiency virus (HIV) infection and increased use of chemotherapeutic agents, the last decade has seen an increase in the number of patients with life-threatening pneumonia or resistant microorganisms.

Community acquired pneumonia

The role of bronchoscopy for community acquired pneumonia (CAP) is not clearly defined. Bronchoscopy help to retrieve specimens from the lower airway in those patients not able to produce sputum and, in addition, can identify endobronchial obstructions and other processes mimicking pneumonia.(Gross et al., 1991; Lynch & Sitrin,1993; Wintrbauer, 1995)

In community acquired pneumonia the causative organism is not identified in more than 40% of cases despite an aggressive search. The use of early bronchoscopy, especially prior to the initiation of antibiotics, has been shown to increase the identification of a specific microorganism. One study reported a yield of 54% to 85% with PSB for potential pathogens. (Jimenez et al., 1993) The use of BAL may be useful in the evaluation of pneumonia with quantitative cultures of specimens correlating well with PSB results. However, a more accurate diagnosis may not significantly change antibiotic or clinical management.

Patients who present with severe pneumonia or who fail to improve or worsen during their hospitalization despite treatment with antibiotics may require further testing with bronchoscopy. Delayed resolution of pneumonia or suspicion of neoplasm should prompt the physician to perform a FFB. (Jimenez et al., 1993; Bates et al., 1992; Torres et al., 1991)

Progressive or non-resolving pneumonias

Majority of patients with CAP recover after appropriate antimicrobial therapy with about 10-15% of cases having no clinical improvement and they are categorized as non-responding or progressive pneumonia. (Arancibia et al., 2000)

Progressive pneumonias are defined as actual clinical deterioration, with acute respiratory failure requiring ventilatory support and/or septic shock, usually occurring within the first 72 h of hospital admission. Non-resolving pneumonias refer to absence of clinical stability after 3 days of antibiotics. (Mandell et al., 2007)

Causes include host factors, inappropriate microbiological therapy (uncommon pathogens) and non infective causes mimicking pneumonia. Non infective differential diagnosis includes acute eosinophilic pneumonia, acute cryptogenic organizing pneumonia, acute sarcoidosis, acute hypersensitivity pneumonitis, pulmonary alveolar proteinosis and others. (Gross et al., 1991; Lynch & Sitrin,1993; Wintrbauer, 1995) Bronchoscopy can establish the diagnosis in many of the infections as well as in non-infectious etiologies like acute eosinophilic pneumonia, diffuse alveolar hemorrhage or damage, pulmonary alveolar proteinosis, lipoid pneumonia, eosinophilic granulomas, and rarely rapidly progressing neoplasms. The use of TBBx can add additional diagnosis in selected patients. (Bulpa et al.,2003)

Ventilator associated pneumonia

Ventilator associated pneumonia (VAP) is a common health care associated infection, that develops in patients on mechanical ventilation and complicates the hospital course in 8-28% of patients on mechanical ventilation. (Haley et al., 1981; Pennington, 1990; Chastre & Fagon, 1994; Centers for Disease Control and Prevention [CDC] MMWR 2000; National Nosocomial Infections Surveillance [NNIS] System.1999)

The crude mortality ranges from 30 to 50%; however attributable mortality ranges widely from 5.8% to 18.8%. (Esperatti et al., 2010; Nguile-Makao et al., 2010; Muscedere et al., 2008)

Early and appropriate antimicrobial therapy has been advocated to decrease complication rates and mortality. (Celis et al., 1988; Luna et al., 1997; Kollef & Ward 1998)

Chest radiographic abnormalities are common in ventilated patients and some of the differential diagnosis includes atelectasis, pneumonia, drug reactions, and pulmonary embolism. Diagnosis of VAP remains a diagnostic challenge with a potential for overuse of antibiotics. To aid in decision making, Pugin et al. suggested the clinical pulmonary infection score (CPIS); a score higher than 6 having a high predictive value for the diagnosis of VAP.(Pugin et al., 1991; Alvarez-Lerma, 1996; Fabregas et al., 1999; Fischer et al., 1998; Flanagan et al., 2000; Singh et al., 2000) A subsequent trial comparing inter observer variability of CPIS score for the diagnosis of VAP, revealed a sensitivity of 83% and specificity of 17% with a area under receiver operating characteristic (AROC) of 0.55 ,when CPIS score was compared with qualitative BAL fluid cultures. (Schurink et al., 2004)

Fagon et al. reported reduced 14-day mortality with the use of a bronchoscopic bacteriologic strategy compared with a clinical strategy alone. (Fagon et al., 2000)

The use of TBBx could increase the diagnostic yield especially in patients with unexplained pulmonary infiltrates. Bronchoscopy can aid to distinguish between colonization and infection in those patients. (Pechkam & Elliott, 2002)

Aspiration pneumonia

Aspiration of stomach contents is a major cause of morbidity and mortality in adults and is a risk factor for acute respiratory distress syndrome. Bronchoscopy is indicated in patients with chemical pneumonia and when aspiration of a foreign body or food material is suspected. Aspirated material is frequently liquid in nature and disperses rapidly. Hence, routine FFB with lavage is not indicated. However, in the event that the aspirate is predominantly particulate in nature with radiographic evidence of lobar collapse or major atelectasis, therapeutic bronchoscopy is helpful.

Bronchoscopy has an important role in diagnosing airway injury and confirming tracheobronchial damage secondary to orally aspirated caustic material. Bronchoscopy may be helpful in guiding antibiotic therapy. This procedure is useful when ruling out the presence of an obstructing neoplasm in anaerobic bacterial pneumonia with lung abscess; however, bronchoscopy is not useful in the treatment of community-acquired aspiration pneumonia. (Kollef et al., 1995; Raghavendran et al., 2011)

Tuberculosis

Tuberculosis (TB) remains a threat with the increased traveling, globalization, HIV epidemic, and immigration. Those patients suspected to have TB and who have no sputum or sputum smear negative for acid fast bacilli seem to benefit the most from bronchoscopy.

Comparison of various bronchoscopic techniques showed that the yield of bronchoalveolar lavage for tuberculosis is superior to bronchial washings. Transbronchial biopsy and bronchial brushing cultures provided little additional diagnostic yield. Bronchoscopy can give immediate diagnosis when there is a positive smear from BAL fluid or caseating granulomas in the TBBx. Occasionally an alternative diagnosis can be found. (Venkateshiah & Mehta, 2003; Kobashi et al., 2007)

Fungal infections

Fungal infections contribute to significant morbidity and mortality in immunocompromised patients and bronchoscopy is useful in the diagnosis of these infections. PJP is a common infection in the immunocompromised and the diagnostic yield for BAL is up to 98 %. (Huang et al., 2006)

Aspergillus is a colonizer of the tracheobronchial tree and tissue diagnosis is necessary for the diagnosis. BAL fluid may suggest the development of invasive disease (Cahill et al., 1997), but does not establish the diagnosis. Newer techniques like BAL galactomannan levels which have a good sensitivity and specificity for the detection of invasive disease could be promising for the diagnosis (Meersseman et al.,2008; Hsu et al., 2010; Maertens et al., 2009); however, false-positive results are seen. (Digby et al., 2003)

Candida is a frequent colonizer and their presence in BAL fluid may represent colonization rather than infection in the immunocompetent host.(el-Ebiary et al.,1997)

In patients with non-resolving pneumonias in endemic areas, morphological and cytological analysis may aid in therapy of endemic mycoses like histoplasmosis, blastomycosis, coccidioidomycosis and paracoccidioidomycosis; however culture is diagnostic.

4.1.3 Diffuse lung diseases

Interstitial lung diseases

The interstitial lung diseases (ILDs), are a diverse group of pulmonary disorders classified together because of similar clinical, radiological, physiologic, or pathologic characteristics. The patient with suspected ILD presents a diagnostic challenge to physicians.

The role of bronchoscopy for the diagnosis of ILD's is limited due to the small size of the biopsies. Several studies have shown that the accuracy of TBBx for the diagnosis of ILD's is only 7 to 37% in immunocompetent patients. (Wall et al., 1981)

The role of FFB with BAL and TBBX in patients with diffuse lung disease is limited to the exclusion of infections, malignancy, sarcoidosis, eosinophilic pneumonias and occasionally cryptogenic organizing pneumonia. Analysis of BAL fluid can show certain cellular profiles that suggest specific disease processes; for example, sarcoidosis has lymphocytosis characterized by an increase in T-helper cells and a high CD4/CD8 ratio; hypersensitivity pneumonitis has T lymphocytosis, with predominance of the suppressor subset CD8; and idiopathic pulmonary fibrosis is characterized by increases in neutrophils and eosinophils. Unfortunately, the BAL findings have limited clinical utility for the diagnosis, prognosis or as a guide to therapy in patients with ILD's. Using TBBx to diagnose idiopathic ILD's is not recommended. Surgical lung biopsy remains the investigation with the greatest overall diagnostic sensitivity for ILD's. (ATS/ERS, 2002; Talmadge, 2005)

Diffuse infiltrative pulmonary disorders in immunocompromised patients

Immunocompromised hosts include patients with AIDS, bone marrow and other transplant recipients, patients on chemo or radiation therapy, and patients on immunosuppressive therapy. These patients can be acutely ill and present often with progressive hypoxia. (Pechkam & Elliott, 2002). Differential diagnosis in this group includes both infective and non infective causes. Infective causes are viral and PJP infections, atypical pathogens, fungal and parasitic infections. Non-infective causes include graft rejection, toxicity secondary to radiation or chemotherapy, diffuse alveolar damage and diffuse alveolar hemorrhage. Rapid progression of the illness is not uncommon with the need for mechanical ventilation. Diagnostic delay in this group increases mortality and bronchoscopy can be very useful in the early diagnosis and management of these patients.

Lung transplant recipients

The number of transplant patients continues to grow and their care is not limited to specialized centers. They can present with a wide range of pulmonary disorders and causes of respiratory deterioration in transplant patients include rejection or infections. Bronchoscopy remains a valuable tool in this setting. FFB with BAL and TBBx has high sensitivity for the diagnosis of PJP, CMV and rejection. (Bulpa et al., 2003) The presence of Aspergillus in BAL fluid though non-diagnostic is predictive of development of invasive disease. (Cahill et al., 1997) Therapeutic bronchoscopic interventions include dilatation and stenting of stenotic lesions and laser ablation of granulation tissue. (Wahidi & Ernst, 2004)

4.1.4 Miscellaneous

Retained secretions and atelectasis

Atelectasis is a frequent complication seen in the ICU and retained secretions and atelectasis remains a common therapeutic indication for bronchoscopy. Although the use of FFB in situations of whole lung collapse associated with hypoxia is well established, there are no definitive guidelines in other situations. Bronchoscopy is usually performed when suctioning and chest physiotherapy fails to result in aeration of involved lungs. Stevens et al reported that 93 (79 %) of 118 bronchoscopies performed for atelectasis resulted in improvement compared with 31 (44%) of 70 patients with retained secretions. (Stevens et al., 1981) Other studies have reported a success rate between 19% to 81%. (Weinstein et al., 1977; Lindholm et al., 1974; Snow& Lucas, 1984)

In a prospective study Marini et al reported that the presence of air bronchograms on the initial chest roentgenogram predicted delayed resolution of atelectasis. (Marini et al., 1979).In this situation bronchoscopy may not be beneficial.

Bronchoalveolar lavage may aid in the resolution of atelectasis and identify some pathogenic microorganisms. In addition, bronchoscopy allows the instillation of mucolytic agents. We suggest bronchoscopy in critically ill patients with lobar or whole lung collapse without air bronchograms if chest physiotherapy is unsuccessful.

Removal of foreign bodies

Foreign body (FB) aspiration is frequently suspected in children with acute or recurrent pulmonary symptoms, but it is rarely considered in adults with acute or chronic respiratory symptoms unless a clear history of aspiration can be obtained. Food items are the most common aspirated FB with peanuts and animal or fish bones being the most common ones. The most common presentation is chronic cough, hemoptysis, dyspnea, and fever. If the FB is not removed, then more persistent findings may be seen such as atelectasis, post obstructive pneumonia, bronchiectasis, or lung abscess, and/or emphysema. The exact incidence of FB aspiration in adults is not known. Some studies report that only 7% of patients present with a history of choking (Chen et al., 1997).

Any condition leading to diminished swallowing reflex places the patients at risk for FB aspiration. Bronchoscopy is a valuable tool for the diagnosis and retrieval of the FB. Instruments used in retrieval include alligator and biopsy forceps, wire baskets and retrieval forceps. Overall success rates for retrieval of FBs ranges from 61 to 89% for both flexible and rigid bronchoscopies. (Limper &Prakash, 1990; Debeljak et al., 1999; Cunanan, 1978; Lan et al., 1989) FFB is probably more useful for FB in distal segments beyond the reach of rigid bronchoscope. In some cases, flexible and rigid bronchoscopy are complementary, with FFB assisting in the localization of the FB and then retrieval done with the rigid bronchoscope. Significant tissue reaction with inflammation is commonly seen in the delayed cases at bronchoscopy. Innovative anecdotal use of cryotherapy instruments to remove some foreign bodies have also been described.

Difficult intubation

Approximately 1% to 3% of tracheal intubations prove to be difficult with standard techniques. This is especially true as all invasive airway maneuvers can be considered difficult in a critically ill patient, either in the ICU or other setting. (Schwartz et al.,1995)

Fiberoptic intubation is a key aspect in the management of difficult intubations and forms part of several difficult airway algorithms (Benumof, 1991; American Society of Anesthesiologists, 2003; Crosby et al., 1998; Henderson et al., 2004) Intubation in these instances is performed using the bronchoscope as an obturator. Care must be taken to use a bite guard or an oral airway as damage to the scope by patient bites should be avoided.

Hemoptysis

Massive hemoptysis, defined as the volume of expectorated blood that is life-threatening due to hypoxia from airway obstruction or hemodynamic instability from blood loss, accounts for 4.8% to 14% of all patients with hemoptysis. (Dweik & Stoller, 1999)

Massive hemoptysis remains an emergent indication for bronchoscopy. The primary intention is to locate the source of bleeding and if possible to control it by use of topical or endobronchial tamponade. Control of bleeding can be achieved by topical application of cold saline or diluted 1: 1000 epinephrine; other agents include application of thrombin or fibrinogen–thrombin combination. (Tsukamoto et al., 1989)

Endobronchial tamponade can be achieved using a Fogarty balloon or rarely a pulmonary artery catheter. In rare instances bronchoscopic guided contralateral lung intubation is life saving. Localization of the bleed helps in the planning of bronchial artery embolization or thoracotomy.

Bronchopleural fistula

In patients with persistent air leaks and suspected broncho-pleural fistula (BPF), bronchoscopy can help define the extent of the broncho-pleural fistula and differentiate between stump dehiscence and a distal parenchymal leak. In addition, BPF associated with pneumonectomy or lobectomy can be directly visualized. In patients with suspected distal BPF a careful sequential inspection of each bronchopulmonary segment should be performed; this usually requires the use of balloons to occlude the bronchial segments to locate the one leading to the fistula and then apply sealants. (Lan et al., 1987; Regel et al. 1989; Lois & Noppen,2005; Oren et al., 2011)

Other indications include confirmation of endotracheal tube (ETT) placement, double lumen ETT placement, diagnosis of bronchial rupture or bronchial stump dehiscence. Less common indications include inspection of upper airway prior to extubation when edema or other anatomical problems are expected in an intubated patient. In such instances, extubation can be attempted under bronchoscopic guidance and reintubation if necessary can be easily done using the bronchoscope as a guide wire. Bronchoscopy in indicated in patients with smoke inhalation to categorize the extent of injury and the need for intubation and in the presence of glottic and subglottic edema, intubation can be performed safely under bronchoscopic guidance.

4.1.5 Bronchoscopy in special circumstances

Bronchoscopy in patients with renal impairment

Uremia has been reported to be associated with an increased risk of bleeding, mainly due to platelet dysfunction. (Cordasco et al., 1991)A 45% incidence of pulmonary hemorrhage after bronchoscopic lung biopsy was documented in immunosuppressed uremic patients.(Cunningham et al., 1977) A more recent study looking at 72 patients with renal insufficiency reported a much lower rate of bleeding complications with TBBx. There were no complications in the hemodialysis (HD) group and only one of 25 (4%) patients not on HD had a bleeding complication. (Mehta et al., 2005)

These findings suggest the possibility that the risk of bleeding in patients with renal insufficiency undergoing TBBx is lower than initially reported. Those patients should be screened for coagulation abnormalities and, if receiving HD, the TBBx should be done after HD with pre-bronchoscopy administration of 1-deamino-8-D-arginine vasopressin (DDAVP).Platelet transfusions, infusion of cryoprecipitate or DDAVP, administration of analogues or derivatives of vasopressin and administration of estrogen are some of the strategies implemented to decrease bleeding complications during FFB. (Cordasco et al., 1991)

Bronchoscopy in patients with cardiac ischemia

Hypoxia is a relatively common complication of FFB, which may predispose to cardiac arrhythmias. (Katz et al., 1981) Cardiovascular stress and hypertension are common and can result in cardiovascular changes during bronchoscopy especially if they have cardiac risk factors.(Davies et al.,1997) Acute myocardial infarction (AMI) is generally considered to increase the risk of FFB. A retrospective study concluded that bronchoscopy is safe in the immediate post-AMI period as long as the patient does not have active ischemia at the time of the procedure; the mean period between the AMI and FFB was 11.7 days. The risks of bronchoscopy are thought to be reduced 4–6 weeks after myocardial infarction. (Dweik et al., 1996; Kvale, 1996; American College of Cardiology and American Heart Association Taskforce, 1996; Dunagan et al., 1998; Bein &Pfeifer, 1997)

Bronchoscopy in patients with obstructive airway disease

Asthma has been associated with laryngospasm or bronchospasm complicating bronchoscopy. The reported incidence of bronchoscopy induced bronchospasm ranges from 0.02% to 8%. Decrease in FEV_1 is seen during FFB and this is more pronounced in asthmatics compared to non asthmatics. In patients with mild asthma, pre procedure use of bronchodilator has not been associated with a decrease in the postoperative FEV_1, however, the use of pre-bronchoscopy bronchodilator is associated with blunting of the post bronchoscopy decrease in FEV_1 in asthmatics with more severe disease.(Fish & Peterman 1979; Djukanovic et al., 1991;Van Vyve et al., 1992; Rankin et al., 1984; Mavritsyn & Lifshits, 1980) In a large multicenter study of over 20,000 bronchoscopies, bronchospasm was reported in 0.004% of all the procedures.(Facciolongo et al., 2009) In general, it is recommended that patients with asthma receive bronchodilator nebulizers before the procedure; taking in consideration that the benefit have been reported mainly in the most severe asthmatic.

The presence of severe chronic obstructive pulmonary disease (COPD) has been shown to increase the complication rate of bronchoscopy. The complication rate is as high as 3% to 5% in severe COPD (FEV_1 /FVC <50% or FEV_1 <1.2 L) when compared with 0.6% of patients with normal lung function. An arterial blood gas should be considered prior to bronchoscopy for those patients with severe COPD. The judicious use of sedation and monitoring of oxygenation and ventilation permit the safe performance of FFB in selected patients with COPD.(BTS, 2001; Peacock et al., 1994; Hattotuwa et al., 2002) Although there is no data regarding the use of pre-procedure bronchodilators in COPD, we routinely use bronchodilators prior to the bronchoscopy and monitoring is done with pulse oximetry and end tidal CO_2 ($ETCO_2$).

Bronchoscopy in the elderly

Epidemiologic studies have shown a trend in the increase of the "oldest old" or those 85 years of age or older from the absolute number of 3.5 million as measured in 1990 to approximately 15.3 million persons in the year 2050. Proportionately to this trend, this age group might comprise a portion of the population that could need diagnostic and therapeutic bronchoscopy.

A study of FFB in 107 octogenarians revealed no difference in procedural indications, complication rates, or diagnostic yield between octogenarians and non-octogenarians. Despite a significantly lower doses of sedation used in octogenarians, they experienced a predominant complication of oversedation. (Patrick et al., 2003; Knox et al., 1988)

Raised intracranial pressure

In patients with head injuries, brain tumor or massive stroke, the increase in the intracranial pressure (ICP) can be significant; (Snow& Lucas, 1984, Lee, 1994; Peerless et al., 1995) raising concerns about the safety of bronchoscopy in this setting. A potential complication of bronchoscopy includes an increase in the ICP due to the manipulation of the airways especially during suctioning and excessive coughing. (Rudy et al., 1991) Kerwin et al reported an increase in ICP during bronchoscopy, the concomitant increase in MAP maintained CPP but the increase in MAP was not linear and there was no persistent increase in ICP after the procedure. (Kerwin et al 2000) They suggested that pharmacologic paralysis and heavy sedation should be used and that the bronchoscopy should be performed in the minimum amount of time possible. In general, bronchoscopy carries a low risk in patients with raised ICP in patients with intracranial space occupying lesions. (Bajwaet al., 1993)

Bronchoscopy in pediatric population

Although the availability of bronchoscopy has been a major advance in adult pulmonary medicine, the role of FFB in pediatrics has remained less well defined. The last 20 years has seen an increase in the use of FFB for the evaluation of respiratory disorders in children. (Nicolai, 2001; Barbato et al., 1997) The main indications for bronchoscopy in children includes the evaluation of stridor, persistent wheezing, or a suspected foreign body, abnormal chest roentgenogram, airway evaluation in patients with tracheostomy, airway obstruction , hoarseness, recurrent pneumonia , chronic cough and hemoptysis.

Overall, the diagnostic yield in this population has been reported in the range of 75% to 88% of cases. (Brown et al., 1983; Wood, 1985; Martinot et al., 1997)

Several studies looking at the safety of bronchoscopy in the pediatric population have reported a low complication rate of less than 2%. De Blic study in 1328 children that underwent FFB under conscious sedation reported 5.2% of minor complications which included moderate and transient episodes of desaturation, excessive coughing and nausea, transient laryngospasm and epistaxis. Major complications were seen in 1.7% of cases and included oxygen desaturation to less than 90%, laryngospasm and bronchospasm, and pneumothorax.(J. de Blic et al 2002) The high diagnostic yield and low complication rate strongly support the use of the FFB in the diagnostic evaluation of infants and children who have a variety of pulmonary problems.(Wood, 1984, 1985)

5. Bronchoscopy in the intensive care unit

Respiratory involvement is common in the critically ill patient in the intensive care unit (ICU) with 30 to 50% of the admissions requiring the use of mechanical ventilation. Fiberoptic bronchoscopy remains a very valuable tool in the evaluation and management of these patients as well as to evaluate complications of mechanical ventilation especially atelectasis and ventilator associated pneumonias (VAP). Bronchoscopy in the ICU plays a role as a diagnostic and therapeutic tool. Many of the indications for bronchoscopy in the ICU overlap with the general indications for the procedure as discussed above.

Bronchoscopy on patients on mechanical ventilation

The routine FFB with BAL is frequently performed in patients on mechanical ventilation (MV). Use of transbronchial biopsy in this group of patient's remains low and underutilized probably due to the lack of fluoroscopy in the ICU setting.

In a non intubated patient a regular 5.7 mm bronchoscope usually occupies 10 % of the tracheal cross sectional area and is of no physiological consequence. The consequences on the respiratory mechanics have been described in detail by Jollier and Chevrolet. (Jolliet & Chevrolet 1992) . A 5.7 mm internal diameter bronchoscope occupies 40% of the total cross-section of a 9 mm internal diameter ETT, 51 % of an 8 mm ETT, and 66% of a 7 mm ETT. This results in the development of intrinsic PEEP and as described, smaller the tube, higher the development of PEEP with the consequent increase in airway pressures. Additionally, functional residual capacity increases by 30% and forced expiratory volume in one second (FEV_1) decreases by 40%.(Matsushima et al.,1984) The decrease in the delivered tidal volume leads to hypoventilation and gas exchange abnormalities resulting in hypoxia and hypercapnea. Suctioning during bronchoscopy limits the delivered tidal volume further and up to 200 to 300 ml of delivered volume can be removed with each suctioning. It is therefore recommended that an ETT of at least size 8 or 8.5 mm be used when performing bronchoscopy in intubated patients. (Grossman& Jacobi, 1974; Jolliet & Chevrolet 1992))

Cardiovascular consequences of bronchoscopy include arrhythmias secondary to vagotonic effects, hypoxia or hypercapnea. Increased intrinsic PEEP can result in impaired preload and hypotension. Adjustments needed prior to bronchoscopy in a patient on MV include preoxygenation with 100% oxygen and increase in the tidal volume by 30%. Bronchoscopy should be performed on 100% FIO_2 and this should be continued into the post bronchoscopy period. Peak airway pressure alarm limit should be increased before the procedure to account for the increase in pressure on introduction of the scope and ensure delivery of adequate tidal volume and adequate ventilation. It is our personal experience to withdraw the scope and allow for ventilation when the SpO_2 reaches 90%. In patients who have acute or chronic pre-procedure hypercapnia, the use of $ETCO_2$ monitoring is helpful.

Bronchoscopic techniques used for procedures done at the bedside of the patient in the ICU are similar to the ones done in the bronchoscopy suite.

Bronchoscopy in mechanically ventilated patients – A bed side approach

1. Review the indication for bronchoscopy and review imaging before the procedure
2. Obtain informed consent

3. Inspect the ETT or tracheostomy size. If ≥ 8mm then a standard 5.7mm outer diameter bronchoscope can be used. If the artificial airway tube is smaller, then a smaller size scope is needed. Shorten the ETT by cutting the distal end to facilitate inspection of the distal tracheobronchial tree. Attach Portex adapter to facilitate ventilation during bronchoscopy. Oral airway or bite guard is recommended to prevent trauma to the scope.
4. Increase FiO_2 to 100 percent 15 minutes before the procedure and make ventilator adjustments. In volume assist modes the peak pressure limit is increased and in pressure control assist mode the pressure control needs to be increased to compensate for the increased resistance generated due to the insertion of the scope.
5. Time out and sedation as per hospital policies. On patients with sedative infusion drips, an initial bolus is recommended
6. Document peak air way pressure before procedure
7. Patient should be monitored with continuous EKG, SpO_2 and $ETCO_2$ for those with hypercapnea. Blood pressure should be monitored every 5 minutes during the procedure
8. Lubricate bronchoscope and insert into the ETT/tracheostomy via the adapter. Topical anesthesia is achieved with topical lidocaine application into the trachea, carinal and main stem bronchi. Recommended maximal dose of lidocaine is 4-5 ml/kg ideal body weight or 300 mg per procedure. Minimal use of suction to prevent loss of tidal volume. Restrict suctioning to less than 3 seconds.
9. After inspection of the tracheobronchial tree, BAL is performed. The exception to this rule is suspected infection, in which case locate the bronchopulmonary segment of interest and perform lavage. This decreases the chances of contamination of the specimen.
10. The BAL is performed as described under bronchoscopic techniques.
11. To perform the TBBx, apply topical lidocaine to the segment of interest and perform biopsy as described under techniques. We take special care that the patient is well sedated and not fighting the ventilator or coughing excessively. We routinely disconnect patient from the respirator for a couple of seconds during initial part of forceps withdrawal. If there is any instability pull out the scope and ventilate patient. Bronchoscopy can be continued after the situation resolves.
12. Post procedure check peak airway and plateau pressure and obtain a chest roentgenogram to evaluate for complications.

Diagnostic yield of bronchoscopy in mechanically ventilated patients

The diagnostic yield of FFB depends on the indication and the comorbid clinical status. Different bronchoscopic techniques are associated with different diagnostic yield in this group of patients.

Protected brush

Pooled results of 18 studies of PSB technique was evaluated in a total of 795 critically ill patients. The overall accuracy of this diagnostic method for diagnosing health care associated pneumonia (HCAP) was high, with a sensitivity of 89% and a specificity of 94%. Prior anti microbial therapy decreases the diagnostic yield. (Chastre & Fagon, 2002)

BAL

Torres & el-Ebiary reviewed 23 studies that evaluated the accuracy of BAL to diagnose VAP in a total of 957 patients. In this review, BAL had a mean sensitivity of 73% (range 22 to 100%) and mean specificity of 82%. The presence of intracellular organisms in BAL was specific for VAP. (Torres & El-Ebiary 2000)

In patients with AIDS, BAL had a diagnostic accuracy of 89 to 98% in the diagnosis of PJP. (Huang et al., 2006) In a prospective multicentre trial in hematology and oncology patients there was no difference between bronchoscopic BAL versus other strategies in establishing diagnosis. (Azoulay et al., 2008) However, FFB-BAL was the only conclusive investigation in a third of patients and induced respiratory deterioration in about half of these cases. A subsequent study by the same investigators showed that noninvasive testing alone was not inferior to noninvasive testing plus FFB-BAL within 24 hours of admission for the identification of the cause for acute respiratory failure. (Azoulay et al., 2010)

In neutropenic patients with pulmonary infiltrates, the diagnostic yield of BAL was 49% with low complication rates; there were infrequent treatment changes and there was improved survival.(Gruson et al., 2000)

TBBx

In patients with diffuse unexplained pulmonary infiltrates, combined BAL and TBBx resulted in diagnosis in 74% of patients and the authors concluded that the benefits of the procedure exceeded the risks. (Bulpa et al 2003) TBBx is useful in distinguishing infections from rejection in lung transplant patients.

Management of critically ill patient on mechanical ventilation with unclear lung findings represents a challenge to the clinician. In cases where FFB-BAL and all noninvasive studies have been non diagnostics, TBBx or surgical lung biopsy is recommended. This is compounded by the fact that there are few studies looking into the role of TBBx in ventilated patients. (Papazian et al., 1998)

6. Safety and contraindications of bronchoscopy

Flexible bronchoscopy is an extremely safe procedure with a low incidence of complications.(Dweik et al., 1996; BTS, 2001;Prakash at al., 1991;ATS,1987) One study reported a mortality rate of 0.01% and a major complication rate of 0.08% in a series of 24521 procedures, and another a mortality of 0.02% and a 0.3% rate of major complications in a series of around 48 000 cases. (Kvale, 1996; Zavala, 1975; Credle et al., 1974; Pue & Pacht, 1995; Surrat et al., 1979)

A multicenter, prospective study describing the practice of bronchoscopy in the United States revealed adverse events in 35% of cases, most of them mild (sore throat 10%, hemoptysis 8%, bleeding 4%, cough 3%). Severe adverse events occurred in 10% and included hospitalizations for cardiac arrhythmias, exacerbation of chronic obstructive pulmonary disease, and hypoxia. The mortality rate was 2% , a rate higher than previously reported. (Bechara et al., 2005)

Major life threatening complications include respiratory depression, pneumonia, pneumothorax, airway obstruction, cardio-respiratory arrest, arrhythmias, and pulmonary edema. Major complications are partly because of the cardiovascular effects of bronchoscopy, leading to an increase in blood pressure and heart rate causing arrhythmias and cardiovascular ischemia. Oxygen desaturation can occur because of the procedure itself or respiratory depression by sedative drugs leading to hypoxemia and increased risk of arrhythmias and ischemia. Bronchoscopy is performed in different settings, varying from local to general anesthesia with intubation; the choice of the way in which the bronchoscopy is performed is more a matter of personal experience and choice than of evidence-based medicine. Comparison of rigid bronchoscopy under general anesthesia and flexible fiberoptic bronchoscopy reveals that FFB with topical anesthesia has a safer profile than rigid bronchoscopy. (BTS, 2001; Hattotuwa et al., 2002; Surrat et al., 1979; Pereira et al., 1978; Lundgren et al.,1982; Davies et al.,1997)

Minor non-life threatening complications include, in order of frequency, vasovagal reactions, fever, cardiac arrhythmias, hemorrhage, nausea and vomiting. Post-bronchoscopy fever occurs in approximately 5% to 16% of the patients, with pulmonary infiltrate occurring in 0.6% of all cases. The self-limiting fever is usually not indicative of pneumonia and may be due to transient bacteremia, translocation of endotoxins or release of inflammatory mediators. (BTS, 2001; Pereira et al., 1978; de Castro & Violan,1996)

Complication rates that are related specifically to the procedure of transbronchial biopsies are higher, with pneumothorax reported in 1 to 5% of cases and mild hemorrhage in 9%. (Bechara et al., 2005; Zavala, 1978; Hanson et al., 1976)

6.1 Pneumothorax

Pneumothorax is very uncommon after FFB; however, a major pneumothorax requiring drainage has been reported to occur in 3.5% of FFB with TBBx. The incidence of pneumothorax with TBBx is as high as 14% for patients on mechanical ventilation. Symptoms and/or signs of a pneumothorax may be delayed after TBBx but it is very uncommon for a pneumothorax to develop after an hour of TBBX. (Lindholm et al., 1974) About 50% of patients who develop pneumothorax will require drainage.

6.2 Fluoroscopy for bronchoscopy

The use of fluoroscopy does not appear to reduce the frequency of pneumothorax, especially in non-mechanically ventilated patients. (Zink et al., 2007; O'Brien et al., 1997; Milman et al., 1993) Literature regarding non fluoroscopy guided transbronchial biopsy in patients on mechanical ventilation is scarce. In most of the ICU's fluoroscopy is not available which limits the use of TBBx in mechanically ventilated patients. In smaller series, the rate of pneumothorax varies from 12 to 27% (Bulpa et al.,2003; Pincus et al., 1987;) and 10.4% in larger series (O'Brien et al., 1997). Risk of pneumothorax is directly proportional to the number of biopsies attempted; Descombes et al reported 38% and 69% yields with 1–3, and 6–10 specimens, respectively. (Descombes et al., 1997)

At our institution, we perform 1-3 biopsies on patients on mechanical ventilation without the use of fluoroscopy; otherwise, to obtain more biopsies we do the procedure in the operating room under fluoroscopic guidance.

In general, the use of fluoroscopy increases the diagnostic yield from TBBx in focal lung lesions. Fluoroscopy carries the limitation of being time consuming, requires some experience, and is not readily available in all centers. (Gasparini, 1997; Cortese & McDougall 1979; Yung, 2003; Liam et al., 2007)

6.3 Bleeding complications

Several studies have shown that patients with uremia, immunosuppression, pulmonary hypertension, liver disease, coagulation disorders, or thrombocytopenia have a higher risk for hemorrhage with transbronchial biopsy(TBBx). (Papin et al., 1985; Zavala, 1976; Borchers & Beamis 1996)

The risk of bleeding during TBBx seems to be unrelated to the size of forceps and is slightly higher in those being mechanically ventilated. (Loube et al., 1993; O'Brien et al., 1997)

In patients with a potential increased risk of bleeding, coagulation profile should be checked before bronchoscopy. There is no information about what constitutes a "safe" level for clotting in this context. Transfusion guidelines and expert opinions recommend platelet counts of 20,000–50,000/mm^3 for FFB with BAL and greater than 50,000/mm^3 for TBBx. It is recommended that platelets be transfused following those guidelines. (Rebulla, 2001)

Thrombocytopenia (platelet count <150.000 mm^3) is seen in 35 to 40% of critically ill medical patients (Vanderschueren et al., 2000; Strauss et al., 2002), with surgical and trauma patients having a higher incidence of thrombocytopenia. ((Stephan et al., 1999)

Patients with coagulopathy are at a high risk for bleeding with brushings and biopsy; Weiss et al., reported 12% of complications in patients with significant thrombocytopenia after bronchoscopy with BAL, but serious complications were rare. (Weiss et al., 1993)

In patient taking oral anticoagulants, published guidelines for managing anticoagulation in the perioperative period are relevant. These state that "the short term risk of thromboembolism in patients with mechanical heart valves when not anticoagulated is very small". (Brickey & Lawlor, 1999; British Committee for Standards in Haematology, 1998)

In patients on anticoagulation undergoing transbronchial biopsy, unfractionated heparin drips should be stopped 6 hours prior and low molecular weight heparin should be held the evening prior and on the day of the procedure

The use of aspirin alone in humans has not been associated with an increase in bleeding complications from TBBx and therefore there are no recommendations to stop the medication before this procedure. (Herth et al., 2002)

The data from aspirin cannot be generalized to clopidogrel use because its mechanism of action differs from that of aspirin. Several studies indicate an increased risk of bleeding when clopidogrel is combined with other antiplatelet drugs. (Hongo et al., 2002; Yende & Wunderink, 2001) A study in 604 patients without underlying coagulation problems who underwent TBBx while on clopidogrel with or without aspirin revealed an increased risk of bleeding after the lung biopsy. Marked bleeding was observed in most patients receiving clopidogrel and in all patients receiving clopidogrel combined with aspirin. On the basis of these results, it is recommended that clopidogrel should be stopped 5 to 7 days before TBBx to ensure patient safety. The indications for TBBx need to be clearly defined, as it means stopping a beneficial medication for patients with cardiovascular diseases. (Ernst et al., 2006)

6.4 Contraindications

The contraindications to bronchoscopy must always be considered in relationship to the expected benefits and clinical consequences. The determining factors are, in addition to the clinical status and prognosis of the patient, the technical difficulties of the procedure, and the skills and experience of the endoscopist. There are no controlled studies of the factors which may make a patient totally unfit for the procedure, so a decision to perform a bronchoscopy is a balance between the likely benefit of obtaining diagnostic material (including therapeutic benefit) and an assessment of the likely risk for complications in that individual patient. (BTS, 2001; ATS, 1987; Ernst et al.,2003; Wood-Baker et al., 2001)

Relative contraindications to bronchoscopy include severe respiratory insufficiency when bronchoscopy will be non-therapeutic, inability to maintain a patent airway and severe cardiovascular instability. Coagulopathy when biopsy is considered and severe generalized debilitated status are other relative factors to be considered prior to bronchoscopy.

Careful planning and taking all appropriate precautions prior to the bronchoscopy cannot be overemphasized in those patients with myocardial infarction within the last 4 weeks and patients with severe hypoxemia who could benefit from intubation prior to the bronchoscopy.

For those patients with severe renal or coagulation impairment, transmissible infection (e.g. active pulmonary tuberculosis) and the very uncooperative patient the benefit of the procedure must be weighed carefully.

Additionally caution is advised in patients on mechanical ventilation with high PEEP, hypoxia requiring high supplemental oxygen and electrolyte abnormalities. In unstable patients it is recommended to stabilize the respiratory status before FFB and this may include intubation and mechanical ventilation. (Crosby et al.,1998; Henderson et al.,2004; Alamoudi et al.,2000;Becker at al., 1991)

7. Conclusion

The development of flexible bronchoscopy in the late 1960s revolutionized the care of patients with lung and airway problems. The flexible bronchoscope has almost completely supplanted the rigid scope for the routine diagnostic evaluation of lung diseases. The technique is acceptable to the patient, is safe and allows a more complete examination of the bronchial tree and is ideal for a variety of other diagnostic procedures such as transbronchial biopsy, bronchial lavage and needle aspiration. Bronchoscopy remains a very valuable tool for both diagnostic and therapeutic procedures for a variety of respiratory conditions encountered in clinical practice including in critically ill patients. Bronchoscopy has a definite diagnostic role in those patients suspected of having pulmonary malignancy or some diffuse lung diseases like sarcoidosis and infections in the immunosuppressed host. In experienced hands, the bronchoscope is an invaluable diagnostic and therapeutic tool in the ICU that at present is probably underused.

Appropriate indication, experience of the bronchoscopist and careful attention to detail results in a high diagnostic yield with a low complication rate even with the inclusion of needle aspiration and biopsies. The current advances in technology, imaging and information processing continue to improve the ability to perform minimally invasive, accurate evaluations of the tracheobronchial tree and to perform an ever-increasing array of diagnostic, staging, therapeutic, and palliative interventions.

We believe that a well trained pulmonologist should continue using the bronchoscope in order to diagnose the most commonly encountered pulmonary conditions. The idea of having an "optimal bronchoscopist" who is highly skilled in all the bronchoscopic techniques and able to handle flexible and rigid scope in adults and pediatric population as Prakash and Stubbs discussed in their 1994 publication is probably not feasible at this point on time. (Prakash & Stubbs 1994) Pulmonologists need to be able to identify those patients that could benefit from more invasive or sophisticated bronchoscopic procedures and refer them to centers of excellence with an interventional pulmonologist.

8. References

Alamoudi OS, Attar SM, Ghabrah TM & Kassimi MA. (2000). Bronchoscopy, indications, safety and complications. Saudi Med J. 2000 Nov; 21(11):1043-7

Alvarez-Lerma F. (1996). Modification of empiric antibiotic treatment in patients with pneumonia acquired in the intensive care unit. ICU-acquired Pneumonia Study Group. Intensive Care Med 1996; 22:387–394.

American College of Cardiology and American Heart Association Taskforce. Guidelines for peri-operative cardiovascular evaluation for non cardiac surgery. (1996). Circulation 1996; 93:1278–317.

American Society of Anesthesiologists Task Force on Management of the Difficult Airway. (2003). Practice guidelines for management of the difficult airway. An updated report. (2003). Anesthesiology 2003; 95: 1269–77.

American Thoracic Society/European Respiratory Society international multidisciplinary consensus classification of the idiopathic interstitial pneumonias. (2002) Am J Respir Crit Care Med 2002; 165:277–304.

Anders GT, Johnson JE, Bush BA & Matthew JI. Transbronchial biopsy without fluoroscopy. (1998). A seven year perspective. Chest 1988; 94:557-560

Arancibia F, Ewing S, Martinez JA, Ruiz M, Bauer T, Angeles Marcos M, Mensa J, & Torres A. (2000). Antimicrobial treatment failures in patients with community-acquired pneumonia. Causes and prognostic implications. Am J Respir Crit Care Med 2000; 162:154–60.

Azoulay E, Mokart D, Lambert J, Lemiale V, Rabbat A, Kouatchet A, Vincent F, Gruson D, Bruneel F, Epinette-Branche G, Lafabrie A, Hamidfar-Roy R, Cracco C, Renard B, Tonnelier JM, Blot F, Chevret S, & Schlemmer B. (2010). Diagnostic strategy for hematology and oncology patients with acute respiratory failure: randomized controlled trial. Am J Respir Crit Care Med 2010; 182:1038–1046

Bajwa MK, Henein S, & Kamholz SL. (1993). Fiberoptic bronchoscopy in the presence of space-occupying intracranial lesions. Chest. 1993;104:101–103

Barbato A, Magarotto M, Crivellaro M, Novello Jr A, Cracco A, de Blic J, Scheinmann P, Warner JO & Zach M. (1997). Use of the paediatric bronchoscope, flexible and rigid, in 51 European centers. Eur Respir J 1997; 10: 1761–1766.

Bates, J. H. , G. D. Campbell, A. L. Barron, G. A. McCracken, P. N. Morgan, E. B. Moses & C. M. Davis. (1992). Microbial etiology of acute pneumonia in hospitalized patients. Chest 1992. 101:1005-1112.

Baughman R. P. (2007) Technical Aspects of Bronchoalveolar Lavage: Recommendations for a Standard Procedure. Semin Respir Crit Care Med 2007; 28: 475–485.

Bechara R, Beamis J, Simoff M, Mathur P, Yung R, Feller-Kopman D & Ernst A. (2005). Practice and Complications of Flexible Bronchoscopy with Biopsy Procedures. J Bronchol 2005; 12:139–142

Becker H. D, Kayser K, Schulz V, Tuengerthal S & Vollhaber HH. (1991). Atlas of Bronchoscopy. B. C. Decker Inc. 1991

Bein T & Pfeifer M. (1997) Fiberoptic bronchoscopy after recent acute myocardial infarction. Stress for the heart? Chest 1997; 112:295.

Bellomo R, Tai E & Parkin G. (1992) Fiberoptic bronchoscopy in the critically ill: A prospective study of its diagnostic and therapeutic value. Anaesth Intensive Care 1992; 20:464–469.

Benumof JL. (1991). Management of the difficult adult airway with special emphasis on awake tracheal intubation. Anesthesiology 1991; 75: 1087–110.

Borchers S & Beamis J. (1996). Flexible bronchoscopy. Chest Surg Clin North Am 1996; 6:169–92.

Brickey DA & Lawlor DP. (1999). Transbronchial biopsy in the presence of profound elevation of the international normalized ratio (INR). Chest 1999; 115:1667–71.

British Committee for Standards in Haematology. Guidelines on oral anticoagulation: third edition. (1998). Br J Haematol1998;101:374–87

British Thoracic Society Bronchoscopy Guidelines Committee. BTS guidelines on diagnostic flexible bronchoscopy. (2001). Thorax. 2001; 56 (suppl I):i1–i2.

Brown Fitzpatrick S, Marsh B, Stokes D & Wang KP. (1983). Indications for Flexible Fiberoptic Bronchoscopy in Pediatric Patients. Am J Dis Child. 1983; 137(6):595-597.

Bulpa PA, Dive AM, Mertens L, Delos MA, Jamart J, Evrard PA, Gonzalez MR & Installe EJ. (2003). Combined bronchoalveolar lavage and transbronchial lung biopsy: Safety and yield in ventilated patients. Eur Respir J 2003;21:489–494.

Cahill BC, Hibbs JR, Savik K, Juni BA, Dosland BM, Edin-Stibbe C & Hertz MI. (1997). Aspergillus airway colonization and invasive disease after lung transplantation. Chest 1997;112(5):1160–4

Celis R, Torres A, Gatell JM, Almela M, Rodriguez-Roisin R & Agustı´- Vidal A. (1998). Nosocomial pneumonia: a multivariate analysis of risk and prognosis. Chest 1988; 93:318–324.

Centers for Disease Control and Prevention. Monitoring hospital acquired infections to promote patient safety: United States, (2000). 1990– 999. MMWR 2000; 49:149–153.

Ceron L, Michieletto L, Pagan V & Zamperlin A. (2007). Transbronchial Needle Aspiration in Patients With Mediastinal and Hilar Disease. J Bronchol 2007;14:6–9

Chastre J & Fagon JY. (1994). Pneumonia in the ventilator-dependent patient. Editor -Tobin MJ : Principles and practice of mechanical ventilation. New York: McGraw-Hill; 1994. p. 857–890.

Chastre J & Fagon JY. (2002) Ventilator-associated pneumonia. Am J Respir Crit Care Med 2002;165(7):867– 903

Chen CH, Lai CL, Tsai TT, Lee YC & Perng RP. (1997). Foreign body aspiration into the lower airways in Chinese adults. Chest 1997; 112:129–33

Cordasco E M Jr, Mehta A C & Ahmad M. (1991). Bronchoscopically Induced Bleeding. A Summary of Nine Years' Cleveland Clinic Experience and Review of the literature. Chest 1991;100;1141-114

Cortese DA & McDougall JC. (1979) Biopsy and brushingof peripheral lung cancers with fluoroscopic guidance. Chest 1979; 75:141–5.
Credle W, Smiddy J & Elliott R. (1974). Complications of fiberoptic bronchoscopy. Am Rev Respir Dis 1974; 109:67–72.
Crosby ET, Cooper RM, Douglas MJ, Doyle JD,Hung OR,Labrecque P,Muir H,Murphy MF,Preston RP,Rose DK & Roy L. (1998). The unanticipated difficult airway with recommendations for management. Can J Anaesth 1998; 45: 757-76.
Cunanan OS. (1978)The flexible fiberoptic bronchoscope in foreign body removal. Experience in 300 cases. Chest 1978;73:725–6.
Cunningham JH, Zavala DC, Corry RJ, & Keim LW. (1977). Trephine air drill, bronchial brush, and fiberoptic transbronchial lung biopsies in immunosuppressed patients. Am Rev Respir Dis. 1977; 115:213–220.
Dasgupta A & Mehta AC. (1999). Flexible Bronchoscopy in the 21st Century. Transbronchial Needle Aspiration An Underused Diagnostic Technique. Clin Chest Med 1999; Volume 20, Issue 1: 39-51
Davies L, Mister R, Spence DP, Calverley PMA, Earis JE & Pearson MG. (1997). Cardiovascular consequences of fiberoptic bronchoscopy. Eur Respir J. 1997; 10:695–698.
Davenport RD. (1990). Rapid on-site evaluation of transbronchial aspirates. Chest 1990; 98:59 61.
de Blic J, Marchac V & Scheinmann P. (2002). Complications of flexible bronchoscopy in children: prospective study of 1,328 procedures. Eur Respir J 2002; 20: 1271–1276
De Castro F R & Violan J S. (1996). Flexible bronchoscopy in mechanically ventilated patients. J Bronchol 1996; 3:64-8.
de Gracia J, Bravo C, Miravitlles M, Tallada N, Orriols R, Bellmunt J, Vendrell M, & Morell F. (1993). Diagnostic value of bronchoalveolar lavage in peripheral lung cancer. Am Rev Respir Dis 1993; 147:649–52.
Debeljak A, Sorli J, Music E & Kecelj P. (1974). Bronchoscopic removal of foreign bodies in adults: experience with 62 patients from 1974–1998. Eur Respir J 1999;14:792–5.
Descombes E, Gardiol D & Leuenberger P: Transbronchial lung biopsy: An analysis of 530 cases with reference to the number of samples. Monaldi Arch Chest Dis 1997; 52:324–329.
Digby J, Kalbfleisch J, Glenn A, Larsen A, Browder W & Williams D. Serum glucan levels are not specific for presence of fungal infections in intensive care unit patients. Clin Diagn Lab Immunol 2003; 10: 882–5
Djukanovic R, Wilson J, Lai C, Holgate ST &Howarth PH. (1991). The safety aspects of fiberoptic bronchoscopy, bronchoalveolar lavage, and endobronchial biopsy in asthma. Am Rev Respir Dis 1991;143:772–7.
Dunagan DP, Burke HL, Aquino SL, Chin R Jr, Adair NE & Haponik EF. (1998). Fibreoptic bronchoscopy in coronary care unit patients. Chest 1998; 114: 1660–7.
Dweik RA, Mehta A. C. , Meeker D. P & Arroliga A. C. (1996). Analysis of the Safety of Bronchoscopy After Recent Acute Myocardial Infarction. Chest 1996; 110:825-28)
Dweik RA & Stoller JK. Role of bronchoscopy in massive hemoptysis. (1999). Clin Chest Med 1999; 20:89-105.
El-Ebiary M, Torres A, Fabregas N, de la Bellacasa JP, González J, Ramirez J, del Baño D, Hernández C & Jiménez de Anta M . (1997). Significance of the isolation of Candida species from respiratory samples in critically ill, non-neutropenic patients. An

immediate postmortem histologic study. Am J Respir Crit Care Med 1997; 156:583–90

El-Bayoumi E & Silvestri GA. (2008). Bronchoscopy for the diagnosis and staging of lung cancer. Semin Respir Crit Care Med 2008;29(3):261–70.

Esperatti M, Ferrer M, Theessen A, Liapikou A, Valencia M, Saucedo LM, Zavala E, Welte T & Torres A. (2010). Nosocomial pneumonia in the intensive care unit acquired by mechanically ventilated versus nonventilated patients. Am J Respir Crit Care Med 2010; 182:1533–9.

Ernst A, Eberhardt R, Wahidi M, Becker H D & Herth FJF. (2006). Effect of Routine Clopidogrel Use on Bleeding Complications after Transbronchial Biopsy in Humans. Chest 2006; 129; 734-737.

Ernst, A, Silvestri, GA & Johnstone, D. (2003). Interventional pulmonary procedures. Guidelines from the American College of Chest Physicians. Chest 2003; 123, 1693-1717

ERS/ATS statement on interventional pulmonology. (2002). Eur Respir J 2002; 19: 356–373

Fabregas N, Ewig S, Torres A, El-Ebiary M, Ramirez J, de La Bellacasa JP, Bauer T & Cabello H. (1999) . Clinical diagnosis of ventilator-associated pneumonia revisited: comparative validation using immediate post-mortem lung biopsies. Thorax 54:867–873

Fabin E, Nagy M & Meszaros G. (1975). Experiences with bronchial brushing method. Acta Cytol 1975;19: 320–1.

Facciolongo N, Patelli M, Gasparini S, Lazzari Agli L, Salio M, Simonassi C, Del Prato B & Zanoni P. (2009). Incidence of complications in bronchoscopy. Multicentre prospective study of 20,986 bronchoscopies. Monaldi Arch Chest Dis 2009; 71: 8-14

Fagon JY, Chastre J, Wolff M, Gervais C, Parer-Aubas S, Stephan F, Similowski T, Mercat A, Diehl JL, Sollet JP & Tenaillon A. (2000). Invasive and noninvasive strategies for management of suspected ventilator-associated pneumonia: a randomized trial. Ann Intern Med 2000; 132:621–630.

Fedullo AJ & Ettensohn DB. (1986). Bronchoalveolar lavage in the lymphangitic spread of adenocarcinoma to the lung. Chest 1985;87:129–31.

Fish JE and Peterman VI. (1979). Effects of inhaled lidocaine on airway function in asthmatic subjects. Respiration 1979; 37:201–7.

Fischer JE, Janousek M, Nadal D & Fanconi S (1998) Diagnostic techniques for ventilator associated pneumonia. Lancet 1988; 352:1066–1067

Flanagan PG, Findlay GP, Magee JT, Ionescu A, Barnes RA & Smithies M (2000) The diagnosis of ventilator-associated pneumonia using non- bronchoscopic, non-directed lung lavages. Intensive Care Med 2000; 26:20–30.

Garg S, Handa U, Mohan H & Janmeja AK. (2007). Comparative analysis of various cytohistological techniques in diagnosis of lung diseases. Diagn Cytopathol 2007; 35(1):26–31.

Gasparini S. (1997). Bronchoscopic biopsy techniques in the diagnosis and staging of lung cancer. Monaldi Arch Chest Dis 1997; 4:392–8.

Gasparini S, Ferrety M, Such E, Baldelli S, Zuccatosta L & Gusella P. (1995). Integration of transbronchial and percutaneous approach in the diagnosis of peripheral pulmonary nodules or masses: experience with 1027 consecutive cases. Chest 1995;108:131–7

Gomez M & Silvestri G. A. (2009)Endobronchial Ultrasound for the Diagnosis and Staging of Lung Cancer. Proc Am Thorac Soc 2009; Vol 6. pp 180–186.

Gross TJ, Chavis AD & Lynch JP III. (1991). Non-infectious pulmonary diseases masquerading as community-acquired pneumonia. Clin Chest Med 1991;12:363–93.

Grossman E & Jacobi AM. (1974) Minimal optimal endotracheal tube size for fiberoptic bronchoscopy. Anesth Analg 53:475-76, 1974.

Gruson, D. , Hilbert, G. , Valentino, R. , Vargas, F. , Chene, G. , Bebear, C. , Allery, A. , Pigneux, A. , Gbikpi-Benissan, G. & Cardinaud, J. P. (2000) Utility of fiberoptic bronchoscopy in neutropenic patients admitted to the intensive care unit with pulmonary infiltrates. Crit Care Med 2000; 28, 2224–2230

Guidelines for fiberoptic bronchoscopy in adults. American Thoracic Society. Medical Section of the American Lung Association. (1987)Am. Rev Respir Dis 1987; 136:1066

Haley RW, Hooton TM, Culver DH, Stanley RC, Emori TG, Hardison CD, Quade D, Shachtman RH, Schaberg DR, Shah BV & Schatz GD. (1981). Nosocomia infections in US hospitals, 1975–1976: estimated frequency by selected characteristics of patients. Am J Med 1981; 70:947–959.

Hanson RR, Zavala DC, Rhodes ML, Keim LW & Smith JD. (1976). Transbronchial biopsy via flexible fiberoptic bronchoscope: results in 164 patients. Am Rev Respir Dis 1976; 114:67–72.

Hattotuwa K, Gamble E, O'Shaughnessy T, Jeffery PK & Barnes NC. (2006). Safety of bronchoscopy, biopsy and BAL in research patients with COPD. Chest 2002; 122:1909–1912.

Hautmann H, Henke MO & Bitterling H. (2010). High diagnostic yield from transbronchial biopsy of solitary pulmonary nodules using low-dose CT-guidance. Respirology. May 2010; 15(4):677-82.

Henderson JJ, Popat MT, Latto IP & Pearce AC. (2004). Difficult Airway Society. Difficult Airway Society guidelines for management of the unanticipated difficult intubation. Anaesthesia 2004; 59: 675-94.

Herth FJ, Becker HD & Ernst A. (2002)Aspirin does not increase bleeding complications after transbronchial biopsy. Chest 2002; 122:1461–1464

Herth FJ, Eberhardt R, Vilmann P, Krasnik M & Ernst A. (2006). Real-time endobronchial ultrasound guided transbronchial needle aspiration for sampling mediastinal lymph nodes. Thorax. 2006; 61: 795–798.

Hongo RH, Ley J, Dick SE & Yee RR. (2002). The effect of clopidogrel in combination with aspirin when given before coronary artery bypasses grafting. J Am Coll Cardiol 2002; 40:231–237

Hsu LY, Ding Y, Phua J, Koh LP, Chan DS, Khoo KL & Tambyah PA. (2010). Galactomannan testing of bronchoalveolar lavage fluid is useful for diagnosis of invasive pulmonary aspergillosis in hematology patients. BMC Infect Dis. 2010; 10:44.

Huang L, Morris A, Limper AH, Beck JM & ATS Pneumocystis Workshop Participants. (2006). An Official ATS workshop summary: recent advances and future directions in Pneumocystis pneumonia (PCP). Proc Am Thorac Soc 2006; 3:655–64.

Jimenez, P. , F. Saldias, M. Meneses, M. E. Silva, M. G. Wilson & L. Otth. (1993). Diagnostic fiberoptic bronchoscopy in patients with community-acquired pneumonia. Chest 1993. 103:1023-1027.

Jolliet P & Chevrolet JC. (1992). Bronchoscopy in the intensive care unit. Intensive Care Med 1992; 18:160-69

Joos L, Patuto N, Chhajed P. N & Tamm M. (2006). Diagnostic yield of flexible bronchoscopy in current clinical practice. Swiss Med Wkly 2006; 136:155–159

Katz AS, Michelson MD, Stawicki J & Holford FD. (1981). Cardiac arrhythmias: frequency during bronchoscopy and correlation with hypoxemia. Arch Intern Med 1981; 141: 603–606

Kerwin AJ, Croce MA, Timmons SD, Maxwell RA, Malhotra AK & Fabian TC. (2000). Effects of fiberoptic bronchoscopy on intracranial pressure in patients with brain injury: A prospective clinical study. J Trauma 2000; 48:878–83

Knox AJ, Mascie-Taylor BH & Page RL. (1988). Fiberoptic bronchoscopy in the elderly: four years' experience. Br J Dis Chest. 1988; 82:290–3.

Kobashi Y, Mouri K, Fukuda M, Yoshida K & Oka M. (2007). The Usefulness of Bronchoscopy for the Diagnosis of Pulmonary Tuberculosis. J Bronchol 2007; 14:22–25

Kollef MH, Bock KR, Richards RD & Hearns ML (1995). The safety and diagnostic accuracy of minibronchoalveolar lavage in patients with suspected ventilator-associated pneumonia. Ann Intern Med 1995; 122:743–748

Kollef MH & Ward S. (1998). The influence of mini-BAL cultures on patient outcomes: implications for the antibiotic management of ventilator associated pneumonia. Chest 1998; 113:412–420.

Kozak E & Brath L. (1994). Do "screening" coagulation tests predict bleeding in patients undergoing fiberoptic bronchoscopy with biopsy? Chest 1994;106:703–5.

Kvale P. (1996). Is it really safe to perform bronchoscopy after a recent acute myocardial infarct? Chest 1996; 110:591–2.

Lan RS, Lee CH, Tsai YH, Wang WJ & Chang CH. (1987). Fiberoptic bronchial blockade in a small bronchopleural fistula. Chest 1987; 92:944–946

Lan RS, Lee CH, Chiang YC & Wang WJ. (1989). Use of fiberoptic bronchoscopy to retrieve bronchial foreign bodies in adults. Am Rev Respir Dis 1989;140:1734–7.

Lee T. (1994). Fiberoptic bronchoscopy and intracranial pressure. Chest. 1994; 105:1909.

Limper AH & Prakash UB. (1990). Tracheobronchial foreign bodies in adults. Ann Intern Med 1990;112:604–9.

Liam CK, Pang YK & Poosparajah S. (2007). Diagnostic yield of flexible bronchoscopic procedures in lung cancer patients according to tumour location. Singapore Med J 2007;48(7):625–31.

Lindholm CE, Ollman B, Snyder J, Millen E & Grenvik A. (1974). Flexible fiberoptic bronchoscopy in critical care medicine: diagnosis, therapy, and complications. Crit Care Med 1974; 2:250–261

Lois M & Noppen M. (2005). Bronchopleural fistulas: an overview of the problem with special focus on endoscopic management. Chest. 2005 ; 128 (6): 3955–3965

Loube D, Johnson J, Wiener D, Anders GT, Blanton HM & Hayes JA. (1993). The effect of forceps size on the adequacy of specimens obtained by transbronchial biopsy. Respir Dis 1993; 148:1411–3.

Luna CM, Vujacich P, Niederman MS, Vay C, Gherardi C, Matera J &Jolly EC. (1997). Impact of BAL data on therapy and outcome of ventilator associated pneumonia. Chest 1997; 111:676–687

Lundgren R, Haggmark S & Reiz S. (1982). Hemodynamic effects of flexible fiberoptic bronchoscopy performed under topical anaesthesia. Chest 1982; 82:295–299.

Lynch JP III & Sitrin RG. (1993). Noninfectious mimics of community acquired pneumonia. Semin Respir Infect 1993;8:14–45.

Maertens J, Maertens V, Theunissen K, Meersseman W, Meersseman P, Meers S, Verbeken E, Verhoef G, Van Eldere J & Lagrou K. (2009): Bronchoalveolar lavage fluid galactomannan for the diagnosis of invasive pulmonary aspergillosis in patients with hematologic diseases. Clin Infect Dis 2009, 49:1688-93

Mandell LA, Wunderink RG, Anzueto A, Bartlett JG, Campbell GD, Dean NC, Dowell SF, File TM Jr, Musher DM, Niederman MS, Torres A & Whitney CG. (2007). Infectious Diseases Society of America/American Thoracic Society consensus guidelines on the management of community-acquired pneumonia in adults. Clin Infect Dis 2007;44 (Suppl 2):S27–72

Marini JJ, Pierson DJ & Hudson LD. (1979) Acute lobar atelectasis: a prospective comparison of fiberoptic bronchoscopy and respiratory therapy. Am Rev Respir Dis 1979, 119:971-978.

Martinot A, Closset M, Marquette C H, Hue V, Deschildre A, Ramon P, Remy J & Leclerc F. (1997). Indications for flexible versus rigid bronchoscopy in children with suspected foreign-body aspiration Am. J. Respir. Crit. Care Med 1997; 155:1676-1679.

Matsushima Y, Jones R, King E, Moysa G & Alton J. (1984) . Alterations in pulmonary mechanics and gas exchange during routine fiberoptic bronchoscopy. Chest 86:184 188

Mavritsyn LE & Lifshits NA. (1980). Complications in the fiber bronchoscopy of bronchial asthma patients. Klinicheskaia Meditsina 1980;58:37–40.

Mazzone P, Jain P, Arroliga AC & Matthay RA. (2002). Bronchoscopy and needle biopsy techniques for diagnosing and staging of lung cancer. Clin Chest Med 2002; 23(1):137–58.

Meersseman W, Lagrou K, Maertens J, Wilmer A, Hermans G, Vanderschueren S, Spriet I, Verbeken E & Van Wijngaerden E. (2008). Galactomannanin bronchoalveolar lavagefluid:a tool for diagnosing aspergillosis in intensive care unit patients. Am J Respir Crit Care Med 2008;177(1):27–34.

Mehta NL, Harkin TJ, Rom WN, Graap W, Addrizzo-Harris & Doreen J. (2005). Should Renal Insufficiency Be a Relative Contraindication to Bronchoscopic Biopsy? J Bronchol 2005; 12:81–83

Milman N, Munch E, Faurschou P, Grode G, Peterson BN, Struve-Christensen E & Svendsen UG. (1993). Fiberoptic bronchoscopy in local anaesthesia. Indications, results and complications in 1323 examinations. Acta Endosc 1993;23:151–62

Muscedere JG, Martin CM & Heyland DK. (2008). The impact of ventilator-associated pneumonia on the Canadian health care system. J. Crit. Care 2008; 23(1), 5–10.

National Nosocomial Infections Surveillance (NNIS) System. National Nosocomial Infections Surveillance (NNIS) System report, data summary from January 1990–May 1999, issued June 1999. Am J Infect Control 1999; 27:520–532.

Nicolai T. (2001). Pediatric bronchoscopy. Pediatr Pulmonol 2001; 31: 150–164.

Nguile-Makao M, Zahar JR, Français A, Tabah A, Garrouste-Orgeas M, Allaouchiche B, Goldgran-Toledano D, Azoulay E, Adrie C, Jamali S, Clec'h C, Souweine B & Timsit JF (2010): Attributable mortality of ventilator-associated pneumonia: respective impact of main characteristics at ICU admission and VAP onset using

conditional logistic regression and multi-state models. Intensive Care Med 2010, 36:781-789.
O'Brien JD, Ettinger NA, Shevlin D, & Kollef MH. (1997). Safety and yield of transbronchial biopsy in mechanically ventilated patients. Crit Care Med 1997; 25:440-6.
Oren Fruchter, Mordechai R. Kramer & Tamir Dagan. (2011). Endobronchial Closure of Bronchopleural Fistulae Using Amplatzer Devices Our Experience and Literature Review. Chest 2011;139;682-687
Papazian L, Thomas P, Bregeon F, Garbe L, Zandotti C, Saux P, Gaillat F, Drancourt M, Auffray JP & Gouin F . (1998). Open-lung biopsy in patients with acute respiratory distress syndrome. Anesthesiology 1998; 88: 935-94
Papin T, Lynch J & Weg J. (1985). Transbronchial biopsy in the thrombocytopenic patient. Chest 1985; 88:549-52.
Patrick F. Allan PF & Ouellette D. (2003). Bronchoscopic Procedures in Octogenarians. J Bronchol . 10:112-117, 2003.
Peacock M, Johnson J & Blanton H. (1994). Complications of flexible bronchoscopy in patients with severe obstructive pulmonary disease. J Bronchol 1994; 1:181-6.
Pechkam D & Elliott MW. (2002). Pulmonary infiltrates in the immunocompromised: Diagnosis and management. Thorax 2002;57(suppl 2):II3- II7
Peerless JR, Snow N, Likavec MJ, Pinchak AC & Malangoni MA. (1995). The effect of fiberoptic bronchoscopy on cerebral hemodynamics in patients with severe head injury. Chest. 1995;108:962-965.
Pennington JE. (1990). Nosocomial respiratory infection. : Editors - Mandell GL, Douglas RG Jr, Bennet JE : Principles and practice of infectious diseases. St. Louis, MO: Churchill Livingstone; 1990. p. 2199-2205.
Pereira W, Kovnat D & Snider G. (1978). A prospective cooperative study of complications following flexible fiberoptic bronchoscopy. Chest 1978; 73:813-6.
Pincus P S, Kallenbach J M, Hurwitz M D, Clinton C, Feldman C, Abramowitz J A, & Zwi S. (1987). Transbronchial biopsy during mechanical ventilation. Crit Care Med 1987; 15:1136-9.
Prakash UBS, Stubbs SE. Optimal Bronchoscopy. Journal of Bronchology. 1994; 1; 44-62
Prakash UBS, Offord KP & Stubbs SE. (1991). Bronchoscopy in North America: The ACCP Survey. Chest 1991; 100:1668-75
Pue C & Pacht E. (1995). Complications of fiberoptic bronchoscopy at a university hospital. Chest 1995; 107:430-2.
Pugin J, Auckenthaler R, Mili N, Janssens JP, Lew PD, Suter PM (1991) Diagnosis of ventilator-associated pneumonia by bacteriologic analysis of bronchoscopic and nonbronchoscopic "blind" bronchoalveolar lavage fluid. Am Rev Respir Dis 143:1121-1129
Raghavendran K, Nemzek J, Napolitano LM & Knight PR. (2011). Aspiration-induced lung injury. Crit Care Med 2011; 39:818-826
Rankin J, Snyder P, Schachter E & Matthay RA. (1984). Bronchoalveolar lavage. Its safety in subjects with mild asthma. Chest 1984; 85: 723-8.
Rebulla P: (2001). Platelet transfusion trigger in difficult patients. Transfus Clin Biol 2001;8:249- 254.
Regel G, Sturm JA, Neumann C, Schueler S & Tscherne H. (1989). Occlusion of broncopleural fistula after lung injury: a new treatment by bronchoscopy. J Trauma 1989; 29:223-226

Rennard SI. (1990). Bronchoalveolar lavage in the diagnosis of cancer. Lung 1990;168:1035–40.

Rudy EB, Turner BS, Baun M, Stone KS & Brucia J. (1991). Endotracheal suctioning in adults with head injury. Heart Lung. 1991;20:667- 674.

Schreiber G & McCrory DC. (2003). Performance characteristics of different modalities for diagnosis of suspected lung cancer: summary of published evidence. Chest 2003; 123(Suppl 1):115S–28S.

Schurink CA, Van Nieuwenhoven CA, Jacobs JA, Rozenberg-Arska M, Joore HC, Buskens E, Hoepelman AI & Bonten MJ (2004) Clinical pulmonary infection score for ventilator-associated pneumonia: accuracy and inter-observer variability. Intensive Care Med 2004; 30:217–224

Schwartz DE, Matthay MA & Cohen NH. (1995). Death and other complications of emergency airway management in critically ill adults. A prospective investigation of 297 tracheal intubations. Anesthesiology. 1995;82:367–376. .

Semenzato G, Spatafora M, Feruglio C, Pace E & Dipietro V. (1990). Bronchoalveolar lavage and the immunology of lung cancer. Lung 1990;168:1041–9.

Singh N, Rogers P, Atwood CW, Wagener MM & Yu VL. (2000). Shortcourse empiric antibiotic therapy for patients with pulmonary infiltrates in the intensive care unit. A proposed solution for indiscriminate antibiotic prescription. Am J Respir Crit Care Med 2000;162:505–511

Snow N & Lucas A. (1984). Bronchoscopy in the critically ill surgical patient. Am Surg 1984; 50:441–445

Spiro S. G & Porter J. C. (2002). Lung Cancer—Where Are We Today? Current Advances in Staging and Nonsurgical Treatment Am J Respir Crit Care Med Vol 166. pp 1166–1196, 2002

Stephan F, Hollande J, Richard O, Cheffi A, Maier-Redelsperger M & Flahault A. (1999). : Thrombocytopenia in a surgical ICU. Chest 1999, 115:1363-1370.

Stevens RP, Lillington GA & Parsons G. (1981) Fiberoptic bronchoscopy in the intensive care unit. Heart Lung 1981; 10:1037- 1045

Strauss R, Wehler M, Mehler K, Kreutzer D, Koebnick C & Hahn EG. (2002). Thrombocytopenia in patients in the medical intensive care unit: bleeding prevalence, transfusion requirements, and outcome. Crit Care Med 2002, 30:1765-1771.

Surrat PM, Smiddly JF & Gruber B. (1979). Death and complications associated with fiberoptic bronchoscopy. Chest. 1979; 69:747–751.

Talmadge E. King, Jr. (2005). Clinical Advances in the Diagnosis and Therapy of the Interstitial Lung Diseases. Am J Respir Crit Care Med 2005;Vol 172. pp 268–279

Torres A & El-Ebiary M. (2000). Bronchoscopic BAL in the diagnosis of ventilator-associated pneumonia. Chest 2000;117(4 Suppl 2):198S- 202.

Torres, A. , Serra-Batlles J, Ferrer A, Jimenez P, Celis R, Cobo E & Rodriquez-Roisin R. (1991). Severe community-acquired pneumonia: epidemiology and prognostic factors. Am. Rev. Respir. Dis. 1991. 144:312-318

Tsushima K, Sone S, Hanaoka T, Takayama F, Honda T & Kubo K. (2006). Comparison of bronchoscopic diagnosis for peripheral pulmonary nodule under fluoroscopic guidance with CT guidance. Respir Med. Apr 2006;100(4):737-45.

Tsukamoto T, Sasaki H & Nakamura H: (1989). Treatment of hemoptysis patients by thrombin and fibrinogen-thrombin infusion therapy using a fiberoptic bronchoscope. Chest 96:473–476, 1989

Uchida J, Imamura F, Takenaka A, Yoshimura M, Ueno K, Oda K, Nakayama T, Tsukamoto Y, Higashiyama M & Kusunoki Y. (2006). Improved diagnostic efficacy by rapid cytology test in fluoroscopy- guided bronchoscopy. J Thorac Oncol 2006; 1(4):314–8.

Van Vyve T, Chanez P, Bousquet J, Lacoste JY, Michel FB & Godard P. (1992). Safety of bronchoalveolar lavage and bronchial biopsies in patients with asthma of variable severity. Am Rev Respir Dis 1992; 146: 116–21.

Vanderschueren S, De Weerdt A, Malbrain M, Vankersschaever D, Frans E, Wilmer A & Bobbaers H. (2000). Thrombocytopenia and prognosis in intensive care. Crit Care Med 2000, 28:1871-1876.

Venkateshiah S. B & Mehta A. C. (2003). Role of Flexible Bronchoscopy in the Diagnosis of Pulmonary Tuberculosis in Immunocompetent Individuals. J Bronchol 2003;10: 300–308

Wahidi MM & Ernst A. (2004). The role of bronchoscopy in the management of lung transplant recipients. Respir Care Clin 2004;10: 549–562

Wall CP, Gaensler EA, Carrington CB & Hayes JA. (1981). Comparison of Transbronchial and open biopsies in chronic infiltrative lung diseases. Am Rev Respir Dis 1981; 123:280–285.

Wang KP, Brower R, Haponik EF & Siegelman S. (1983). Flexible Transbronchial needle aspiration for staging of bronchogenic carcinoma. Chest 1983; 84:571–576

Wang KP, Wise RA, Terry PB, Kaplan J, Britt EJ, Haponik EF, Summer WR & Marsh B. (1980). Comparison of standard and large forceps for transbronchial lung biopsy in the diagnosis of lung infiltrates. Endoscopy. Jul 1980;12(4):151-4.

Weinstein HJ, Bone RC & Ruth WE. (1977). Pulmonary lavage in patients treated with mechanical ventilation. Chest 1977; 72:583–587

Weiss SM, Hert RC, Gianola FJ, Clark JG & Crawford SW: Complications of fiberoptic bronchoscopy in thrombocytopenic patients. Chest 1993, 104: 4. 1025-1028.

Wintrbauer RH. (1995). Mimics of pneumonia. Semin Respir Infect 1995;10:63–120.

Wood RE. (1984). Spelunking in the pediatric airways: explorations with the flexible fiberoptic bronchoscope. Pediatr Clin North Am 1984; 31: 785–799.

Wood RE. (1985). The diagnostic effectiveness of the flexible bronchoscope in children Pediatric Pulmonology. 1985; 1:188–192 DOI: 10. 1002/ppul. 1950010404

Wood-Baker R, Burdon J, McGregor A, Robinson P & Seal P. (2001). Fiber-optic bronchoscopy in adults: a position paper of The Thoracic Society of Australia and New Zealand. Intern Med J 2001;31:479–87

Yende S & Wunderink RG. (2001). Effect of clopidogrel on bleeding after coronary artery bypass surgery. Crit Care Med 2001; 29:2271–2275

Yung RC. (2003). Tissue diagnosis of suspected lungcancer: selecting between bronchoscopy, transthoracic needle aspiration, and resectional biopsy. Respir Care Clin N Am 2003;9(1):51–76.

Zavala DC. (1975). Diagnostic fiberoptic bronchoscopy: techniques and results of biopsy in 600 patients. Chest 1975; 68:12–9.

Zavala DC. (1976). Pulmonary hemorrhage in fiberoptic transbronchial biopsy. Chest 1976; 70:584–8.

Zavala DC. (1978). Complications following fiberoptic bronchoscopy. Chest 1978; 73:783–5.

Zink A, Fritsch K, Eich C & Thurnheer R. (2007). Pneumothorax after Transbronchial Biopsy or Fine Needle Aspiration: Can it be Predicted? A Prospective Study of 94 Cases. J Bronchol 2007; 14:162–164.

2

Monitoring, Sedation, and Anesthesia for Flexible Fiberoptic Bronchoscopy

Michael J. Morris[1], Herbert P. Kwon[2] and Thomas B. Zanders[3]
[1]Brooke Army Medical Center, Fort Sam Houston, Texas
[2]Womack Army Medical Center, Fort Bragg, North Carolina
[3]Brooke Army Medical Center, Fort Sam Houston, Texas
USA

1. Introduction

Since the advent of flexible fiberoptic bronchoscopy (FFB) in the 1970's, the use of sedation and topical anesthesia has allowed the practice of bronchoscopy, specifically FFB, to evolve from the operating room to the outpatient setting. Early techniques of general anesthesia and regional blockade of nerves innervating the airway have been largely replaced by improved techniques of patient monitoring, intravenous conscious sedation, and application of topical anesthetics in the airway. Today the bronchoscopist, in addition to basic FFB techniques such as bronchoalveolar lavage and transbronchial biopsy, can also perform complicated procedures such as removal of foreign bodies, ablation of airway tumors, and endobronchial stenting, all in the outpatient bronchoscopy suite. A continued emphasis has been placed on improvements in patient safety due to the complexities of the procedure itself, but also the role of conscious sedation and topical anesthetics to ensure maximal performance by the bronchoscopist to achieve the desired goal of successful biopsy or other interventions while the patient remains comfortable throughout the entire procedure. A full understanding of the patient's medical history, underlying risk factors such as cardiovascular and pulmonary disease, and medication use is required to plan the requirements for the FFB.

1.1 Guidelines for bronchoscopy

There is some expert consensus guidance published on the use of sedation and topical anesthesia during FFB. The National Institutes of Health published a workshop summary on the investigational use of FFB in patients with asthma in 1985 (National Institutes of Health [NIH], 1985). Further recommendations for investigational FFB in asthmatics was provided in 1991 and commented on potential hazards, high risk and unsuitable patients, and

---

The opinions or assertions contained herein are the private views of the authors and are not to be construed as reflecting the Department of the Army, Department of the Air Force, or the Department of Defense.

No outside funding from any source was received during conduct of this research or preparation of this manuscript. Dr. Morris is a paid speaker for Spiriva by Boehringer-Ingelheim/Pfizer. The other authors have no financial conflicts to disclose.

procedural limitations (NIH, 1991). The American Thoracic Society (ATS) published a concise one-page guideline in 1987 which outlined diagnostic and therapeutic uses, research applications, conditions with increased risk, and contraindications for FFB (American Thoracic Society [ATS], 1987). It did not, however, provide any specific guidance on the optimal use of topical anesthesia or intravenous sedation. In 2001, the British Thoracic Society published a more complete guideline and made several major recommendations related to sedation and topical anesthesia for all patients undergoing FFB (British Thoracic Society [BTS], 2001). All of the following recommendations had level B evidence (except for #8 with level C) to support their use.

1. Sedation should be offered to patients where there is no contraindication.
2. Atropine is not required routinely before bronchoscopy.
3. Patients should be monitored by pulse oximetry.
4. Oxygen supplementation should be used to achieve an oxygen saturation of at least 90% to reduce the risk of significant arrhythmias during the procedure and also in the postoperative recovery period.
5. The total dose of lidocaine should be limited to 8.2 mg/kg in adults (approximately 29 ml of a 2% solution for a 70 kg patient) with extra care in the elderly or those with liver or cardiac impairment.
6. The minimum amount of lidocaine necessary should be used when instilled through the bronchoscope.
7. Sedatives should be used in incremental doses to achieve adequate sedation and amnesia.
8. Routine ECG monitoring during bronchoscopy is not required but should be considered in those patients with a history of severe cardiac disease and those who have hypoxia despite oxygen supplementation.

A survey of BTS pulmonologists was conducted after the publication of these guidelines (Pickles et al., 2003). A variety of lidocaine (or lignocaine) preparations to include gel, spray, and nebulized were used in 97% of patients with rare use of other anesthetics such as cocaine or amethocaine lozenges. Interestingly, sedation was most commonly done with midazolam but was not used by 27% of respondents citing age, frailty, and medical co-morbidities. Assessment of sedation during FFB was most frequently done by measurements of oxygen saturations (98%) and observation of patient response (57%). Similar findings on the lack of standardization were noted in a separate survey of BTS pulmonologists (Smyth et al., 2002).

1.2 Contraindications

The American Thoracic Society (ATS) 1987 guidelines presented four absolute contraindications to the performance of FFB that included: 1) operator inexperience, 2) lack of adequate facilities, 3) absence of informed consent, and 4) inability to maintain adequate oxygenation. Other significant contraindications thought to confer a high risk to patients during FFB included: 1) profound refractory hypoxemia; 2) severe bleeding diathesis uncorrectable prior to the procedure, and 3) malignant cardiac arrhythmias (ATS, 1987). Other medical conditions that also increased the risk of FFB and were listed as relative contraindications included: 1) lack of patient cooperation, 2) recent myocardial infarction or unstable angina, 3) respiratory insufficiency or failure, 4) uremia, 5) unstable asthma, 6) unstable cardiac arrhythmias, and 7) significant debilitation or malnutrition. The 2001 BTS guidelines do not present any specified contraindications but noted there are no controlled studies of the patient risk factors and each patient must be individually assessed based on the risk-benefit ratio (BTS, 2001).

2. Preparation for bronchoscopy

The goal of patient assessment for any invasive procedure such as FFB is to forewarn of potential complications or to identify complications that occur as a result of the procedure. Possible bronchoscopic complications may include a variety of respiratory, cardiac, and other conditions (Pereira et al., 1978, Suratt et al., 1976). Reported respiratory complications include hypoxia, hypercapnea, laryngospasm, bronchospasm, pulmonary edema, aspiration, airway obstruction, pneumomediastinum and pneumothorax (Facciolongo et al., 2009). Cardiac complications can include vasovagal reactions, tachycardia, bradycardia, dysrhythmias, and myocardial infarction. Other reported complications are airway trauma, hemorrhage, epistaxis, infection, nausea and vomiting, adverse reactions to topical anesthesia, exposure to radiation, and death. In an attempt to avoid these possible events, preparation of the patient begins with the initial assessment and evaluation, and monitoring continues through all phases of FFB.

2.1 Patient evaluation

All patients with an indication for FFB should undergo a historical assessment to identify potential bleeding, respiratory, medication, neurologic, or cardiovascular risks. These could potentially include blood dyscrasias, uremia, anti-coagulant or anti-platelet medications, surgical or dental history, a history of asthma, cervical spine disease, interstitial pneumonia, upper airway obstructions, congenital defects, cardiac history, epilepsy, neoplastic mass or therapies. A previous history of bronchoscopy complications, adverse reactions to sedation, drug or alcohol abuse history may also prove useful (American Society of Anesthesiologists [ASA], 2002). Additionally, a family history for clotting complications or bleeding disorders may suggest when a patient is at higher risk for complication. The airway exam should include an assessment of potential bronchoscope entry points in either nares or mouth for potential risks such as small lumens, excessive deviation, congenital deformities or loose dentition. As some patients require intubation due to procedural complications a Mallampati score, exam of habitus, neck, jaw, and oral structures as they affect direct laryngoscopic intubation are also recommended. Pulmonary exams should include an assessment for tachypnea, increased effort or asymmetry, "barrel-chest", auscultation, cyanosis or clubbing. As bleeding and cardiovascular events have also been reported to complicate bronchoscopy a focused exam to identify potential risk factors in these systems should also be performed. Finally, an American Society of Anesthesiologist's Physical Status Classification should also be recorded (ASA, 2002).

All patients undergoing FFB with sedation should undergo a thorough evaluation to include medical and surgical history, current medications, drug allergies, and amount and type of alcohol and illicit drug use. Medical and surgical history should focus on evaluating the patient's degree of cardiac and respiratory compromise and reserve physiology. Close attention and consideration should be given to those with obstructive lung disease, obstructive sleep apnea, neuromuscular disorders, renal and hepatic impairments. Physical exam should focus on upper airway abnormalities, assessment of potential difficult airway anatomy, pulmonary system focusing on active airway obstruction, and gross neurologic function.

2.2 Pulmonary function testing

Pulmonary function testing should be performed if there is clinical suspicion for severe obstruction. The BTS guideline suggests testing be performed when forced expiratory volume at one second (FEV_1) is less than 40% predicted or oxygen saturation (SaO_2) is less than 93% (BTS, 2001). One small prospective trial reported a drop of 13.8% in FEV_1 (baseline $1.37 \pm 0.16L$) approximately 15 minutes into bronchoscopy (Salisbury et al., 1975). A slightly larger retrospective review reported patients who had a FEV_1/forced expiratory volume (FVC) ratio less than 50% or an FEV_1 less than one liter with an FEV_1/FVC ratio less than 69% had a bronchoscopic complication rate of 5% compared to 0.6% of controls with normal spirometric function (Peacock et al., 1994). If the patient requires additional procedures such as bronchoalveolar lavage or transbronchial biopsy and there are concerns for possible respiratory compromise, screening spirometry may also be useful. Lima reported that patients with diffuse lung disease have a decrease of approximately 12.7% in FEV_1 following bronchoalveolar lavage (Lima et al., 2009).

2.3 Radiographic studies

It is assumed that a patient who is scheduled to undergo FFB has already had a chest radiograph performed given the minimal risk and ability to non-invasively assess the thorax. However, if a computed tomography (CT) scan of the chest has not already been performed, it should be considered for patients with hemoptysis or undergoing a neoplastic evaluation. A higher diagnostic sampling yield for malignancy has been reported if the patient had a CT performed prior to bronchoscopy (Bungay et al., 2000; Laroche et al., 2000). Additionally, in cases of hemoptysis, pre-procedural CT was able to improve sampling in patients who were at higher risk for neoplastic associated hemoptysis, obviate the need for invasive evaluation, or help identify areas of bronchiectasis for sampling (McGuinness et al., 1994; Tsoumakidou et al., 2006).

2.4 Laboratory testing

A large number of practitioners empirically order coagulation tests prior to performing FFB. The ability of these tests to predict bleeding risks prior to FFB is controversial and several sources recommend against routine testing (Bjørtuft et al., 1998; Kozak & Brath, 1994; Segal et al., 2005). Additionally, Weiss reported bleeding risks in a group of thrombocytopenic patients with platelet counts less than 100,000 who underwent a total of 58 FFB procedures. There were seven occurrences of epistaxis and/or hemorrhage but only one patient experienced severe epistaxis despite an oral approach and a platelet count of 18,000 (Weiss et al., 1993). Thus, routine testing without significant suspicion for bleeding risk is not recommended. A pre-procedural arterial blood gas is recommended in the 2001 BTS guidelines for the same patients who may benefit from a pre-procedural PFT, FEV_1 less than 40% predicted or SaO2 $<93\%$ (BTS, 2001). There is scant available data to support this recommendation except for the report by Salisbury in which one patient whose PaO2 plummeted from 60 mm Hg to 38 mm Hg intra-procedurally and resolved with removal of the bronchoscope (Salisbury et al., 1975).

2.5 Anti-platelet medications and anticoagulants

Anti-platelet agents and non-steroidal anti-inflammatory (NSAID) medications are commonly used by patients who have an indication for FFB. While there is a potential for bleeding complications from biopsy, there are few reported cases of complications related to NSAID medication use. Aspirin is not reported to increase the rate of bleeding bronchoscopic complications when compared to controls (Herth et al., 2002). However, the continued use of clopidogrel prior to bronchoscopy has been associated with a bleeding rate of 89% and up to 100% of patients who continued to take both aspirin and clopidogrel together (Ernst et al., 2006). In patients who can tolerate the cessation of antiplatelet therapy, the 2008 American College of Chest Physicians (ACCP) clinical practice guidelines recommend stopping clopidogrel seven to ten days before FFB while Ernst, et al. recommended stopping five to seven days before FFB.(Douketis et al., 2008; Ernst et al., 2006) While the ACCP additionally recommends that NSAID medications be stopped five half-lives prior to a planned procedure with bleeding risk, there is no specific data on FFB to support this statement. Direct thrombin inhibitors and vitamin K antagonists such as warfarin are also commonly used by patients who require bronchoscopy. The 2008 ACCP Clinical Practice guidelines recommend cessation of warfarin for at least five days prior to a procedure with an INR assessment 1-2 days before the procedure for an INR < 1.5. Certain patients, i.e. those with mechanical valves, may also require bridging on other anticoagulants (Douketis et al., 2008).

3. Monitoring during bronchoscopy

3.1 Pre-procedure assessment

Immediately prior to FFB, the patient should be re-evaluated for recent medical events or other changes in condition such as infection or flare of respiratory disease (ASA, 2002; BTS, 2001). Patients who have experienced a recent myocardial infarction are recommended to have the procedure delayed for up to 6 weeks (BTS, 2001). The patient history of oral intake should be confirmed. In healthy patients without modifiers such as delayed gastric emptying, the ASA Pre-Procedure Fasting Guidelines recommend fasting for two hours for clear liquids, four hours for breast milk, and six hours for formula or light meals to decrease the risk of aspiration (ASA, 2002) The BTS guidelines for FFB lower the time limit for light meals to four hours (BTS, 2001). In all patients, intravenous access should be obtained and maintained throughout the procedure. Routine vital signs to confirm systemic and hemodynamic stability are recommended. If the patient has a high risk for cardiovascular disease, consideration should be given to obtain a 12-lead electrocardiogram (Shrader & Lakshminarayan, 1978).

3.2 Intraprocedural monitoring

For patients who will receive a moderate level of sedation (able to maintain spontaneous ventilation and respond to verbal or tactile stimuli), continuous hemodynamic monitoring should be used at five minute intervals (ASA, 2002). While it is uncertain that all patients undergoing FFB would benefit from intra-procedural continuous electrocardiographic monitoring, both societies recommend continued monitoring in patients who are at high cardiovascular risk. (ASA, 2002; BTS, 2001) A study of continuous electrocardiographic monitoring demonstrated evidence of myocardial ischemia in 17% of 29 patients above the age of 50 undergoing FFB (Matot et al., 1997).

3.3 Supplemental oxygen

The routine use of supplemental oxygen during FFB has previously been a point of disagreement with some authors. Given the known risks for cardiac arrhythmia during periods of hypoxia, both supplemental oxygen administration and monitoring with pulse oximetry are recommended for all patients. The sensitivity of pulse oximetry to detect hypoxia compared to clinical exam should make this a routine part of FFB even in healthy or research patients, especially with the use of conscious sedation (ASA, 2002; BTS, 2001; Shrader & Lakshminarayan, 1978). Ghio et al. demonstrated evidence of hypoxia in healthy volunteers during the initiation of bronchoalveolar lavage (Ghio et al., 2007). Nearly 25% of patients in a study of 1,051 FFB required the use of supplemental oxygen for desaturations (Jones & O'Driscoll, 2000). The BTS recommends using supplemental oxygen to maintain a goal of SaO2 greater than 89% during and after FFB (BTS, 2001). Patients who undergo FFB are frequently at increased risk for hypercapnea due to intravenous sedation or underlying lung disease (Salisbury et al., 1975). While capnography is also more sensitive to hypercapnea than physical exam, there is no clear recommendation or evidence to support the routine use of capnography during FFB with moderate levels of sedation.

3.4 Post-procedure assessment

After FFB is completed, patients should continue to receive oximetry and be monitored until they are near their baseline state of consciousness and interaction (ASA, 2002). Supplemental oxygen should also be continued until the patient can spontaneously maintain a SaO2 greater than 89%. The return of the gag reflex and the ability to safely swallow clear liquids should be confirmed (BTS, 2001). If the patient has received transbronchial biopsies with or without fluoroscopic guidance, a chest radiograph should be performed one hour following the procedure (BTS, 2001). Transthoracic ultrasound has recently come to prominence for the ability to identify the presence of pneumothorax, but its routine use following FFB is not yet well established.

4. Sedation

Persons undergoing FFB can experience significant degree of anxiety, sense of asphyxiation, and severe coughing. Sedative and analgesic agents are frequently administered to patients undergoing bronchoscopy to reduce these noxious sensations. Both the ATS and the BTS guidelines recommend the use of sedation during bronchoscopy (ATS, 1987; BTS, 2001). Despite this, debate has continued regarding the necessity of sedation during FFB. Surveys have revealed increased physician comfort and use of sedation during bronchoscopy (McLean et al., 1998; Prakash et al., 1991). Patient satisfaction and willingness to pursue repeat FFB procedures if required has been shown to be higher in those receiving sedative and systemic analgesic agents (Gonzales et al., 2003; Hirose et al., 2008; Putinati et al., 1999; Steinfort & Irvin, 2010). Tolerance to FFB was clearly decreased in a prospective study of 357 patients who received no sedation for their procedure (Lopez et al., 2006). Putinati et al. also demonstrated improved procedural success in those receiving sedative agents. Bronchoscopy was aborted prior to completion in six of fifty patients in the placebo group

(Putinati et al., 1999). Interestingly, Hatton et al. described decreased patient satisfaction and willingness to undergo repeat procedure when comparing midazolam to placebo (Hatton et al., 1994). Subsequent editorial comments highlight the difficulty in evaluating these studies as the results were criticized for insufficient medication dosing and administration sequence (Hanley, 1995).

Previous reviews reveal wide variation in the practice patterns for sedation use during FFB (Matot & Kramer, 2000; Vincent & Silvestri, 2007). No single regimen has been found to be superior and previous guidelines did not have recommended regimens (BTS, 2001). Recently, the American College of Chest Physicians released a consensus statement on topical anesthesia, analgesia and sedation during FFB. The consensus statement suggested the use of lidocaine for topical anesthesia and the combination of a benzodiazepine and opiate administration for sedation and analgesia during the procedure, with propofol as an effective alternative agent (Wahidi et al., 2011). Multiple factors must be taken into consideration when selecting an analgesic and sedative regimen. Patient characteristics include age, co-morbidities, and baseline respiratory physiology. The procedure complexity and time required must be considered as an airway survey and bronchoalveolar lavage invariably requires less time and sedation than more complex procedures such as transbronchial biopsies, mediastinal lymph node sampling, debulking and stenting of endobronchial lesions. The degree of sedation required can vary greatly from mild sedation to general anesthesia (ASA, 2002). Increasingly complex FFB procedures are being performed without the assistance of general anesthesia including mediastinal lymph node staging with endobronchial ultrasound guidance with good patient satisfaction (Steinfort & Irvin, 2010). Finally one must be familiar with the degree of support staff able to provide pre and post-procedural care and monitoring during the recovery process.

4.1 Degree of sedation

The desired degree of sedation and analgesia should be determined for individual patients and follow American Society of Anesthesiologists (ASA) definitions:

1. Minimal Sedation (Anxiolysis): A drug induced state with normal response to verbal stimulation with unaffected airway, spontaneous ventilation and cardiovascular function
2. Moderate Sedation/Analgesia (Conscious Sedation): A drug induced state with purposeful response to verbal or tactile stimulation, no airway interventions required, maintains adequate spontaneous ventilation, and cardiovascular function typically maintained.
3. Deep Sedation/Analgesia: A drug induced state with purposeful response after repeated or painful stimuli, airway intervention may be required, spontaneous ventilation may be inadequate and cardiovascular function typically maintained.
4. General Anesthesia: A drug induced state in which patients are not arousable even with painful stimulus, airway intervention required, spontaneous ventilation frequently inadequate, and cardiovascular function may be impaired.

The level of sedation required for FFB is typically minimal to moderate depending upon the type of procedure planned and is often performed by a non-anesthesiologist. When greater than moderate sedation is desired, those patients with limited cardiovascular or pulmonary reserve, or prolonged procedure anticipated, it is recommended the expertise of an anesthesiologist be obtained.

4.2 Sedative and analgesic agents

Favorable agent profiles include relatively rapid onset of action, rapid and predictable recovery, with minimal hemodynamic instability and lack of significant respiratory depression at doses achieving desired level of sedation. For these reasons benzodiazepines, opioids, and more recently propofol have been increasingly used for sedation during FFB (Vincent & Silvestri, 2007). Other intravenous agents to improve patient comfort such as atropine are not currently recommended and limited studies have failed to demonstrate a significant benefit (Hasanoglu et al., 2001; Korteweg et al., 2004; Triller et al., 2004)

4.2.1 Benzodiazepines

Benzodiazepines have sedative-hypnotic, anxiolytic, and amnestic effects by interacting on GABA receptors. Frequently used agents include diazepam, midazolam, lorazepam, and temazepam (Greig et al., 1995; Leite et al., 2008; Vincent & Silvestri, 2007; Watts et al., 2005). Oral use of temazepam and diazepam has been described and appear to offer an appropriate degree of mild sedation/anxiolysis (Matot & Kramer, 2000; Watts et al., 2005). The advent of midazolam, a water soluble, short-acting benzodiazepine able to be given intravenously has made it the primary agent in many bronchoscopy suites. The metabolites of midazolam have minimal subsequent effects. Midazolam can be given via intermittent intravenous doses and tailored to patient responses. Caution should be used when administrating to the elderly and those with obstructive airway physiology. Sedation is typically effective for 20-40 minutes. Midazolam can be safely given in 0.5mg to 1mg increments at five minute intervals until desired level of sedation achieved. Another desirable attribute to benzodiazepines is the availability of a reversal agent. The competitive antagonist, flumazenil can rapidly reverse the effects of benzodiazepines. Though not standard practice, a study of 22 patients demonstrated successful reversal FB sedation using flumazenil (Williamson et al., 1997). Flumazenil use is typically reserved for benzodiazepine reversal in those patients experiencing sedation related hypoxia, need for improved airway clearance, or increasing hypercarbia. Flumazenil use should be avoided in those patients on chronic benzodiazepines due to possible seizure provocation.

4.2.2 Opiates

Opiates have both sedative and analgesic properties as well as antitussive effects. Frequently used opiate agents include fentanyl, alfentanil, remifentanil, meperidine and less frequently morphine. Many studies have evaluated opiate agents in combination with other sedatives including benzodiazepines and propofol (Greig et al., 1995; Hwang et al., 2005; Leite et al., 2008; Matot & Kramer, 2000; Vincent & Silvestri, 2007; Yoon et al., 2011). Greig et al. demonstrated that a lone opiate agent in combination with a benzodiazepine resulted in a reduced number of coughs and reduced topical lidocaine dose (Greig et al., 1995). Fentanyl and related agents are desired due to rapid onset of action, high potency, and short duration of action. A study of alfentanil with standard dose topical lidocaine revealed improved composite score of sedative effects and adverse events when compared to lidocaine alone or midazolam combined with topical lidocaine. The propofol combination composite score was slightly superior to alfentanil combination (Leite et al., 2008). All opiates can produce respiratory depression and this is amplified when given in combination with another sedative agent (Yoon et al., 2011). If severe respiratory depression occurs, reversal of opiate agents can be obtained with naloxone use. Due to potential adverse hemodynamic effects of naloxone and sudden opiate reversal, this should be reserved for those patients with clinically significant respiratory depression.

4.2.3 Propofol

Propofol is an alkyl-phenol sedative-hypnotic agent in a lipid emulsion capable of producing a dose-dependent degree of sedation from conscious sedation to general anesthesia. It has a rapid onset of action (less than two minutes) and rapid recovery (less than 15 minutes) (Matot & Kramer, 2000; Vincent & Silvestri, 2007). When compared to alfentanil and midazolam as well as topical lidocaine, propofol had the lowest composite score indicating the lowest complication index (Leite et al., 2008). Propofol has been demonstrated to have improved patient neuropsychometric recovery with no difference in physician procedural sedation satisfaction when compared to midazolam (Clark et al., 2009). Propofol has also been reported to be a safe option for sedation in pediatric patients (Berkenbosch et al., 2004; Larsen et al., 2009). In a retrospective study, it must be noted however that fifty percent of pediatric patients were classified as having minor complications which included the need for supplemental oxygen, oropharyngeal suctioning or jaw-thrust to improve oxygen saturation (Larsen et al., 2009). Propofol in separate combinations with alfentanil and ketamine has been demonstrated to provide patient controlled sedation via a patient-controlled-analgesia device (Hwang et al., 2005). Fospropofol, a water-soluble prodrug of propofol, has been demonstrated to be a safe agent during FFB in a phase three trial (Silvestri et al., 2009). Mild to moderate hypoxia was noted in 15% of the patients given the described optimal sedative dose. One must be aware of and recognize the typically dose dependent hemodynamic effects (hypotension, decreased cardiac output) as well as the rare development of propofol infusion syndrome.

5. Topical anesthesia

Along with sedation, topical airway anesthesia is an important component of FFB as it provides the patient additional comfort and tolerability that sedation alone will not provide. Local anesthesia of the nares, oropharynx, and hypopharynx allows comfortable passage of the bronchoscope to the upper airway. More importantly, topical anesthesia of the airways beyond the glottis blunts the cough reflex and allows the bronchoscopist to visualize the airways and perform necessary procedures. Selected patients such as healthy volunteers with adequate topical anesthesia can tolerate FFB without the need for intravenous sedation (Ghio et al., 1998). There have been a variety of studies that have explored issues of patient comfort, tolerability of FFB and dosing regimens. While patient comfort is the primary goal, the ability for the bronchoscopist to complete the procedure is likewise paramount.

5.1 Administration

There is significant variation in the administration of topical anesthesia during FFB. The optimal preparation largely depends on the patient, the experience of the technician, and the estimated length of the procedure. A typical airway preparation for FFB in our institution includes the application of 2% viscous lidocaine for the nasal mucosa, nebulized 4% topical lidocaine for oral inhalation prior to the FFB, and application of 1% topical lidocaine during the procedure for additional upper and lower airway mucosal anesthesia to control coughing. This airway preparation uses approximately 500 mg of topical lidocaine. The amount of 1% lidocaine used is highly variable and physician dependent with approximately 100 mg used for direct application to the vocal cords and carina and additional lidocaine used for lower airway anesthesia to suppress coughing. There are relatively few studies examining the optimal lidocaine dosing for patient comfort and safety during FFB. A study examining various lidocaine amounts (mg/kg) and strengths ranging from 1% to 2% in 96 patients found no differences between the six groups in terms of patient comfort (Mainland et al., 2001). The author recommended use of 1% lidocaine for topical airway anesthesia based on similar amounts of supplemental lidocaine doses and serum lidocaine levels. An earlier 1985 study demonstrated there was no effect on patient comfort scores when a fixed dose of 370 mg of lidocaine was compared with higher lidocaine doses with as needed dosing (mean lidocaine dose=512 mg) (Sutherland et al., 1985). Notably, the airway preparation in the fixed dose group used 1% lidocaine versus 2% in the uncontrolled group. A 2008 prospective study evaluating the equivalence of 1% versus 2% topical lidocaine during FFB demonstrated no difference in cough frequency or as needed doses of lidocaine by the bronchoscopist. The 2% lidocaine group received twice the mg/kg dose as the 1% lidocaine without increasing patient comfort (Hasmoni et al., 2008). Finally, the use of nebulized lidocaine during the FFB preparation is equivocal (Keane & McNicholas, 1992). Several studies have demonstrated less cough and safety when comparing nebulized lidocaine with other preparations (Gove et al., 1985; Graham et al., 1992) However, other studies were unable to demonstrate a benefit for nebulized lidocaine compared with saline placebo in terms of cough perception, patient discomfort, or use of supplemental lidocaine doses (Charalampidou et al., 2006; Stolz et al., 2005).

5.2 Agents

Lidocaine (or lignocaine) is the most commonly used topical anesthetic applied to the airway mucosa during FFB. Other agents that may be used include tetracaine (2%), benzocaine (10-20%), and cocaine (4-10%). Lidocaine is preferred as it is less toxic, more widely available to the bronchoscopist, and shorter acting than cocaine or tetracaine. Lidocaine is metabolized by the liver and may have side effects at serum levels greater than 5 microgram/ml. Benzocaine has duration of action of only five to ten minutes and is not ideal for FFB; its use is limited by potential toxicity due to methemoglobinemia. Tetracaine has a longer duration of action but a very narrow margin of safety and is not advocated for use in FFB. Use of cocaine is limited due to excess sympathetic nervous system activity and possible toxicity and potential for abuse. However, direct comparisons of lidocaine with other preparations such as cocaine have shown equivalence in terms of patient tolerance (Teale et al., 1990)

5.3 Dosing of topical anesthesia

Initial guidelines for lidocaine dosing published by the National Institutes of Health (NIH) in 1985 recommended no more than 400 mg cumulative dose of lidocaine for healthy asthmatics undergoing FFB. This recommendation was primarily based on expert opinion (NIH, 1985). The updated 1991 NIH guidelines for FFB in asthmatics simply stated the lowest topical anesthetic dose possible should be used (NIH, 1991). When the BTS published general guidelines for topical anesthesia in the routine clinical practice of FFB, their recommendation was based primarily on two recently published studies (BTS, 2001). A study of 48 asthmatics undergoing research FFB demonstrated safety with a mean dose of 8.2 mg/kg of lidocaine as the upper limit of normal (Langmack et al., 2000). Another smaller study by Milman et al. of 16 patients undergoing FFB recommended a maximum dosage of 6-7 mg/kg (Milman et al., 1998).

The current medical literature contains a substantial collection of studies evaluating serum lidocaine levels during FFB. These studies evaluating lidocaine dosing have been done to evaluate a variety of techniques in application of topical anesthesia (Ameer et al., 1989; Amitai et al., 1990, Berger et al., 1989; Boye & Bresden, 1979; Efthimiou et al., 1982; Gjonaj et al., 1997; Gomez et al., 1983; Jones et al., 1982; Karvonen et al., 1976; Korttila et al., 1981; Langmack et al., 2000; Le Lorier et al., 1979; Loukides et al., 2000; Mainland et al., 2001; McBurney et al., 1984; Milman et al., 1998; Patterson et al., 1975; Smith et al., 1985; Sucena et al., 2004; Sutherland et al., 1985). These twenty studies were reviewed by Frey et al. in their study of lidocaine dosing (Frey et al., 2008). This compilation of studies included a total of 457 patients whose mean age was 47.4 ± 23.7 years and the mean total dose of lidocaine was 488 ± 463 mg. The mean lidocaine dose (reported as adjusted for weight) was 9.7 ± 5.0 mg/kg. Only six of these studies gave a lidocaine dose greater than 8.2 mg/kg or total dose greater than 600 mg. None of the studies reported an average peak lidocaine level > 5.0 mg/kg, while only three of the 21 studies reported a maximum lidocaine level > 5.0 mg/kg. This cumulative data of nearly 500 patients did not suggest a trend towards lidocaine toxicity despite higher lidocaine levels than the BTS recommendations (Frey et al., 2008) The Frey study collected measured lidocaine dosing and serum levels for 154 patients with a mean age of 64.7 years undergoing FFB. Mean lidocaine usage was 15.4 ± 4.5 mg/kg (1.17±0.20 gm), mean serum lidocaine level was 1.6 ± 0.7 mg/mL, and mean blood methemoglobin level was 0.7 ± 0.3%. No clinical toxicity was noted and the authors adequately demonstrated the safety of higher doses of topical lidocaine (Frey et al., 2008).

Other studies have also demonstrated the safety of higher doses of lidocaine during FFB (Ameer et al., 1989; Gjonaj et al., 1997; Sucena et al., 2004]. In the earliest study in 1979, 12 FOB patients received an average of 600 mg of topical lidocaine. The maximum lidocaine level was found to be 3.79 µg/ml in a patient with hepatic metastases who only received 420 mg topical lidocaine (LeLorier et al., 1979). A follow-up study in 1982 by Efthimiou et al. of 41 FOB patients used a similar mean lidocaine dose (9.3 ± 0.5 mg/kg); mean peak levels were 2.9 ± 0.5 µg/ml and two patients had a lidocaine level > 5 µg/ml with no complications (Efthimiou et al., 1982). Ameer et al. compared an elderly group of 14 patients (mean age of 67 years) with a young group of five patients (mean age of 42 years). Both groups received total lidocaine doses of nearly 1200 mg without significant toxicity. No difference in mean or peak serum lidocaine was found between groups (Ameer et al., 1989). As part of a study evaluating the effect of lidocaine on endobronchial cultures, Berger et al. studied eight patients who received an average total lidocaine dose greater than 2000 mg. The mean serum level was 2.7 µg/ml and the peak level in one patient was 5.5 µg/ml; no toxicity was reported (Berger et al., 1989). In 1997, Gjonaj et al. evaluated 8 mg/kg vs. 4 mg/kg of nebulized 2% lidocaine in a pediatric population and found no evidence of toxicity. The total lidocaine dose for the high-dose group was 10.13 ± 1.26 mg/kg with mean serum lidocaine levels of 1.17 ± 0.54 µg/ml and peak levels of 2.27 µg/ml [Gjonaj et al.,

1997). The most recent studies by Loukides (mean lidocaine dose of 622 ± 20 mg) and Sucena (mean lidocaine dose of 11.6 ± 3.1 mg/kg) also found no toxicities with these doses (Loukides et al., 2000; Sucena et al., 2004). Notably, five of 30 patients studied by Sucena et al. had serum levels greater than 5 µg/ml but no clinical toxicity (Sucena et al., 2004).

5.4 Complications

Serious effects of lidocaine toxicity (seizures, methemoglobinemia, respiratory failure, and cardiac arrhythmias) are reported to begin at serum levels > 5 µg/ml (Fahimi et al., 2007; Rodins et al., 2003; Sutherland et al., 1985; Wu et al., 1993). At lower serum concentrations, milder side effects such as drowsiness, dizziness, euphoria, paresthesias, nausea, and vomiting may occur. Consideration should also be given to allergic reactions due to lidocaine administration (Bose & Colt, 2008). Serum lidocaine clearance can be decreased in the elderly, patients with cardiac or liver disease, and those patients taking certain medications such as beta-blockers, cimetidine, or verapamil (Abernethy et al., 1983, Smith et al., 1985, Thomson et al., 1973). Despite these potential toxicities, there are few reports of significant complications related to topical anesthetic administration. An early survey of nearly 25,000 FFB only noted six patients with complications (respiratory arrest, seizures) related to airway anesthesia and only one patient with methemoglobinemia (Credle et al., 1974). Additional concern was raised about volunteer FFB and the use of topical anesthesia was noted when a 19-year-old healthy volunteer died from lidocaine toxicity after undergoing a research FFB (Day et al., 1998).

Although elevated methemoglobin levels are another potential concern with the use of higher lidocaine doses, there is scant information supporting this as a significant clinical issue. The 1974 bronchoscopy survey only noted symptoms related to methemoglobinemia in a single patient who received tetracaine (Credle et al., 1974). Recently, Karim et al. reported three patients who received topical lidocaine who developed clinical evidence of methemoglobinemia; one patient was undergoing FOB and was taking trimethoprim-sulfamethoxazole (Karim et al., 2011). Most reported methemoglobinemia cases have been in association with benzocaine used in combination with lidocaine or as the sole topical anesthetic (Kern et al., 2000; Kucshner et al., 2000; O'Donohue & Moss, 1980; Rodriguez et al., 1994).

6. Bronchoscopy in the ICU

The 2001 BTS guidelines comment specifically on the differences for FFB performed in the intensive care unit (ICU) (BTS, 2001). There are a significant range of diagnostic (endobronchial cultures, lung collapse, hemoptysis, acute inhalation injury) and therapeutic (excess secretions, treatment of hemoptysis, foreign body removal) indications reported in the ICU setting (Anzueto et al., 1992; Shennib & Baislam, 1996). Intensive care units should be able to provide urgent and timely FFB to carry out these indications. From a safety perspective, these critically ill patients should be considered high risk for complications and absolutely require physiological monitoring during and after the procedure. In ventilated patients, the bronchoscopist can achieve higher levels of sedation and/or anesthesia to complete the diagnostic or therapeutic requirements for FFB. However, the bronchoscope must be able to pass easily through the endotracheal tube and the technique must allow adequate ventilation and oxygenation throughout (BTS, 2001). Hertz et al. demonstrated that bronchoalveolar lavage could be performed successfully in ventilated patients without complications by using specific bronchoscopy techniques and proper ventilator management (Hertz et al., 1991)

7. Conclusion

Flexible fiberoptic bronchoscopy is a very important and useful tool for the pulmonologist to diagnose and treat various pulmonary disorders. Overall, it is a very safe procedure with low complication rates reported. There are several published guidelines to provide general guidance on the conduct of FFB. With proper preparation of the patient and close monitoring of the patient's condition, FFB can be performed with the desired outcome. An important component of the overall process is to ensure that the patient is both as safe and comfortable as possible. Choosing the proper agent and level of sedation along with adequate topical anesthesia can make the experience better for the patient and the bronchoscopist. This chapter has provided a broad delineation of the studies in the medical literature that address the role of monitoring, oxygen supplementation, intravenous sedation, and topical anesthesia.

8. References

Abernethy, DR. & Greenblatt, DJ. (1983). Impairment of Lidocaine Clearance in Elderly Male Subjects. Journal of Cardiovascular Pharmacology, Vol.5, No.6, (November-December 1983), pp.1093-1096, ISSN 0160-2446

Ameer, B.; Burlingame, MB. & Harman, EM. (1989). Systemic Absorption of Topical Lidocaine in Elderly and Young Adults Undergoing Bronchoscopy. Pharmacotherapy, Vol.9, No.2, (March-April 1989), pp.74-81, ISSN 0277-0008

American Society of Anesthesiologists Task Force on Sedation and Analgesia by Non-Anesthesiologists. (2002). Practice Guidelines for Sedation and Analgesia by Non-Anesthesiologists. Anesthesiology, Vol.96, No.4, (April 2002), pp.1004-1017. ISSN 0003-3022

American Thoracic Society. (1987). Guidelines for Fiberoptic Bronchoscopy in Adults. American Review of Respiratory Disease, Vol.136, No.4, (October 1987), p.1066, ISSN 0003-0805

Amitai, Y.; Zylber-Katz, E.; Avital, A.; Zangen, D. & Noviski N. (1990). Serum Lidocaine Concentrations in Children during Bronchoscopy with Topical Anesthesia. Chest, Vol.98, No.6, (December 1990), pp. 1370-1373, ISSN 0012-3692

Anzueto, A.; Levine, SM. & Jenkinson, SG. (1992). The Technique of Fiberoptic Bronchoscopy. Diagnostic and Therapeutic Uses in Intubated, Ventilated Patients. Journal of Critical Illness, Vol.7, No.10, (October 1992), pp. 1657-64, ISSN 1040-0257

Berger, R.; McConnell, JW.; Phillips, B. & Overman. TL. (1989). Safety and Efficacy of Using High-Dose Topical and Nebulized Anesthesia to Obtain Endobronchial Cultures. Chest, Vol. 95, No.2, (February 1989), pp.299-303, ISSN 0012-3692

Berkenbosch, JW.; Graff, GR.; Stark, JM.; Ner, Z. & Tobias, JD. (2004). Use of a Remifentanil-Propofol Mixture for Pediatric Flexible Fiberoptic Bronchoscopy Sedation. Pediatric Anaesthesia,Vol.14, No.11, (November 2004), pp. 941-946, ISSN 1155-5645

Bjørtuft, Ø.; Brosstad, F. & Boe, J. (1998). Bronchoscopy with Transbronchial Biopsies: Measurement of Bleeding Volume and Evaluation of the Predictive Value of

Coagulation tests. European Respiratory Journal, Vol. 12, No.5, (November 1998), pp.1025–1027, ISSN 0903-1936

Bose, AA. & Colt, HG. (2008). Lidocaine in Bronchoscopy, Practical Use and Allergic Reactions. Journal of Bronchology, Vol.15, No.3, (July 2008), pp.163-166, ISSN 1984-6586

Boye, NP. & Bredesen, JE. (1979). Plasma Concentrations of Lidocaine during Inhalation Anaesthesia for Fiberoptic Bronchoscopy. Scandanavian Journal of Respiratory Diseases, Vol. 60, No.3, (June 1979), pp. 105-108, ISSN 0336-5572

British Thoracic Society Bronchoscopy Guidelines Committee. (2001). British Thoracic Society Guidelines on Diagnostic Flexible Bronchoscopy. Thorax, Vol.56, No. Suppl 1, (March 2001), pp. i1–i21, ISSN 0040-6376

Bungay, HK.; Pal, CR.; Davies, CWH.; Davies, RJO. & Gleeson, FV. (2000). An Evaluation of Computed Tomography as an Aid to Diagnosis in Patients Undergoing Bronchoscopy for Suspected Bronchial Carcinoma. Clinical Radiology, Vol.55, No.7, (July 2000), pp.554-560, ISSN 0033-8419

Charalampidou, S.; Harris, E.; Chummun, K.; Hawksworth, R.; Cullen, JP. & Lane, SJ. (2006). Evaluation of the Efficacy of Nebulised Lignocaine as Adjunctive Local Anaesthesia for Fibreoptic Bronchoscopy: a Randomised, Placebo-Controlled Study. Irish Medical Journal, Vol.99, No.1, (January 2006), pp. 8-10, ISSN 0332-3102

Clark, G.; Licker, M.; Younissian, AB.; Soccal, PM.; Frey, JG.; et al. (2009), Titrated Sedation with Propofol or Midazolam for Flexible Bronchoscopy: a Randomised Trial. European Respiratory Journal, Vol.34, No.6, (December 2009), pp1277-1283, ISSN 0903-1936

Credle, WF.; Smiddy, JF. & Elliot, RC. (1974). Complications of Fiberoptic Bronchoscopy. The American Review of Respiratory Disease, Vol.109, No.1, (January 1974), pp. 67-72. ISSN 0003-0805

Day, RO.; Chalmers, DR.; Williams, KM. & Campbell, TJ. (1998). The Death of a Healthy Volunteer in a Human Research Project: Implications for Australian Clinical Research. Medical Journal of Australia, Vol. 168, No.9, (May 1998); pp. 449-451, ISSN 0025-729X

Douketis, JD.; Berger, PB.; Dunn, AS.; Jaffer, AK.; Spyropoulos, AC.; Becker, RC. & Ansell J. (2008). The Perioperative Management of Antithrombotic Therapy: American College of Chest Physicians Evidence-Based Clinical Practice Guidelines (8th Edition). Chest, Vol.133, No.6, (June 2008), pp.299S-339S. ISSN 0012-3692

Efthimiou, J.; Higenbottam, T.; Holt, D. & Cochrane, GM. (1982). Plasma Concentrations of Lignocaine during Fibreoptic Bronchoscopy. Thorax, Vol.37, No.1, (January 1982), pp.68-71, ISSN 0040-6376

Ernst, A.; Eberhardt, R.; Wahidi, M.; Becker HD. & Herth, FJF. (2006). Effect of Routine Clopidogrel Use on Bleeding Complications after Transbronchial Biopsy in Humans. Chest, Vol.129, No.3, (March 2006), pp.734-737, ISSN 0012-3692

Facciolongo, N.; Patelli, M.; Gasparini, P.; Lazzari Agli, L.; Salio, M.; Simonassi, C.; Del Prato, B. & Zanoni, P. (2009). Incidence of Complications in Bronchoscopy: Multicentre Prospective Study of 20,986 Bronchoscopies. Monaldi Archives for Chest Disease, Vol.71, No.1, (March 2009), pp.8-14, ISSN 1122-0643

Fahimi, F.; Baniasadi, S. & Malekmohammad, M. (2007). Neurologic and Psychotic Reaction Induced by Lidocaine. Journal of Bronchology, Vol.14, No.1, (January 2007), pp.57-58, ISSN 1944-6586

Frey, WC.; Emmons, EE. & Morris, MJ. (2008). Safety of High Dose Lidocaine in Flexible Bronchoscopy. Journal of Bronchology, Vol.15, No.1, (January 2008), pp.33-37, ISSN 1984-6586

Ghio, AJ.; Bassett, M.; Chall, AN.; Levin, DG. & Bromberg, PA. (1998). Bronchoscopy in Healthy Volunteers. Journal of Bronchology, Vol.5, No.3, (July 1998), pp.185-194, ISSN 1944-6586

Ghio, AJ.; Bassett, MA.; Levin, D. & Montilla, T. (2007). Oxygen Supplementation is Required in Healthy Volunteers during Bronchoscopy with Lavage. Journal of Bronchology, Vol.14, No.1, (January 2007), pp.19-21, ISSN 1944-6586

Gjonaj, ST.; Lowenthal DB. & Dozor, AJ. (1997). Nebulized Lidocaine Administered to Infants and Children Undergoing Flexible Bronchoscopy. Chest, Vol.112, No. 6, (July 1997), pp.1665-1669, ISSN 0012-3692

Gomez, F.; Barrueco, M.; Lanao, JM.; Vicente, MT. & Dominguez-Gil, A. (1983). Serum Lidocaine Levels in patients Undergoing Fibrobronchoscopy. Therapeutic Drug Monitoring Vol.5, No.2, (June 1983), pp. 201-203, ISSN 0163-4356

Gonzalez, R.; De La Rosa-Ramirez I.; Maldonado-Hernandez A. & Dominguez-Cherit G. (2003). Should Patients Undergoing a Bronchoscopy be Sedated? Acta Anaesthesiologica Scandinavica, Vol.47, No.4, (April 2003), pp.411-415, ISSN 0001-1572

Gove, RI.; Wiggins, J. & Stableforth, DE. (1985). A Study of the Use of Ultrasonically Nebulized Lignocaine for Local Anaesthesia During Fibreoptic Bronchoscopy. British Journal of Diseases of the Chest, Vol.79, No.1, (January 1985), pp.49-59, ISSN 0007-0971

Graham, DR.; Hay, JG.; Clague, J.; Nisar, M. & Earis, JE. (1992). Comparison of Three Different Methods Used to Achieve Local Anesthesia for Fiberoptic Bronchoscopy. Chest, Vol.102, No.3, (September 1992), pp.704-707, ISSN 0012-3692

Greig, JH.; Cooper, SM.; Kasimbazi, HJ.; Monie, RD.; Fennerty, AG. & Watson, B. (1995). Sedation for Fibre Optic Bronchoscopy. Respiratory Medicine, Vol.89, No.1, (January 1995), pp.53-56, ISSN 0954-6111

Hanley, SP. (1995). Sedation in Fibreoptic Bronchoscopy. No Grounds for Abandoning Sedation. British Medical Journal, Vol.310, No.6983, (April 1995), p.873, ISSN 0959-8138

Hasanoglu, HC.; Gokirmak, M.; Yildirim, Z.; Koksal, N. & Cokkeser,Y. (2001). Flexible Bronchoscopy. Is Atropine Necessary for Premedication? Journal of Bronchology, Vol.8, No.1, (January 2001), pp.5-9, ISSN 1944-6586

Hasmoni, MH.; Adbul Rani, MF.; Harun, R.; Manap, RA.; Ahamd Tajudin, NA. & Anshar, FM. (2008). Randomized-Controlled Trial to Study the Equivalence of 1% Versus 2% Lignocaine in Cough Suppression and Satisfaction during Bronchoscopy. Journal of Bronchology, Vol.15, No.2, (April 2008), pp.78-82, ISSN 1944-6586

Hatton, MQ.; Allen, MB.; Vathenen, AS.; Mellor, E. & Cooke, NJ. (1994). Does Sedation Help in Fibreoptic Bronchoscopy? British Medical Journal, Vol.309, No.6963, (November 1994), pp.1206-1207, ISSN 0959-8138

Herth, FJF.; Becker, HD. & Ernst, A. (2002). Aspirin Does Not Increase Bleeding Complications After Transbronchial Biopsy. Chest, Vol.122, No.4, (October 2002), pp.1461-1464, ISSN 0012-3692

Hertz, MI.; Woodward, ME.; Gross, CR.; Swart, M.; Marcy, TW. & Bitterman, PB. (1991). Safety of Bronchoalveolar Lavage in the Critically Ill, Mechanically Ventilated Patient. Critical Care Medicine, Vol.19, No.12, (December 1991), pp.1526-1532, ISSN 0090-3493

Hirose, T.; Okuda, K.; Ishida, H.; Sugiyama, T.; Kusumoto, S.; Nakashima, M.; Yamaoka, T. & Adachi, M. (2008). Patient Satisfaction with Sedation for Flexible Bronchoscopy. Respirology, Vol.13, No.5, (September 2008), pp.722-727, ISSN 1440-1843

Hwang, J.; Jeon, Y.; Park, HP.; Lim, YJ. & Oh, YS. (2005). Comparison of Alfetanil and Ketamine in Combination with Propofol for Patient-Controlled Sedation during Fiberoptic Bronchoscopy. Acta Anaesthesiologica Scandinavica, Vol.49, No.9, (October 2005), pp.1334-1338, ISSN 0001-5172

Jones, AM. & O'Driscoll, R. (2000). Do All Patients Require Supplemental Oxygen During Flexible Bronchoscopy? Chest, Vol.119, No.6, (June 2000), pp.1906-1909, ISSN 0012-3692

Jones, DA.; McBurney, A.; Stanley, PJ.; Tovey, C. & Ward, JW. (1982). Plasma Concentrations of Lignocaine and its Metabolites during Fibreoptic Bronchoscopy. British Journal of Anaesthesia, Vol.54, No.8, (August 1982), pp.853-857, ISSN 0007-0912

Karim, A.; Ahmed, S.; Siddiqui, R. & Mattana, J. (2001). Methemoglobinemia Complicating Topical Lidocaine Used During Endoscopic Procedures. American Journal of Medicine, Vol.111, No.2, (August 2001), pp.150-153, ISSN 0002-9343

Karvonen, S.; Jokinen, K.; Karvonen, P. & Hollmen, A. (1976). Arterial and Venous Blood Lidocaine Concentrations after Local Anaesthesia of the Respiratory Tract Using an Ultrasonic Nebulizer. Acta Anaesthesiologica Scandinavica, Vol.20, No.2, (April 1976), pp.156-159, ISSN 0001-5172

Keane, D. & McNicholas, WT. (1992). Comparison of Nebulized and Sprayed Topical Anaesthesia for Fibreoptic Bronchoscopy. European Respiratory Journal, Vol.5, No.9, (October 1992), pp.1123-1125, ISSN 0903-1936

Kern, K.; Langevin, PB. & Dunn BM. (2000). Methemoglobinemia after Topical Anesthesia with Lidocaine and Benzocaine for a Difficult Intubation. Journal of Clinical Anesthesia, Vol.12, No.2, (March 2000), pp.167-172, ISSN 0952-8180

Korteweg, C.; van Mackelenbergh, BA.; Zanen, P. & Schramel, FM. (2004). Optimal Premedication for Diagnostic Flexible Fiberoptic Bronchoscopy without Sedation. Journal of Bronchology, Vol.11, No.1, (January 2004), pp.12-16, ISSN 1984-6586

Korttila, K.; Tarkkanen, J. & Tarkkanen, L. (1981). Comparison of Laryngotracheal and Ultrasonic Nebulizer Administration of Lidocaine in Local Anaesthesia for Bronchoscopy. Acta Anaesthesiologica Scandinavica, Vol.25, No.2, (April 1981), pp.161-165, ISSN 0001-5172

Kozak, EA. & Brath LK. (1994). Do "Screening" Coagulation Tests Predict Bleeding in Patients Undergoing Fiberoptic Bronchoscopy With Biopsy? Chest, Vol.106, No.3, (September 1994), pp.703-705, ISSN 0012-3692

Kuschner, WG.; Chitkara, RK.; Canfield, J Jr.; Poblete-Coleman, LM.; Cunningham, BA. & Sarinas, PS. (2000). Benzocaine-Associated Methemoglobinemia Following

Bronchoscopy in a Healthy Research Participant. Respiratory Care, Vol.45, No.8, (August 2000), pp.953-956, ISSN 0020-1324

Langmack, EL.; Martin, RJ.; Pak, J. & Kraft, M. (2000). Serum Lidocaine Concentrations in Asthmatics Undergoing Research Bronchoscopy. Chest, Vol.117, No.4, (April 2000), pp.1055-1060, ISSN 0012-3692

Laroche, C.; Fairbairn, I.; Moss, H.; Pepke-Zaba, J.; Sharples, L.; Flower, C. & Coulden R. (2000). Role of computed tomographic scanning of the thorax prior to bronchoscopy in the investigation of suspected lung cancer. Thorax, Vol.55, No.5, (May 2000), pp.359-363, ISSN 0040-6376

Larsen, R.; Galloway, D.; Wadera, S.; Kjar, D.; Hardy, D.; Mirkes, C.; et al. (2009). Safety of Propofol Sedation for Pediatric Outpatient Procedures. Clinical Pediatrics, Vol.48, No.8, (October 2009), pp.819-823, ISSN 0009-9228

Le Lorier, J.; Larochelle, P.; Bolduc, P.; Clermont, R.; Gratton, J.; Knight, L et al. (1979). Lidocaine Plasma Concentrations During and After Endoscopic Procedures. International Journal of Clinical Pharmacology and Biopharmacy, Vol.17, No.2, (February 1979), pp.53-55, ISSN 0340-0026

Leite, AG.; Xavier, RG.; Moreira, JD. & Wisintainer, F. (2008). Anesthesia in Flexible Bronchoscopy, Randomized Clinical Trial Comparing the Use of Topical Lidocaine Alone or in Association with Propofol, Alfentanil , or Midazolam. Journal of Bronchology, Vol.15, No.4, (October 2008), pp.233-239, ISSN 1944-6586

Lima, VP.; Jardim, JR. & Ota, LH. (2009). Immediate Spirometric Alterations after Bronchoscopy in Diffuse Lung Disease. Journal of Bronchology & Interventional Pulmonology, Vol.16, No.2, (April 2009), pp.81–86, ISSN 1944-6586

Lopez, FJR.; Salas, MDV.; Perez, JL.; Lucas, JAR.; Suarez, BF.; Gascon, FS. & Cruz, ML. (2006). Flexible Bronchoscopy with Only Topical Anesthesia. Journal of Bronchology, Vol.13, No.2, (April 2006), pp.54-57, ISSN 1984-6586

Loukides, S.; Katsoulis, K.; Tsarpalis, K.; Panagou, P. & Kalogeropoulos, N. (2000). Serum Concentrations of Lignocaine Before, During and After Fiberoptic Bronchoscopy. Respiration; International Review of Thoracic Diseases, Vol.67, No.1, (2000), pp.13-17, ISSN 0025-7931

Mainland, PA.; Kong, AS.; Chung, DC.; Chan, CH. & Lai, CK. (2001). Absorption of Lidocaine during Aspiration Anesthesia of the Airway. Journal of Clinical Anesthesia, Vol.13, No.6, (September 2001), pp.440-446, ISSN 0952-8180

Matot, I. & Kramer, MR. (2000). Sedation in Outpatient Bronchoscopy. Respiratory Medicine, Vol.94, No.12, (December 2000), pp.1145-1153, ISSN 0954-6111

Matot, I.; Kramer, MR.; Glantz, L.; Drenger, B. & Cotev, S. (1997). Myocardial Ischemia in Sedated Patients Undergoing Fiberoptic Bronchoscopy. Chest, Vol.112, No.6, (December 1997), pp.1454-1458, ISSN 0012-3692

McBurney, A.; Jones, DA.; Stanley, PJ. & Ward, JW. (1984). Absorption of Lignocaine and Bupivacaine from the Respiratory Tract during Fibreoptic Bronchoscopy. British Journal of Clinical Pharmacology, Vol.17, No.1, (January 1984), pp.61-66, ISSN 0306-5251

McGuinness, G.; Beacher, JR.; Harkin, TJ.; Garay, SM.; Rom, WN. & Naidich, DP. (1994). Hemoptysis: Prospective High-Resolution CT/Bronchoscopic Correlation. Chest, Vol.105, No.4, (April 1994), pp.1155-1162, ISSN 0012-3692

McLean, AN.; Semple, PD'A.; Franklin, DH.; Petrie, G.; Millar, EA. & Douglas JG. (1998). The Scottish Multi-Centre Prospective Study of Bronchoscopy for Bronchial Carcinoma and Suggested Audit Standards. Respiratory Medicine, Vol.92, No.9, (September 1998), pp.1110-1115, ISSN 0954-6111

Milman, N.; Laub, M.; Munch, EP. & Angelo, HR. (1998). Serum Concentrations of Lignocaine and its Metabolite Monoethylglycinexylidide During Fibre-optic Bronchoscopy in Local Anaesthesia. Respiratory Medicine, Vol.92, No.1, (January 1998), pp.40-43, ISSN 0954-6111

National Institutes of Health Workshop Summary and Guidelines. (1991). Investigative Use of Bronchoscopy, Lavage, and Bronchial Biopsies in Asthma and Other Airway Diseases. Journal of Allergy and Clinical Immunology, Vol.88, No.5, (November 1991), pp.808-814, ISSN 0091-6749

National Institutes of Health Workshop Summary. (1985). Summary and Recommendations of a Workshop on the Investigative Use of Fiberoptic Bronchoscopy and Bronchoalveolar Lavage in Individuals with Asthma. Journal of Allergy and Clinical Immunology. Vol.76, No.2 Pt1, (August 1985), pp.145-147, ISSN 0091-6749

O'Donohue, WJ Jr. & Moss, LM.; (1980). Acute Methemoglobinemia Induced by Topical Benzocaine and Lidocaine. Archives of Internal Medicine, Vol. 140, No.11, (November 1980), pp.1508-1509, ISSN 0003-9926

Patterson JR.; Blaschke TF.; Hunt KK. & Meffin PJ. (1975). Lidocaine Blood Concentrations during Fiberoptic Bronchoscopy. American Review of Respiratory Disease, Vol.112, No.1, (July 1975), pp.53-57, ISSN 003-0805

Peacock, MD.; Johnson, JE. & Blanton, HM. (1994). Complications of Flexible Bronchoscopy in Patients with Severe Obstructive Pulmonary Disease. Journal of Bronchology, Vol.1, No.3, (July 1994), pp.181-186, ISSN 1944-6586

Pereira, W.; Kovnat, D. & Snider G. (1978). A Prospective Cooperative Study of Complications Following Flexible Fiberoptic Bronchoscopy. Chest, Vol.73, No.6, (June 1978), pp.813-816, ISSN 0012-3692

Pickles J.; Jeffrey M.; Datta A. & Jeffrey AA. (2003). Is Preparation for Bronchoscopy Optimal? European Respiratory Journal, Vol.22, No.2, (August 2003), pp.203-206, ISSN 0903-1936

Prakash, UBS.; Offord, KP. & Stubbs, SE. (1991). Bronchoscopy in North America: the ACCP Survey. Chest, Vol.100, No.6, (December 1991), pp.1668-1675, ISSN 0012-3692

Putinati, S.; Ballerin, L.; Corbetta, L.; Trevisani, L. & Potena, A. (1999). Patient Satisfaction with Conscious Sedation for Bronchoscopy. Chest, Vol.115, No.5, (May 1999), pp.1437-40, ISSN 0012-3692

Rodins, K.; Hlavac, M. & Beckert, L. (2003). Lignocaine Neurotoxicity Following Fibre-optic Bronchoscopy. The New Zealand Medical Journal, Vol.116, No.1177, (July 2003), p.U500, ISSN 1175-8716

Rodriguez, LF.; Smolik, LM. & Zbehlik, AJ. (1994). Benzocaine-Induced Methemoglobinemia: Report of a Severe Reaction and Review of the Literature. Annals of Pharmacotherapy, Vol.28, No.5, (May 1994), pp.643-649, ISSN 1060-0280

Salisbury, BG.; Metzger, LF.; Altose, MD.; Stanley, NN. & Cherniack, NS. (1975). Effect of Fiberoptic Bronchoscopy on Respiratory Performance in Patients with Chronic Airways Obstruction. Thorax, Vol.30, No.4, (August 1975), pp.441-446, ISSN 0040-6376

Segal, JB.; Dzi, WH. & Transfusion Medicine/Hemostasis Clinical Trials Network. (2005). Paucity of Studies to Support That Abnormal Coagulation Test Results Predict Bleeding in the Setting of Invasive Procedures: an Evidence-Based Review. Transfusion, Vol.45, No. 9, (September 2005), pp.1413-1425, ISSN 0041-1132

Shennib, H. & Baslaim, G. (1996). Bronchoscopy in the Intensive Care Unit. Chest Surgery Clinics of North America, Vol.6, No.2, (May 1996), pp.349-361, ISSN 1052-3359

Shrader, DL. & Lakshminarayan, S. (1978). The Effect of Fiberoptic Bronchoscopy on Cardiac Rhythm. Chest, Vol.73, No.6, (June 1978), pp.821-824, ISSN 0012-3692

Silvestri, GA.; Vincent, BD.; Wahidi, MM.; Robinette, E.; Hansbrough, JR. & Downie, GH. (2009). A Phase 3, Randomized, Double-Blind Study to Assess the Efficacy and Safety of Fospropofol Disodium Injection for Moderate Sedation in Patients Undergoing Flexible Bronchoscopy. Chest, Vol.135, No.1, (January 2009), pp.41-4, ISSN 0012-3692

Smith, MJ.; Dhillon, DP.; Hayler, AM.; Holt, DW. & Collins, JV. (1985). Is Fibreoptic Bronchoscopy in Patients with Lung Cancer and Hepatic Metastases Potentially Dangerous? British Journal of Diseases of the Chest, Vol.79, No.4,(October 1985), pp.368-373, ISSN 0007-0971

Smyth, CM. & Stead, RJ. (2002). Survey of Flexible Fibreoptic Bronchoscopy in the United Kingdom. European Respiratory Journal, Vol.19, No.3, pp. 458-63, (March 2002), ISSN 0903-1936

Steinfort, DP. & Irving, LB. (2010). Patient Satisfaction During Endobronchial Ultrasound-Guided Transbronchial Needle Aspiration Performed Under Conscious Sedation. Respiratory Care, Vol.55, No.6, (June 2010), pp.702-706, ISSN 0020-1324

Stolz, D.; Chhajed, PN.; Leuppi, J.; Pflimlin, E. & Tamm, M. (2005). Nebulized Lidocaine for Flexible Bronchoscopy: a Randomized, Double-Blind, Placebo-Controlled Trial. Chest, Vol.128, No.3, (September 2005), pp.1756-1760, ISSN 0012-3692

Sucena, M.; Cachapuz, I.; Lombardia, E.; Magalhaes, A. & Tiago Guimaraes, J. (2004). Plasma Concentration of Lidocaine during Bronchoscopy. Revista Portuguesa de Pneumologia, Vol.10, No. 4, (July-August 2004), pp.287-296, ISSN 0873-2159

Suratt, P.; Smiddy, J. & Gruber B. (1976). Deaths and Complications Associated with Fiberoptic Bronchoscopy. Chest, Vol.69, No.6, (June 1976), pp.747–751, ISSN 0012-3692

Sutherland, AD.; Santamaria, JD. & Nana, A. (1985). Patient Comfort and Plasma Lignocaine Concentrations during Fibreoptic Bronchoscopy. Anaesthesia and Intensive Care, Vol.13, No.4, (November 1985), pp. 370-374, ISSN 0310-057X

Teale, C.; Gomes, PJ.; Muers, MF. & Pearson, SB. (1990). Local Anaesthesia for Fibreoptic Bronchoscopy: Comparison between Intratracheal Cocaine and Lignocaine. Respiratory Medicine, Vol.84, No.5, (September 1990), pp.407-408, ISSN 0954-6111

Thomson, PD,; Melmon, KL.; Richardson, JA.; Cohn, K.; Steinbrunn, W.; Cudihee, R. & Rowland, M. (1973). Lidocaine Pharmacokinetics in Advanced Heart Failure, Liver Disease, and Renal Failure in Humans. Annals of Internal Medicine, Vol.78, No.4 (April 1973), pp.499-508, ISSN 0003-4819

Triller, N,; Debeljak, A,; Kecelj, P.; Erzen, D.; Osolnik, K. & Sorli, J. (2004). Topical Anesthesia with Lidocaine and the Role of Atropine in Flexible Bronchoscopy. Journal of Bronchology, Vol.11, No.4, (October 2004), pp.242-245, ISSN 1944-6586

Tsoumakidou, M.; Chrysofakis, G.; Tsiligianni, I.; Maltezakis, G.; Siafakas, NM. & Tzanakis N. (2006). A Prospective Analysis of 184 Hemoptysis Cases - Diagnostic Impact of Chest X-Ray, Computed Tomography, Bronchoscopy. Respiration, Vol.73, No.6, (November 2006), pp. 808-814, ISSN 0025-7931

Vincent, BD. & Silvestri, GA. (2007). An Update on Sedation and Analgesia during Flexible Bronchoscopy. Journal of Bronchology, Vol.14, No.3, (July 2007), pp.173-180, ISSN 1944-6586

Wahidi, M.; Jain, P.; Jantz, M.; Lee, P.; Mackensen, G.; Barbour, S.; Lamb, C. & Silvestri, G. (2011). American College of Chest Physicians Consensus Statement on the Use of Topical Anestheisa, Analgesia, and Sedation During Flexible Bronchoscopy in Adult Patients. Chest, Vol. 140, No.5, (November 2011), pp 1342-1350, ISSN 0012-3692

Watts, MR.; Geraghty, R.; Moore, A.; Saunders, J. & Swift, CG. (2005). Premedication for Bronchoscopy in Older Patients: a Double-Blind Comparison of Two Regimens. Respiratory Medicine, Vol.99, No.2 (February 2005), pp.220–226, ISSN 0954-6111

Weiss, SM.; Hert, RC.; Gianola, FJ.; Clark, JG. & Crawford, SW. (1993). Complications of Fiberoptic Bronchoscopy in Thrombocytopenic Patients. Chest, Vol.104, No.4, (October 1993), pp.1025-1028, ISSN 0012-3692

Williamson, BH.; Nolan, PJ.; Tribe, AE.; & Thompson, PJ. (1997). A Placebo Controlled Study of Flumazenil in Bronchoscopic Procedures. British Journal of Clinical Pharmacology, Vol.43, No.1, (January 1997), pp.77-83, ISSN 0306-5251

Wu, FL.; Razzaghi, A. & Souney, PF. (1993). Seizure after Lidocaine for Bronchoscopy: Case Report and Review of the Use of Lidocaine in Airway Anesthesia. Pharmacotherapy, Vol.13, No.1, (January-February 1993), pp.72-78, ISSN 0277-0008

Yoon, HI.; Kim, JH.; Lee, JH.; Park, S.; Lee, CT.; Hwang, JY.; Nahm, SF. & Han, S. (2011). Comparison of Propofol and the Combination of Propofol and Alfentanil during Bronchoscopy: a Randomized Study. Acta Anaesthesiologica Scandinavica, Vol.55, No.1, (January 2011), pp.104-109, ISSN 0001-5172

Section 2

Bronchoscopic Investigations

3

Role of Broncoalveolar Lavage in Diagnosis

Mohammad Shameem
Department of Tuberculosis and Chest Diseases, Jawaharlal Nehru Medical College, Aligarh Muslim University, Aligarh, Uttar Pradesh
India

1. Introduction

The lung is continuously exposed to the external environment and mixtures of complex antigens through the air. It is estimated that the resting human adult inhales 12,000 liters of air per day, while even mild physical activity can double or triple this amount (1). Protective immunity against inhaled antigens is mediated by the lymphocytes that are localized to the surface of the respiratory tract. The compartments in the lung where lymphocytes are present are (i) the epithelium and lamina propria of the air-conducting regions, (ii) the bronchus-associated lymphoid tissue (found commonly in certain animals i.e. rabbit and rats) (iii) the pulmonary interstitium and vascular beds (iv) the bronchoalveolar space. In addition to anatomical barriers, such as airway angulation, mucociliary clearance, and coughing, both humoral and cellular defense mechanisms play an important role in maintaining the viability of the host. One of the first lines of defense against particulate matter is mucociliary clearance and phagocytic activity of alveolar macrophages. Antigens entering the pulmonary tract encounter antigen-presenting cells comprised of alveolar and interstitial macrophages and effector T lymphocytes.

2. Bronchoalveolar lavage for diagnosis of various respiratory disorders

Bronchoscopy with bronchoalveolar lavage (BAL) is an important tool for the diagnosis of pulmonary infections and malignancies. Flexible fiberoptic bronchoscopy is a relatively safe and minimally invasive means by which to obtain bronchoalveolar lavage fluid (BALF). It is usually well tolerated by patients and can be performed safely even on those patients who are quite ill.

The diagnostic and prognostic utility of BAL was first evaluated in the 1980s (2). The investigatory technique of BAL has become one of the most valuable research tools for studying inflammatory mechanisms in a wide range of diseases that affect the lungs and airways in humans. In addition, cytological and microbiological testing of BAL samples are of established value for assisting in clinical diagnosis and management of many lung diseases, and these procedures are available routinely.

Since the introduction of the rigid bronchoscope by Dr. Jackson in 1904, BAL is a diagnostic procedure in which a fiber-optic bronchoscope is passed through the mouth or nose into the lung and fluid is put into a small part of the lung and then recollected for examination.

Bronchoalveolar lavage is typically performed to diagnose lung disease. Primarily, BAL was used as a treatment for patients who suffered from diseases associated with accumulation of purulent secretions such as alveolar proteinosis, cystic fibrosis and bacterial pneumonia (3).

3. Definition

By definition BAL is a method for the recovery of cellular and non-cellular components from the lower respiratory tract (e.g. alveoli) (4). It is a safe technique, with few major complications (5). In many cases (e.g. pulmonary proteinosis, alveolar hemorrhage, eosinophilic pneumonia) BAL can replace lung biopsy (6). Possible uses of BAL in diagnostics are summarized in following table

Non-infectious	Infectious
Sarcoidosis	(Ventilator-associated) pneumonia
Hypersensitivity pneumonitis	Pneumocystis pneumonia
Idiopatic lung fibrosis	Mycobacterial infection
Connective tissue disorders	Aspergillus fumigatus infection
Langerhans cell histiocytosis	Viral pneumonia
Malignancies	Toxoplasma pneumonia
Alveolar hemorrhage	Legionella infection
Alveolar proteinosis	Mycoplasma pneumoniae pneumonia
Eosinophilic pneumonia	Chlamydia pneumoniae pneumonia
Bronchiolitis obliterans with organizing pneumonia	Cryptococcal infection
Asbestosis	Histoplasma infection
Silicosis	Strongyloides infection

Table 1. Pulmonary diseases where BALF can be used to a diagnosis (7, 8, 9).

4. Procedure

Bronchoalveolar Lavage is a minimally invasive technique which is used to obtain cells, inhaled particles, infectious organisms and solutes from the alveolar spaces of the lung. To achieve this, a sufficient volume of lavage fluid must be instilled to ensure a sufficient aspirate. In adults, a minimum of 100 mL of lavage fluid should be instilled. Besides diagnostic BAL, there are other lavage techniques are used and they differ in the following ways: 1) Bronchial lavage (or bronchial washing) requires relatively little instilled fluid (10 - 30 mL) and samples from large airways for bacteriological study and/or tumour cytology; 2) therapeutic lavage usees small volumes and is used to remove sticky bronchial secretions in patients with asthma or cystic fibrosis; and 3) whole lung lavage is performed in order to wash out an entire lung in patients with alveolar proteinosis, which requires repeated instillation of 1 L of fluid (in total 10–40 L for each lung) through a double-lumen endotracheal tube during general anaesthesia.

BAL is usually performed during fibreoptic bronchoscopy with topical anaesthetic after general inspection of the tracheobronchial tree. BAL can also be performed under general anaesthesia and in ventilated patients through a rigid bronchoscope or an endotracheal tube.

5. Site of bronchoalveolar lavage

The site of lavage depends on the localization of the abnormalities. In case of localized disease, for instance an infection with a radiographically apparent infiltrate or a malignancy, the involved segment should be sampled (10). In diffuse lung disease, the middle lobe or lingular lobe is commonly used as a standard site for BAL. This is often the most accessible site and the fluid obtained at one site is representative of the whole lung in diffuse lung diseases (11). If anatomical difficulties are encountered in both lobes the anterior segment of either the upper or lower lobe may be used. Using the method described, approximately 1.5-3% of the lung (approximately 1,000,000 alveoli) are sampled (4).

Usually, the lavage is performed using sterile, unbuffered isotonic saline (0.9% NaCl) solution and preferably the saline is preheated to body-temperature (37°C) to help prevent coughing and increase cellular yield (12). The volume varies between 100 and 300 ml in aliquots of 20 to 50 ml (13). The ERS task force recommended the use of 200-240 ml divided in four aliquots.

5.1 Fluid instillation and recovery

The fluid is instilled with syringes through the biopsy channel of bronchoscope and immediately recovered by applying suction (25-100 mmHg), using a standard number of input aliquots of 20–60 mL (commonly four to five aliquots are recommended) up to a total volume of 100–300 mL. Smaller instilled volumes (<100 mL) increase the likelihood of contamination by the bronchial spaces, including inflammatory cells derived from the larger airways, which may skew the differential cell counts [14].

The first aspirated volume is normally smaller than the following ones. Usually, 40–70% of the instilled volume is recovered. In obstructive airway disease and emphysema the recovery rate is significantly lower and may be <30%. The yield is also reduced in healthy smokers and the elderly. In addition, fluid recovery may be low with a poor wedge position leading to leakage of lavage fluid around the bronchoscope, which is associated with cough. Differential evaluation of the "bronchial" (first aliquot) and "alveolar" (subsequent aliquots) samples may be useful in airway diseases. Siliconised or plastic containers should be used for collection and processing of BAL fluid to avoid loss of cells through adhesion to glass surfaces.

6. Safety aspects

The BAL procedure is practically associated with no mortality and carries a low complication rate of 0–2.3% [15–17]. After BAL procedure there is fever in some hours and a transient decrease in lung function parameters, both usually self-limited and resolving within 24 h. These are the most frequent adverse effects and occur in 3–30% of patients, depending on the instilled volume. Other adverse effects include short-lasting alveolar infiltration, wheezing and bronchospasm in patients with hyper-reactive airways. Major or late complications are only seen in patients with severe lung or heart disease, and bleeding has only been reported in patients with clotting disorders or thrombocytopenia. Risk factors for developing adverse effects are: 1) extensive pulmonary infiltrates, an arterial oxygen tension <8.0 kPa (<60 mmHg) and an oxygen saturation <90%; 2) a forced expiratory volume in 1 s <1.0 L; 3) prothrombin time >50 s and platelet counts <20,000 platelets/mL; 4) significant comorbidity; and 5) bronchial hyperreactivity.

6.1 Quality control of BALF

To ensure that the obtained material represents the situation in the alveoli, a number of criteria have been established. A BALF is regarded non-representative if it fulfills one of the following criteria: i) volume <20 ml, ii) total cell count <60,000 cells/ml, iii) presence of >1% squamous epithelial cells, iv) presence of >5% bronchial epithelial cells, v) presence of extensive amounts of debris, vi) severely damaged cell morphology.

6.2 Specimen processing

The total fluid recovered is kept at room temperature and should be transported to the laboratory within 1 hr because the cells are not well preserved in the saline solution. The fluid should be pooled into a single container and total volume should be measured. The lavage fluid frequently contains large amounts of mucus; therefore, filtration through cotton gauze or nylon mesh is often performed. Filtration leads to a preferential loss of bronchial epithelial cells without a significant effect on the total cell count and cell differentials. After filtration, the fluid is centrifuged for 10 min at 500g and after this the supernatant can be stored at -20°C or -70°C for subsequent analysis of soluble components. The total number of cells is counted in a haemocytometer, either in a sample of the pooled native fluid or in a resuspension of the cells after the first centrifugation. Washing procedures result in a loss of total cell count but lead to an increase in cell viability of the remaining cells. The total cell count is usually expressed as the total number of cells recovered per lavage but also as the concentration of cells per mL of recovered fluid. Cell viability is assessed by trypan blue exclusion and should range from 80% to 95% [18, 19].

For the enumeration of cell differentials, at least 600 cells are counted on cytocentrifuge or cell smear preparations after staining with May-Grunwald-Giemsa stain. A high percentage of epithelial cells (>5%) is indicative of contamination of the alveolar samples by bronchial cells. At least three unstained slides should be stored so that special stains (iron, periodic acid–Schiff (PAS), silver, toluidine blue, fat or Ziehl–Neelsen) can be performed as per need.

Besides these routine investigations, further work-up can be performed as needed. For example, if a tumor is suspected the Papanicolau stain can be applied. If infection is suspected, a complete microbiological assessment, including cultures, should be performed. To document asbestos exposure, quantitative determination of asbestos bodies can be made after vacuum filtration of the native BAL fluid through a 0.45-1.2 μm Millipore membrane. The exact dust composition can be determined by electron microscopy with energy dispersive X-ray spectrometry. Lymphocyte subpopulations can be identified by immunocytochemical methods, immunofluorescence or flow cytometry using monoclonal antibody techniques [20].

These investigations are not recommended as a routine procedure for all BAL specimens. They are indicated in cases with high lymphocyte counts, such as extrinsic allergic alveolitis, or if Langerhans cell histiocytosis is suspected CD3. CD4, CD8, CD20 and markers of T-cell activation can be determined. CD1a or Langerin are very specific markers of Langerhans cell histiocytosis. Flow cytometry is also a useful tool to detect markers of malignant lymphoma [21].

There are some studies also performed for research purposes including functional studies of viable BAL cells, cell cultivation in appropriate culture medium and determination of mediators along with the mechanisms that appear to regulate the mediator release. Cells can also be probed with molecular biology to investigate gene activation and intracellular signaling pathways.

7. Normal values of BAL in healthy volunteers

The BAL fluid obtained from healthy, nonsmoking adults without lung disease contains only small percentages of lymphocytes, neutrophils and other inflammatory cells; alveolar macrophages are the predominant cell population (80–90%) (fig. 1a). Differential cell count in healthy non-smokers have been reported to show macrophages >80%, lymphocytes ≤15%, neutrophils ≤3%, eosinophils ≤0.5%, and mast cells ≤0.5%.

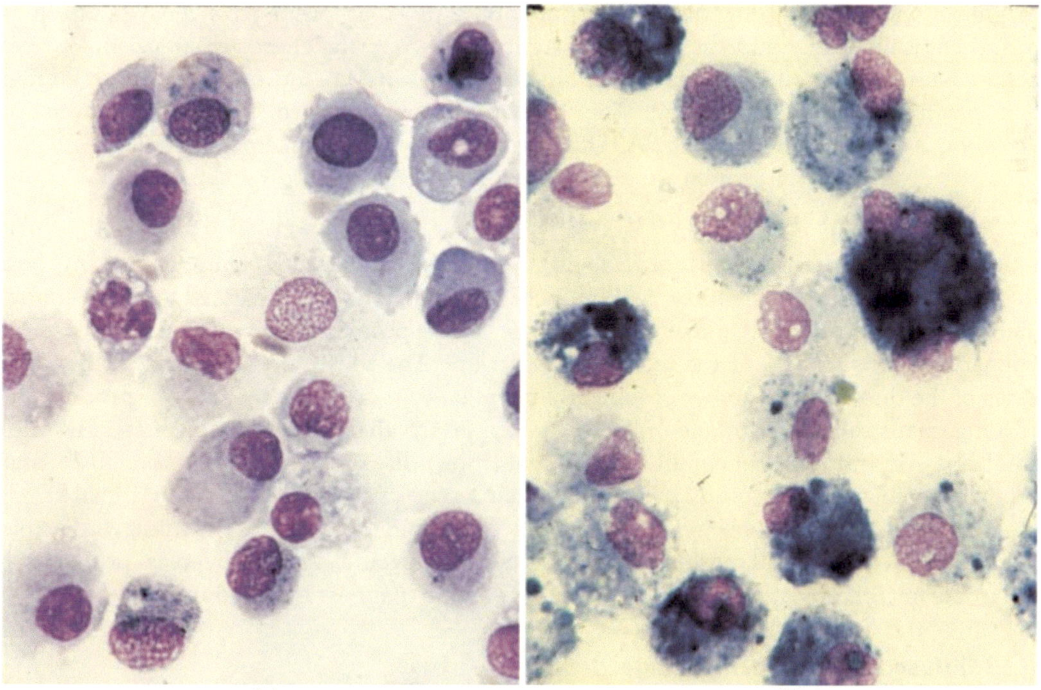

(a) (b)

Fig. 1. Bronchoalveolar lavage in a) a healthy nonsmoker and b) a healthy smoker [22].

Cigarette smoking is a strong confounding factor with significant effects on BAL samples. The alveolar macrophages from smokers show a 3 to 5 fold increase and characteristic morphology: many of them are much larger than those in nonsmokers and contain cytoplasmic inclusion bodies (smoker's inclusion bodies) consisting of tar products, lipids, lipofuscin and other substances (fig. 1b).

7.1 BAL in the diagnosis of diffuse parenchymal lung disease

BAL is indicated in every patient with nuclear pulmonary shadowing or interstitial lung disease (ILD). BAL findings may be very specific, so that they can directly confirm a particular diagnosis. BAL should not be considered as a stand-alone diagnostic test and should be interpreted in the context of clinical, laboratory and radiographical high resolution computed tomography (HRCT) findings. It has been used in diagnostic and prognostic evaluation in diffuse parenchymal lung disease for three decades and has a central role in the diagnosis of a number of rare disorders and in excluding opportunistic infection in treated patients. It also has an important role in the diagnosis of many prevalent disorders, including sarcoidosis, hypersensitivity pneumonitis and idiopathic pulmonary fibrosis.

7.2 Specific BAL findings in rare diseases

7.2.1 Pulmonary alveolar proteinosis

Pulmonary alveolar proteinosis is one of the few diseases in which BAL can confirm the diagnosis and replace lung biopsy. In pulmonary alveolar protienosis the BAL fluid is macroscopically milky and turbid. Under light microscopy the characteristic acellular oval bodies (surfactant derived lipoproteins) are basophilic on May-Grunwald-Giemsa staining and positive with PAS staining. The background is occupied by large amounts of amorphous debris showing weak PAS staining and a few foamy macrophages [21].

7.2.2 Langerhans cell histiocytosis

Pulmonary Langerhans cell histiocytosis is strongly associated with cigarette smoking, and the BAL differential shows the typical smoker's constellation with increased total cell counts and macrophages with smoker's inclusions. The specific finding is an increase in Langerhans cells to >4% of the total BAL cell count. The sensitivity is low because in late cases of the disease the number of Langerhans cells decrease in the tissue. Low proportions of Langerhans cells in the range of 2-4% can be seen in other conditions, such as in healthy smokers, respiratory bronchiolitis/interstitial lung disease (RB/ILD), other ILD and bronchioalveolar carcinoma [21]. The Langerhans cells can be easily identified in BAL by their staining with the monoclonal antibody for CD1a or Langerin [23]. The intracytoplasmic reaction with polyclonal antibody S100 is not as specific. As in alveolar proteinosis, electronic microscopy is not recommended as a routine diagnostic procedure.

7.2.3 Diffuse alveolar haemorrhage

Diffuse alveolar haemorrhage (DAH) is a clinical syndrome with widespread bleeding into the alveolar space as a result of multiple causes. The demonstration of numerous haemosiderin-laden macrophages on BAL cytology enables a diagnosis to be made even in cases with occult bleeding. In patients with fresh bleeding episodes free red blood cells in the fluid and fragments of ingested red blood cells within the cytoplasm of macrophages are pathognomonic.

To asses the severity of bleeding, the percentage of siderophages can easily be counted. It has been shown that a percentage of siderophages ≥20% is sufficient for a diagnosis of DAH.

Many syndromes belong to this group and other clinical and laboratory findings must be investigated to establish the cause of the bleeding. In the clinical setting, chronic left heart failure with pulmonary congestion is one of the most frequent underlying conditions for the finding of DAH in BAL fluid examination. Endogenous bleeding has to be differentiated from exogenous iron load of the lungs. Exogenous siderosis does not show roundish fragments of erythrocytes but irregular shaped dust particles engulfed by macrophages.

7.2.4 Chronic aspiration

In the differential diagnosis of recurrent pneumonia, gastro-oesophageal reflux with aspiration needs to be considered. The BAL cell differential may show a mixed pattern with increase in lymphocytes, neutrophils and eosinophils. The characteristic diagnostic finding is the presence of large numbers of lipid-laden macrophages and is highly suggestive of lipoid pneumonia caused by chronic aspiration.

7.2.5 Pneumoconioses

In ILD due to mineral dust exposure, BAL can confirm exposure by the detection of dust particles in alveolar macrophages. It is of two types:

a. Asbestos-related disease: Asbestos bodies in BAL fluid can be detected by smear technique or cytocentrifuge technique. However quantification of asbestos bodies by a specific Millipore filtration is a more sensitive technique. The results are expressed as number of asbestos bodies per mL of BAL fluid, which shows a relatively good correlation with the asbestos body count in lung tissue analysis. However, 10–15% of subjects with known occupational asbestos exposure may have no detectable asbestos bodies in their BAL fluid. Thus, a negative BAL asbestos body count does not exclude asbestos-related disease.
b. Chronic beryllium disease: This condition is clinically, radiologically and histologically identical to sarcoidosis and in this condition BAL lymphocytes have an increase in the CD4/CD8 ratio . Because the antigen is known, a diagnostic in vitro lymphocyte transformation test can be performed. Lymphocytes from blood or BAL fluid are incubated with beryllium salts and the beryllium-specific proliferation of the lymphocytes is quantified. A positive lymphocyte transformation test of BAL T-cells to beryllium salts is highly sensitive and specific (definitely more sensitive than the blood test) and always recommended in doubtful cases to confirm the diagnosis.

7.2.6 Eosinophilic lung disease

Eosinophilic lung disease can be diagnosed when there are ≥25% eosinophils in BAL of the radiologically affected segment. In both acute and chronic eosinophilic pneumonia the fraction of BAL eosinophils ranges from 20% to 90% and is higher than the neutrophil fraction. In this condition a mild-to-moderate increase in lymphocyte count with a decrease in CD4/CD8 ratio can be observed. In combination with clinical and HRCT findings, eosinophilic lung diseases can be appropriately diagnosed by BAL alone without an open lung biopsy [21].

7.2.7 Opportunistic infections

BAL has achieved the greatest diagnostic value among immunocompromised patients with pulmonary infiltrates. The sensitivity of BAL ranges from 60–90% in the diagnosis of bacterial infections, 70–80% in mycobacterial, fungal and most viral infections, and from 90–95% in Pneumocystis carinii pneumonia. The characteristic cysts of Pneumocystis can be detected on May-Grunwald-Giemsa stained slides.

In cytomegalovirus pneumonia, the characteristic cytomegalic-transformed cell (the owl eye cell) with typical nuclear or cytoplasmic inclusions is highly specific and can be seen on light microscopy in 30–50% of cases.

7.2.8 Malignancies

BAL is not as sensitive for solid tumours as biopsy and cytology techniques. Diffuse malignant infiltrates can be reliably diagnosed in 60–90% of cases. The highest yield is seen in widespread malignancies, such as primary bronchoalveolar carcinoma or lymphangitic carcinomatosis due to adenocarcinoma. It can also provide diagnostic cytological material in haematological malignancies of the lung, including Hodgkin's disease, non-Hodgkin lymphoma, leukaemia, Waldenstrom's macroglobulinaemia, myeloma and mycosis fungoides. In malignant B-cell lymphoma the immunocytological demonstration of a monoclonal B-cell population, expressing only one immunoglobulin type and either kappa or lambda light chains, can confirm the diagnosis of malignancy [24, 25].

8. BAL as an adjunct to diagnosis

There are no specific BAL findings in the more common interstitial lung diseases. However, when BAL cellular analysis is considered in the context of clinical and HRCT findings it may contribute to narrowing the differential diagnosis and to avoiding open lung biopsy. BAL cellular patterns can generally differentiate the fibrosing conditions (characterised by neutrophilia and eosinophilia) from granulomatous diseases (lymphocytosis with or without granulocytosis).

8.1 Sarcoidosis

In sarcoidosis, BAL shows lymphocytic alveolitis in 90% of patients at the time of diagnosis, independent of the stage of sarcoidosis. It was shown that the patients with active sarcoidosis have a tendency to show higher lymphocyte counts than those with inactive sarcoidosis. However, in the late stage of sarcoidosis neutrophils may also be increased, as well as the number of mast cells. Patients with primary extrathoracic sarcoidosis may show typical findings of sarcoidosis on BAL even when imaging findings are normal [26]. The CD4/CD8 ratio also has high variability in sarcoidosis and approximately only 55% of patients show an increased CD4/CD8 ratio at the time of diagnosis. The ratio is even decreased to 1.0 in 15% of patients. The CD4/CD8 ratio is especially high in patients with Lofgren syndrome and acute sarcoidosis. Some studies have demonstrated an increased neutrophil count in BAL obtained from newly diagnosed patients with sarcoidosis.

8.2 Extrinsic allergic alveolitis

This disease shows the highest total cell count and the highest lymphocyte count of all ILD's. The total cell yield is usually >20 million from a 100-mL BAL, with the proportion of lymphocytes exceeding 50%. The number of activated T-cells is also increased. The assessment of the CD4/CD8 ratio has produced contradictory findings. It is a general belief that the CD4/CD8 ratio is decreased. However, more recent studies have demonstrated that the ratio may be decreased, normal or increased [27, 28]. The alveolar macrophages are heterogeneous and often show a foamy cytoplasm. In acute episodes of extrinsic allergic alveolitis, the neutrophil count may increase transiently for approximately one week. A normal cell appearance or an isolated increase in neutrophil or eosinophil count widely excludes extrinsic allergic alveolitis.

8.3 Drug induced pneumonitis

There are a large number of drugs which may induce an ILD, mediated by either toxic or immunological mechanisms (Table 2) [29]. Along with BAL lymphocytosis and/or granulocytosis, cytotoxic reactions with atypical type II pneumocytes or diffuse alveolar haemorrhage may be observed. The most frequent finding is lymphocytic alveolitis with a dominance of CD8+ T-cells. Methotrexate-induced pneumonitis may show an increase in CD4+ cells. Characteristic changes in amiodarone-induced pneumonitis are the presence of alveolar macrophages with a finely vacuolated foamy cytoplasm. These are also seen in patients without clinical signs of ILD. If no foamy macrophages are found, amiodarone-induced pneumonitis can probably be excluded. The BAL findings described are not specific for drug-induced lung disease; therefore, additional assessment including tests like anti-histone antibody is necessary to make the diagnosis.

8.4 Idiopathic pulmonary fibrosis and other idiopathic interstitial pneumonias

The typical BAL findings in idiopathic pulmonary fibrosis (IPF) is a moderately increased neutrophil count (10-30% of the total cells), with or without an increased eosinophil count. In total, 70–90% of the patients show an increased neutrophil count, while 40–60% shows an additionally increased eosinophil count. In 10–20% of the patients, a moderately increased lymphocyte count (proportion <30%) is seen .

In nonspecific interstitial pneumonia (NSIP), a BAL lymphocytosis with a mild increase in the neutrophil and eosinophil count can be seen [30]. A BAL lymphocytosis is likely to be found more frequently in cellular NSIP than in fibrotic NSIP. The BAL findings in cellular NSIP appear to resemble those in bronchiolitis obliterans organizing pneumonia (BOOP).

In acute interstitial pneumonia the histological finding of diffuse alveolar damage shows an extremely unfavourable prognosis. The BAL fluid in acute interstitial pneumonia is mostly bloody and rich in albumin, indicating increased alveolar capillary permeability. The typical

Lymphocytosis	Eosinophilia	Neutrophilia	Cytotoxic reaction	Haemorrhage
Methotrexate	Bleomycin	Bleomycin	Bleomycin	D-Penicillamine
Azathioprine	Nitrofurantoin	Minocycline	Methotrexate	Amphotericin B
Cyclophosphamide	Cotrimazole	Amiodarone	Nitrosoureas	Cytotoxic drugs
Bleomycin	Penicillin		Busulfan	
Busulfan	Sulfasalazine		Cyclophosphamide	
Vincristine	Ampicillin			
Nitrofurantoin	Tetracycline			
Minocycline	Maloprim			
Gold	Minocycline			
Sulfasalazine	L-Tryptophan			
Amiodarone				
Acebutolol				
Atenolol				
Celiprolol				
Propranolol				
Flecainide				
Diphenylhydantoin				
Nilutamide				

Table 2. Bronchoalveolar lavage findings in drug-induced interstitial lung disease

cellular BAL finding is a marked increase in neutrophils and an occasional increase in lymphocytes. Atypical pneumocytes mimicking adenocarcinoma and fragmented hyaline membranes may also be observed [25]. The typical BAL findings in desquamative interstitial pneumonia and RB/ILD are an increase in macrophages with black pigmented inclusions. In this an increase in neutrophils, eosinophils and, occasionally, lymphocytes may also be seen. Idiopathic lymphocytic interstitial pneumonia is rare and is usually associated with collagen vascular diseases, Sjogren's syndrome or lymphoma. The typical BAL finding in lymphocytic interstitial pneumonia is lymphocytosis and CD4/CD8 ratio shows diverse alterations.

8.5 Collagen vascular disease

In collagen vascular diseases (CVD), pulmonary involvement can be associated with various histopathological patterns. The pathology may be similar to IPF with a usual interstitial pneumonia pattern, but many of the cases of CVD-associated pulmonary fibrosis show a pattern that is in the category of NSIP, based on a computed tomography scan or histology [26]. The BAL findings are also somewhat different from IPF. The general pattern is increased neutrophils, with or without eosinophils, but increased lymphocytes are more commonly seen than in IPF [31]. In general, BAL seems to have a limited value in the diagnosis of CVD affecting the lungs because the BAL profile is very nonspecific. However, BAL may be useful in detecting other pulmonary problems that may arise in these disorders, including drug induced toxicity, infection, pulmonary haemorrhage associated with vasculitis and malignancy. The NSIP pattern was the more prevalent pattern. It has previously been shown that increased BAL neutrophils were associated with more extensive changes on HRCT. An abnormal BAL may be the first evidence of pulmonary involvement in CVD. If radiographic signs are absent and pulmonary function tests are normal, this abnormal finding indicates subclinical alveolitis. It is still not clear whether such subclinical alveolitis needs treatment. It is also not clear whether the pattern of BAL cells (increase in neutrophils or lymphocytes) in a setting of subclinical alveolitis reflects the prognosis [32].

9. Role of BAL in the prognosis and activity of disease

It is unclear whether BAL cellularity is useful for assessing the activity of disease processes with respect to obtaining prognostic information. In sarcoidosis, differences were observed for several BAL parameters between clinically active and inactive patient groups, but without predicting long-term outcome in individual patients. It is not proven that BAL or serial BAL is useful to guide therapy or predict treatment response. At present, BAL cannot be routinely recommended for this purpose.

10. Role of BAL in research and development of new drugs

The discovery of new signal pathways and biomarkers between cells and the application of proteomics, gene arrays and metabolomics has contributed many important insights into the pathogenesis of respiratory tract diseases. BAL has been profiled as a fundamental method to obtaining alveolar space and airway specimens for research, and this could lead to more clear-cut longitudinal monitoring of ILD in the future. For example, KL-6, a high-molecular weight glycoprotein predominantly expressed on the surface of alveolar type II cells, is a promising biomarker in the field of ILD. Increased levels of KL-6 in BAL fluid and plasma correlate with the severity of alveolar inflammation and poor survival in acute respiratory distress syndrome [33]. Increased levels of KL-6 in both BAL fluid and blood, with a strong correlation between BAL and blood, also reflect disease severity in patients with idiopathic pulmonary alveolar proteinosis [34]. BAL is suitable for studying the cellular and biological changes induced by drugs. In this view, BAL can be used for concept studies in the clinical development of new drugs.

11. Conclusion

Bronchoalveolar lavage is an easily performed and well tolerated procedure able to provide cellular contents, cellular products, and proteins from the lower respiratory tract.

In the rapidly evolving field of pulmonary diagnostic tests, BAL has a specific value for the diagnosis of certain ILD's, such as alveolar proteinosis, Pneumocystis pneumonia, bronchoalveolar carcinoma, malignant non-Hodgkin lymphoma and alveolar haemorrhage, allowing surgical lung biopsy to be avoided. In other ILD's, BAL findings may be able, in combination with clinical and HRCT findings, to strengthen or weaken a suspected diagnosis. This method is also valid support for research. Genetic and molecular biomarkers, with different diagnostic/prognostic significance, can be detected in BAL.

12. References

[1] Rankin, J. A. 1988. Pulmonary immunology. Clin. Chest Med. 9:387–393.

[2] Klech H, Hutter C. Clinical guidelines and indications for bronchoalveolar lavage (BAL). Report of the European Society of Pneumonology Task Group on BAL. Eur Respir J 1990; 3: 937–974.

[3] Rogers RM, Braunstein MS, Shurman JF. Role of bronchopulmonary lavage in the treatment of respiratory failure: a review. Chest. 1972; 62: Suppl: 95S-106.

[4] Goldstein RA, Rohatgi PK, Bergofsky EH, Block ER, Daniele RP, Dantzker DR, Davis GS, Hunninghake GW, King TE Jr, Metzger WJ, et al. Clinical role of bronchoalveolar lavage in adults with pulmonary disease. Am Rev Respir Dis. 1990; 142:481-6.

[5] Klech H, Hutter C. Side-effects and safety of BAL. Eur Respir J. 1990; 3:939-40, 961-9.

[6] Drent M, Baughman RP, Meyer P. Bronchoalveolar Lavage. In: Costabel U, DuBois R, Egan J, editors. Diffuse Parenchymal Lung Disease. Basel: Karger; 2007.

[7] Reynolds HY. Use of bronchoalveolar lavage in humans--past necessity and future imperative. Lung 2000;178:271-93.

[8] Park DR. The microbiology of ventilator-associated pneumonia. Respir Care. 2005;50(6):742-63; discussion 763-5.

[9] Reynolds HY. Bronchoalveolar lavage. Am Rev Respir Dis. 1987;135:250-63.

[10] Meduri GU, Chastre J. The standardization of bronchoscopic techniques for ventilator-associated pneumonia. Chest 1992;102 (5 Suppl 1):557S-64S.

[11] Haslam PL, Baughman RP. ERS task force report on a-cellular components in BAL. Eur Respir Rev 1999;9:25-7.

[12] Pingleton SK, Harrison GF, Stechschulte DJ, Wesselius LJ, Kerby GR, Ruth WE. Effect of location, pH, and temperature of instillate in bronchoalveolar lavage in normal volunteers. Am Rev Respir Dis. 1983;128:1035-7.

[13] Costabel U, Guzman J. Bronchoalveolar lavage in interstitial lung disease. Curr Opin Pulm Med. 2001;7:255-61.

[14] Lam S, Leriche JC, Kijek K, et al. Effect of bronchial lavage volume on cellular and protein recovery. Chest 1985; 88: 856–859.

[15] Klech H, Pohl W. Technical recommendations and guidelines for bronchoalveolar lavage (BAL). Report of the European Society of Pneumology Task Group. Eur Respir J 1989; 2: 561–585.

[16] Klech H, Hutter C. Clinical guidelines and indications for bronchoalveolar lavage (BAL): report of the European Society of Pneumology Task Force on BAL. Eur Respir J 1990; 3: 937–974.
[17] Bronchoalveolar lavage constituents in healthy individuals, idiopathic pulmonary fibrosis, and selected comparison groups. The BAL Cooperative Group Steering Committee. Am Rev Respir Dis 1990; 141: S169–S202.
[18] Costabel U, eds. Atlas der bronchoalveola¨ren Lavage. Stuttgart, Thieme, 1994.
[19] Costabel U., Guzman J. Bronchoalveolar lavage. In: Gibson GJ, Geddes DM, Costabel U, et al., eds. Respiratory Medicine. 3rd Edn. London, WB Saunders, 2003; pp. 438–448.
[20] Harbeck RJ. Immunophenotyping of bronchoalveolar lavage lymphocytes. Clin Diagn Lab Immunol 1998; 5: 271–277.
[21] Costabel U, Guzman J, Bonella F, et al. Bronchoalveolar lavage in other interstitial lung diseases. Semin Respir Crit Care Med. 2007; 28: 514–524.
[22] Bonella F, Ohshimo S, Bauer P, Guzman J, Costabel U. Bronchoalveolar lavage. Eur Respir Mon, 2010, 48, 59–72.
[23] Smetana K Jr, Mericka O, Saeland S, et al. Diagnostic relevance of Langerin detection in cells from bronchoalveolar lavage of patients with pulmonary Langerhans cell histiocytosis, sarcoidosis and idiopathic pulmonary fibrosis. Virchows Arch 2004; 444: 171–174.
[24] Costabel U, Bross KJ, Matthys H. Diagnosis by bronchoalveolar lavage of cause of pulmonary infiltrates in haematological malignancies. BMJ 1985; 290: 1041.
[25] Poletti V, Poletti G, Murer B, et al. Bronchoalveolar lavage in malignancy. Semin Respir Crit Care Med 2007; 28: 534–545.
[26] Drent M, Mansour K, Linssen C. Bronchoalveolar lavage in sarcoidosis. Semin Respir Crit Care Med 2007; 28: 486–495.
[27] Barrera L, Mendoza F, Zuniga J, et al. Functional diversity of T-cell subpopulations in sub-acute and chronic hypersensitivity pneumonitis. Am J Respir Crit Care Med 2008; 177: 44–55.
[28] Ye Q, Nakamura S, Sarria R, et al. Interleukin 12, interleukin 18, and tumor necrosis factor alpha release by alveolar macrophages: acute and chronic hypersensitivity pneumonitis. Ann Allergy Asthma Immunol 2009; 102: 149–154.
[29] Costabel U, Uzaslan E, Guzman J. Bronchoalveolar lavage in drug-induced lung disease. Clin Chest Med 2004; 25: 25–35.
[30] Ryu YU, Chung MP, Han J, et al. Bronchoalveolar lavage in fibrotic idiopathic interstitial pneumonias. Respir Med 2007; 101: 655–660.
[31] Nagao T, Nagai S, Kitaichi M, et al. Usual interstitial pneumonia: idiopathic pulmonary fibrosis versus collagen vascular diseases. Respiration 2001; 68: 151–159.
[32] Goh NS, Veeraraghavan S, Desai SR, et al. Bronchoalveolar lavage cellular profiles in patients with systemic sclerosis-associated interstitial lung disease are not predictive of disease progression. Arthritis Rheum 2007; 56: 2005–2012.
[33] Nathani N, Perkins GD, Tunnicliffe W, et al. Kerbs von Lungren 6 antigen is a marker of alveolar inflammation but not of infection in patients with acute respiratory distress syndrome. Crit Care 2008; 12: R12.

[34] Lin FC, Chen YC, Chang SC. Clinical importance of bronchoalveolar lavage fluid and blood cytokines, surfactant protein D, and Kerbs von Lungren 6 antigen in idiopathic pulmonary alveolar proteinosis. Mayo Clin Proc 2008; 83: 1344–1349.

4

Lung Cancer – CT Vs Bronchoscopy

António Saraiva and Christopher Oliveira
Escola Superior de Tecnologia da Saúde de Coimbra (ESTeSC), Coimbra
Portugal

1. Introduction

During the recent years was possible to witness significant changes in the incidence and types of lung pathology seen by clinicians. It is important to mention that lung pathologies are some of the most common medical conditions worldwide.

Lung cancer was a rare disease in the early 1900s, but has since become far more prevalent and this lung pathology remains one of the greatest medical challenges with nearly 1.5 million cases worldwide each year and is the most common cause of cancer death in the world (Harewood GC et al., 2002) and (Spiro SG et al., 2010). It is typically a disease of elderly patients, with a peak incidence at around 70-80 years of age (Chen YM et al., 2009).

The incidence and mortality of lung cancer have increased sharply during this century, making it a common cause of death and the most frequent fatal cancer in men and women (Beckett WS, 1993). Clearly, lung cancer is an important and widespread disease that constitutes a major public health problem (Witschi H, 2001).

From all malignant tumors, except for non-melanoma skin cancer, lung cancer is the second most common type among men and the most frequent among women. The most concerning characteristics of this kind of cancer is that it has caused more deaths that the sum of the deaths caused by prostate, breast and rectal cancer in developed countries (Silva AC et al., 2011).

Smoking is estimated to be the cause of 85% of lung cancer deaths (Agarwal A et al., 2003). It is important to remind that the consumption of tobacco is not the only cause of this malignant tumor. Other factors are associated, affecting the incidence of this disease: exposure to arsenic, chromium, nickel and asbestos, cicatricial lesions of tuberculosis, and familiar history of lung cancer (Beckett WS, 1993) and (Figueiredo L et al., 1999).

Studies in molecular biology have elucidated the role that genetic factors play in modifying an individual's risk for lung cancer. Although chemopreventive agents may be developed to prevent lung cancer, prevention of smoking initiation and promotion of smoking cessation are currently the best weapons to fight lung cancer (Bilello Ks et al., 2002).

This malignant pathology, like most other solid tumors, is usually recognized late in its natural history. The five-year mortality from the time of presentation remains at approximately 85 to 90% and more than 90% of the patients with lung cancer will be symptomatic at presentation (Beckles MA et al., 2003).

Most patients with lung cancer present to the clinician in a fairly advanced stage and at best only 25-30% of patients can be offered curative resection (Kamath AV et al., 2006). A minority present with symptoms related to the primary tumor, and most patients present with either nonspecific systemic symptoms, including anorexia, weight loss and fatigue, or specific symptoms indicating metastatic disease (Beckles MA et al., 2003).

One of the causes of the low survival rate from lung cancer is related to difficulty of its precocious diagnosis due to the absence of symptoms and to the poor diagnosis at more advanced stages of the disease (Jamnik S et al., 2002). Prognosis is related to the type of presenting symptoms (Beckles MA et al., 2003).

Patients with lung cancer have a five-year survival rate varying from 13% to 21% in developed countries and varying from 7% to 10% in emerging countries (Silva AC et al., 2011).

However, when lung cancer is found at the early stage I or II, five-year survival rates can be as high as 60-70% (Beadsmoore CJ & Screaton NJ, 2003). The best survival rates are found in the subgroup of patients with lung cancer with surgically resectable tumors. Clinicians, therefore, are vitally interested in recognizing lung cancer early and determining surgical resectability accurately (Colice Gl, 1994).

Symptoms, signs and abnormalities in laboratory tests relating to the lung cancer can be classified as follows: those related to the primary lesion, those related to intrathoracic spread, those related to distant metastasis, and those related to paraneoplastic syndromes (Beckles MA et al., 2003).

Lung cancer is routinely classified as Small Cell Lung Cancer (SCLC) or Non Small Cell Lung Cancer (NSCLC) on the basis of distinctive pathological and molecular features but also for appropriate therapeutic management (Scagliotti GV et al., 2009). The distinction between SCLC and NSCLC came into proeminence when it was realized that SCLC was characterized by widespread metastatic spread at diagnosis and often displayed partial or complete response to conventional cytotoxic therapies (Gazdar AF, 2010).

The NSCLC category encompasses several subtypes having different morphological features generally treated according to similar strategies, so that a clear cut distinction among these types was not considered mandatory and accounts for 80% to 85% of lung carcinoma and determining the prognosis for an individual patient with NSCLC is difficult, in part because of the marked clinical heterogeneity of patients with the disease. Patients with early stage NSCLC have relatively high long-term survival rates after surgical resection, but a substantial majority of patients, approximately 80%, present in advanced stages (Scagliotti GV et al., 2009) and (Wang T et al., 2010).

SCLC is associated with poor diagnosis, with an average two-year survival rate of less than 10%. Patients are usually symptomatic at diagnosis, 30% to 40% report dyspnea and chest pain. Only 4% to 5% of SCLC cases are detected as solitary pulmonary nodule. Therefore, SCLC differs markedly from NSCLC in biologic behavior and clinical behavior. SCLC it is associated with rapid growth, and almost two-thirds of patients have metastatic disease at presentation. The response to the initial phase of the treatment is usually good, with almost 80% of the patients showing a major response (Argiris A & Murren JR, 2001) and (Oliveira C & Saraiva A, 2010).

The main histological types of this malignant disease include: adenocarcinoma, squamous cell carcinoma, SCLC and large-cell carcinoma. Adenocarcinoma accounts for 25 to 30% of NSCLC and is the most common histological type. It is typically classified as acinar, papillary, solid, and bronchioloalveolar varieties (Beckles MA et al., 2003) and (Patz EF Jr, 2000). The incidence of adenocarcinoma has increased in recent decades, while the incidence of squamous cell carcinoma has reached a plateau or has decreased (Chen YM et al., 2009).

A variety of techniques are available as methods of achieving a definitive diagnosis. The diagnostic evaluation of this disease has two main objectives: the definition of the pathological type of the tumor and staging of the disease (Westeel V, 2003). A diagnosis should be obtained by whatever method is easiest in patients who are presumed to have SCLC or who have very clear evidence of advanced NSCLC (*e.g.*, a large pleural effusion or metastatic disease). The most appropriate test is usually determined by the type of lung cancer (SCLC or NSCLC), the size and location of the tumor, and the presumed stage of the cancer (Brundage MD et al., 2002).

The available tools for diagnosing and staging lung cancer patients can be broadly categorized into non-invasive, minimally invasive and invasive (surgical) modalities (Hicks RJ et al., 2007).

Current imaging for lung cancer makes use of chest radiographs, Computed Tomography (CT), Magnetic Resonance Imaging (MRI), and nuclear medicine. Most studies are designed to detect anatomic abnormalities, leading to some problems in sensitivity and especially specificity. In the future, imaging may be directed more at tumor biology, and perhaps then will have a greater impact on this devastating disease (Patz EF Jr, 2000).

Although histology diagnosis is the most accurate detection method in the medical environment, it is an aggressive invasive procedure that involves risks, discomfort and trauma, which restrict it to be used in the clinical practice (Xiuhua G et al., 2011).

A person who is at high-risk for lung cancer and asymptomatic, and who is interested in potentially being screened should be fully apprised of the implications of screening and of the treatment that may result. It is fulcral to mention that the value of screening for early disease is not yet established and trials to see if mortality can be improved as a result are in progress (Henschke CI et al., 2007) and (Spiro SG et al., 2010).

It is important to refer that most symptomatic lung cancer is discovered at advanced stages, with the goal of long-term survival entirely dependent on effective treatment of stage III and IV lung cancer (Wang T et al., 2010).

More accurate staging at the time of initial presentation could improve design of clinical trials and avoid inappropriate surgical decisions in individual patients (Roberts JR et al., 1999). The TNM classification system for the staging of lung cancer has led to important advances in the determination of prognosis and treatment of patients with this disease (McLoud TC, 2006). TNM-staging has important influence on prognosis and therapy (Serke M & Schönfeld N, 2007).

This system takes into account the degree of spread of the primary tumor (represented by T); the extent of regional lymph node involvement (represented by N); and the presence or absence of distant metastases (represented by M). The TNM system is used for all lung carcinomas except SCLCs, which are staged separately. SCLC is staged as limited or extensive disease. Limited disease is localized enough to be included in a radiation port, while extensive disease includes distant metastases.

Staging of extrathoracic disease is very important in providing optimal care for the patient with lung cancer (Shaffer K, 1997). The majority of the patients will have locally advanced or metastatic disease at the time of diagnosis (Stinchcombe TE et al., 2009).

It is fulcral to mention that survival is inversely proportional to the stage, with early detection and diagnosis being the key to achieving surgical cure (Hollings N & Shaw P, 2002).

An early diagnosis is the determining factor in the therapeutic selection. Surgery, Chemotherapy and Radiotherapy are the most frequently utilized types of treatment. It is important to refer that in SCLC surgery has a restricted use in management of this type of lung cancer, as only a few patients with limited disease may be eligible; chemotherapy is the primary form of treatment for both stages, and radiation is included for patients staged with limited disease (Argiris A & Murren JR, 2001).

Surgery has a pivotal role in the treatment of bronchogenic carcinoma. Indeed, resection is the standard treatment of early stages (I and II) non-small cell lung cancer, remains optional for a portion of patients with a locally advanced disease (IIIA and IIIB) and in anecdotal carefully selected patients with an oligometastatic disease (IV) (Thomas PA, 2009). In many situations a combination of two or even three treatment modalities is necessary.

In this chapter the authors will emphasize the role of Bronchoscopy and Computed Tomography in the diagnosis of Lung Cancer.

2. Bronchoscopy

Bronchoscopy is an essential tool in respiratory medicine, which allows visualization and sampling from the main airways and it is a central technique in diagnosing lung cancer, but also in different therapeutic approaches (Herth FJ et al., 2006).

This exam is currently the most commonly employed invasive procedure in the practice of pulmonary medicine. Both the rigid and flexible bronchoscopes are used to diagnose and to treat various pulmonary disorders (Udaya B & Prakash S, 1999).

It is important to emphasize that the most common indication for bronchoscopy is for tissue sampling and determining the extent of lung cancer and it is, also, utilized extensively in the initial evaluation of patients suspected of having this pulmonary malignant pathology (Simon M et al., 2010) and (Aristizabal JF et al., 1998). The indications for the bronchoscopic exam are extensive. The main diagnostic indications include pulmonary involvement by neoplasms, infections, diffuse lung diseases, and airway problems (Table 1) (Plekker D et al., 2010), (Shah PL, 2008) and (Udaya B & Prakash S, 1999).

The principal advantages of flexible bronchoscopy include a more extensive view of the tracheobronchial tree, case of performance, and no requirement for general anesthesia (Suleman A et al., 2008).

Advancements in computer technology and engineering have allowed for the emergence of newer modalities to evaluate endobronchial, parenchymal, and mediastinal pathology (El-

Indications for Bronchoscopy
Diagnostic
Investigation of symptoms – Haemoptysis, Persistent cough, Recurrent Infection
Investigation of abnormal chest imaging - Lung masses, Diffuse infiltrates, Atelectasis or Pleural effusions
Diagnostic sampling of pathological processes - Endobronchial forceps biopsy, Transbronchial lung biopsy, Endobronchial brush, Bronchoalveolar lavage, Transbronchial needle aspiration
Staging of lung cancer - Mediastinal tissue diagnosis and staging
Infection - Identification of organisms (*e.g.* suspected tuberculosis), Evaluate airways if recurrent or persistent infection
Interstitial Lung Disease – Bronchoalveloar lavage for differential cell count and histology
Therapeutic
Foreign body removal, Management of massive haemoptysis, Endobronchial laser ablation, Electrocautery, Cryotherapy, Brachytherapy, Photodynamic therapy, Dilation of airway, Stent placement, Bronchoscopic lung volume reduction, Thermoplasty, Radiofrequency ablation
Research
Endobronchial biopsies in research of airway diseases, Bronchoalveolar lavage in research of diffuse lung diseases

Table 1. Indications for Bronchoscopy

Bayoumi E et al., 2008). Bronchoscopy has an important role in the evaluation of suspected lung cancer, interstitial lung disease, persistent infection and the assessment of new pulmonary infiltrates in immunocompromised patients. Recent developments have ranged from the improvement in image quality to integration of ultrasound (Shah PL, 2008).

Laser therapy, electrocautery, cryotherapy and stenting are well-described techniques for the palliation of symptoms due to airway involvement in patients with advanced stages (Simon M et al., 2010).

The decision about whether to perform a diagnostic bronchoscopy for a lesion that is suspicious for lung cancer depends largely on the location of the lesion (central Vs peripheral) (Rivera MP et al., 2003).

The bronchoscopic procedure requires specific training and experience in both flexible and rigid bronchoscopy. The recent advances in minimally invasive procedures has ultimately included a new array of therapeutic bronchoscopy for diseases which would otherwise not be treated, or offered only surgery, ended up adding a new variety of procedures that demand constant updates for the specialist to keep up with this rapidly evolving technology (Herth FJ et al., 2006).

Various diagnostic accessories can be inserted through the working channel of the flexible bronchoscope. These accessories include biopsy forceps, needles, and brushes, and they have greatly aided in the diagnosis and staging of lung cancers. Their combined effect has greatly improved the ability to obtain pulmonary biopsies, especially of ever smaller lesions (Herth FJ et al., 2006) and (Udaya B & Prakash S, 1999).

Bronchoscopy with Transbronchial Needle Aspiration (TBNA) for cytologic or histologic examination of mediastinal lymph node has been shown to be a safe procedure (Rivera MP et al., 2003).

Flexible bronchoscopy is an extremely safe procedure provided some basic precautions are taken. A recent retrospective analysis of 23.682 patients over a period of 11 years showed a mortality rate of 0.013% with a complication rate of 0.739% (Jin F et al., 2008).

Complications may result from topical anesthesia, agents used for sedation or the procedure itself. Potentially life-threatening complications include respiratory depression, airway obstruction, arrhythmias, haemorrhage, infection and pneumothorax. Patient preparation for elective bronchoscopy includes fasting prior to procedure, informed consent, careful sedation in some cases, and topical anesthesia. Some of the contraindications include totally uncooperative patients, hemodynamically unstable patients, any severe acute illness and those who refuse to undergo the procedure (Plekker D et al., 2010) and (Suleman A et al., 2008).

Diagnostic yield depends on the location, size, character of the border of the lesion, and the ability to perform all sampling methods (Chechani V, 1996). The success rate of bronchoscopy in obtaining diagnostic pathologic material is significantly higher when a third- to fifth-order bronchus can be traced to the pulmonary nodule on a chest CT (positive CT bronchus sign) (Aristizabal JF et al., 1998).

The role of flexible bronchoscopy in lung cancer includes the following: inspection of airways to detect ipsilateral and contralateral endobronchial disease and their biopsy; transbronchial biopsy of the pulmonary nodule or mass; detection of mediastinal and/or hilar adenopathy; and possible transbronchial needle aspiration of the hilar or mediastinal nodes (Aristizabal JF et al., 1998). Bronchoscopy is also important in staging and it is required a careful inspection of the upper airways, superior vocal cords, trachea, carina and bronchi.

The endoscopic signs of lung carcinoma are variable, extending from a simple loss of brightness in a small area of the bronchial mucosa to a typical vegetative mass. Classically, three types of typical lesions or direct signs of tumor are taken into consideration: mass, infiltration and obstruction. However many other endoscopic changes or indirect signs (edema or local vascular fragility, localized inflammation or congestion, stenosis, bronchial stiffness and extrinsic compression) may correspond to a lung cancer so that, especially in patients at risk, these lesions should be investigated by aspiration and/or brushing and/or biopsy (Baughman RP et al., 1999) and (Cook RM et al., 1995).

Central lesions can present as an exophitic endobronchial mass, submucosal spread or a peribronchial tumor causing extrinsic compression. Most studies defined peripheral lesion as lesions that are not visible in the main or lobar airways (Rivera MP et al., 2003).

In central tumors endoscopically visible, studies referred a diagnostic yield of 91% to 94% in central lesions and 83% in peripheral lesions (Shure D, 1996).

The sensitivity of bronchoscopy for peripheral lesions is most affected by the size of the lesion. The False-Negative rate can be estimated to be fairly high in the case of peripheral lesions, especially smaller ones, because of the relatively low sensitivity in this setting (Rivera MP et al., 2003).

A negative initial bronchoscopy in a suspected lung cancer patient implies a greater potential for excessive delays in diagnosis and treatment in spite of a greater chance of curative treatment. Most of the delay occurs in the interval from the outpatient appointment to decision-to-treat. Patients with negative bronchoscopy require a more concerted effort to achieve a timely diagnosis and treatment (Devbhandari MP et al., 2008).

Bronchoscopy has, also, an important role in the diagnosis of benign conditions, but the chance of finding a benign condition in a patient who is clinically suspected of having lung cancer is only 1% (Rolston KVI et al., 1997).

The role of both old and new diagnostic bronchoscopy will continue to evolve as further improvements are made in bronchoscopes, accessory equipment, and imaging technologies (Herth FJ et al., 2010).

It is important to refer that special emphasis has been placed on their role in the early detection and staging of lung cancer. Some technology requires further study to delineate its role in the disease, whereas other modalities are emerging as the new gold standard in evaluation of lung cancer (El-Bayoumi E et al., 2008).

3. Computed tomography

Radiological studies play a fundamental role in every aspect of clinical medicine. Imaging offers invaluable information in establishing a diagnosis, guiding interventional procedures and directing patient management. Thus, imaging techniques play a crucial role in the diagnosis, staging and follow-up of patients with lung cancer. (Hansell DM et al., 2010) and (Wynants J et al., 2007).

Computer aided diagnosis of lung CT image has been a remarkable and revolutionary step, in the early and premature detection of lung abnormalities. CT was introduced into clinical practice in the 1970s as an exciting new method for imaging the thorax. Since then, clinicians have come to rely heavily on CT for evaluating potentially malignant chest lesions and the intrathoracic spread of lung cancer (Colice GL, 1994).

CT scanners can image the entire central airways in only half a second, allowing for dynamic cine imaging of the trachea and bronchi during respiratory manoeuvres (Hansell DM et al., 2010).

High Resolution CT techniques developed in the last decade have become invaluable tools for the detection of subtle diffuse lung disease patterns and for their characterization into multiple possible diseases and they provide detailed information regarding the lung parenchyma and can delineate structures down to the level of the secondary pulmonary lobule. It is particularly useful for image-based diagnosis, since alteration of the lung anatomy, caused by a disease, can be clearly seen in a thin-slice CT image (Tatjana Z & Busayarat S, 2011).

CT is still the basis of imaging studies in the preoperative staging and post- therapeutic evaluation of lung cancer and is currently the best imaging modality for diagnosing lung diseases. The most recent developments in multidetector technology have dramatically improved the temporal and spatial resolution of CT (Lauren F et al., 2006) and (Tatjana Z & Busayarat S, 2011).

A chest CT is obtained in most of the patients with a pulmonary nodule or mass. A large body of imaging literature suggests that CT is a sensitive method to evaluate the proximal bronchi for neoplasm. It is also suggested that CT is helpful in predicting the yield of bronchoscopy in obtaining pathologic diagnosis of a pulmonary nodule or mass. In addition to demonstrating the location of the nodule (lobe, peripheral vs. central location), CT can also demonstrate if a third or fourth-order bronchus leads to or is contained within the pulmonary nodule or mass (Aristizabal JF et al., 1998).

CT plays a relevant role in the determination of presence and extent of lung cancer, demonstrating the size and site of the tumor. However, this exam presents some limitations such as high cost, utilization of ionizing radiation, contrast agent nephrotoxicity, besides the necessity of further procedures to confirm the diagnosis (Oliveira C & Saraiva A., 2010).

The findings of CT scans of the chest and clinical presentation usually allow a presumptive differentiation between SCLC and NSCLC. CT may also predict the yield of bronchoscopy in making a tissue diagnosis of pulmonary nodule or mass, if the predictive value of bronchoscopy is low, an alternate method of diagnosis may be chosen. CT can identify specific features in lung nodules that are diagnostic (e.g. arteriovenous fistulae, rounded atelectasis, fungus balls, mucoid impaction and infarcts) (Aristizabal JF et al., 1998), (Hollings N & Shaw P, 2002) and (Rivera MP et al., 2003).

This imaging modality also assists the implementation of complementary techniques including transthoracic needle aspiration biopsy, mediastinoscopy or video-assisted thoracic surgery (Landreneau RJ et al., 1996).

The CT indispensability in the study of lung cancer is associated with the obligatoriness of endoscopy of the respiratory tract with flexible endoscope (Cordeiro AJA Robalo, 1995).

Computed Tomography can detect tumors as small as 0.5 cm compared to a chest radiography which detects tumors at 3 cm. Yet, it is important to note that smaller tumor size does not necessarily equate to an early stage cancer as each tumor has its own growth pattern and disease development (Read et al., 2006).

It is important to note that pulmonary nodules of lung cancer in CT images share similarity with benign cases to some extent (such as tuberculosis, inflammatory pseudotumor, hamartoma, and aspergillosis) which makes it difficult to distinguish (Jee WC et al., 2008).

The majority of patients who present with lung cancer undergo CT scanning of the chest and liver (adrenal glands should be routinely included if lung cancer is suspected) and it is useful in helping to distinguish vascular structures from lymph nodes as well as in delineating mediastinal invasion by centrally located tumors (Al Jahdali H, 2008). Prediction of lymph node metastasis using combination of gene signatures and chest CT is superior to the CT-only diagnosis (Chang JW et al., 2008).

Morphologic imaging techniques such as CT cannot always differentiate reliably between benign and malignant lesions, as enlarged nodes may also be inflammatory whereas normal-sized lymph nodes may contain malignancy. Thoracic CT is the most commonly used noninvasive staging method of the mediastinum (Harewood GC et al., 2002). CT scanning reliably depicts mediastinal invasion, provided that the tumor surrounds the major mediastinal vessels or bronchi. So it is fulcral to mention that CT of the chest is an important imaging modality that helps in detailed imaging of the primary tumor and its anatomic relationship to other structures, and it provides information with respect to the size of mediastinal lymph nodes and the status of the pleural space.

Currently available results on CT screening for lung cancer show that the work-up on baseline screening can be confined to less than 15% of the individuals and to less than 6% on annual repeat screening, almost all cases are detected by screening with very few diagnoses made between screening on the prompting of symptoms, and over 80% of all the diagnoses are of Stage I (Henschke CI et al., 2005).

Although the introduction of low-dose spiral CT is considered to be one of the most promising clinical research developments, CT screening is used for detecting small peripheral lesions. CT screening is a far more sensitive method than conventional radiography for identifying small, potentially early-stage, lung cancers (Hansell DM et al., 2010) and (Yasufuku K, 2010).

CT scanning of the chest is useful in providing anatomic detail that better identifies the location of the tumor, its proximity to local structures, and whether or not lymph nodes in the mediastinum are enlarged (Silvestri GA et al., 2007). CT enables us to see the lung anatomy in great detail and has been used to accurately diagnose lung diseases and is a remarkable technique for visualizing structures within the thorax (Colice GL, 1994) and (Xu Y et al., 2006).

In the decades, CT has been the main diagnosis tool of lung cancer for its convenience and safety, and widely used in clinical practice. However, it is difficult to distinguish between benign and malignant cases in the CT images of pulmonary nodules, especially for the doctors who were lack of experience. This imaging modality is useful in predicting the likelihood of achieving positive histocytology at Flexible Bronchoscopy. The overall CT prediction is superior to any of the individual CT features taken alone (Bungay HK et al., 2000) and (Xiuhua G et al., 2011).

4. CT Vs bronchoscopy in the diagnosis of lung cancer

4.1 Purpose

The main objective of this study was to analyze the role of Bronchoscopy and CT in the diagnosis of lung cancer by evaluating the effectiveness of these techniques in the presence of this malignant pathology.

It is important to emphasize that the possibility to evaluate two important diagnostic methods in the presence of Lung Cancer is the main factor that justifies this study.

4.2 Methods

This retrospective study was conducted with the approval of the institutional review board of the Hospital Distrital da Figueira da Foz.

This investigation was done in the Department of Pneumology of the Hospital Distrital da Figueira da Foz, between January and July 2009.

To carry out this study, the medical records of 70 patients were analyzed (42 patients were men and 28 patients were women; the mean age was 66 years).

These patients were referred to the Department of Pneumology of the Hospital Distrital da Figueira da Foz (along a four-year period - January 2003 to January 2007) and submitted to Bronchoscopy and Computed Tomography for suspicion of Lung Cancer, confirmed or not by the study of the pathology.

It is fulcral to refer that bronchoscopy and CT exams were considered as either negative or positive according to the information included in the respective reports. Bronchoscopy exams and the subsequent reports were performed by a Pneumologist. A Radiologist performed the chest CT exams and prepared the respective reports.

In this investigation agreements between the results of the exam and the presence or absence of lung cancer were analyzed by calculating Cohen Kappa statistics. Agreements were assessed for both exams in study (Bronchoscopy and Computed Tomography).

4.3 Results and discussion

It is important to mention that among the 70 patients submitted to bronchoscopy and CT, 37 were diagnosed with lung cancer.

The statistical analysis permitted to observe that the relation between the bronchoscopy results and the presence or absence of lung cancer was statistically significant ($p < 0.05$). Also the Kappa Value 0.656 demonstrated a good rate of agreement between the results.

It is primordial to refer that the authors observed that in the 37 positive bronchoscopic studies, 83.8% corresponded to the presence of cancer, and 16.2% to a negative diagnosis of this lung pathology. As regards the 33 negative bronchoscopic exams, 81.8% corresponded to the absence of lung cancer, and 18.2% to the presence of this malignant pathology (Table 2).

The relation between CT results and the presence or absence of lung cancer was considered statistically significant ($p < 0.05$), after the statistical analysis. The kappa value was 0.451, corresponding to a weak agreement between the results.

Among the 42 CT studies interpreted as positive, 71.4% corresponded to the presence of this malignant pathology, and 28.6% corresponded to the absence of this pathology. In the 28 CT studies read as negative, 75% corresponded to a negative diagnosis of lung cancer, and 25% demonstrated the presence of this disease (Table 3).

In Table 4 is possible to observe the sensitivity, specificity, accuracy, false-positive and false-negative of bronchoscopy and CT scans. In this study, Bronchoscopy sensitivity was 83.8%, specificity 81.8%, and accuracy 82.8%. False-positive results corresponded to 18.2%, and false-negative results to 16.2%.

The CT sensitivity was 81.1%, specificity 63.6%, and accuracy 72.8%. False-positive results corresponded to 36.4% and false-negative results to 18.9%.

			Presence or Absence of Lung Cancer		TOTAL
			PRESENT	ABSENT	
Bronchoscopy	POSITIVE	N	31	6	37
		% Bronchoscopy	83.8%	16.2%	100.0%
		% Total	44.3%	8,6%	52.9%
	NEGATIVE	N	6	27	33
		% Bronchoscopy	18.2%	81.8%	100.0%
		% Total	8.6%	38.6%	47.1%
TOTAL		N	37	33	70
		% Bronchoscopy	52.9%	47.1%	100.0%
		% Total	52.9%	47.1%	100.0%

Table 2. Relation between the results of Bronchoscopy and the Presence or Absence of Lung Cancer ($\chi2 = 30.125$; gl = 1; p = 0; Kappa value = 0.656)

			Presence or Absence of Lung Cancer		TOTAL
			PRESENT	ABSENT	
CT	POSITIVE	N	30	12	42
		% CT	71.4%	28.6%	100.0%
		% TOTAL	42.9%	17.1%	60.0%
	NEGATIVE	N	7	21	28
		% CT	25.0%	75.0%	100.0%
		% TOTAL	10.0%	30.0%	40.0%
TOTAL		N	37	33	70
		% CT	52.9%	47.1%	100.0%
		% TOTAL	52.9%	47.1%	100.0%

Table 3. Relation between the results of CT exams and the Presence or Absence of Lung Cancer ($\chi2 = 14,533$; gl=1; p=0; Kappa value =0,451)

	SENSITIVITY	SPECIFICITY	ACCURACY	FALSE-POSITIVE	FALSE-NEGATIVE
Bronchoscopy	83.8%	81.8%	82.8%	18.2%	16.2%
CT	81.1%	63.6%	72.8%	36.4%	18.9%

Table 4. Sensitivity, Specificity, Accuracy, False-Positive and False-Negative of Bronchoscopy and CT Exams

The results of Bronchoscopy confirmed the fact that this is an important test in the diagnosis of lung cancer, by its diagnostical dependence in the pathological examination of tissue or cells obtained by various techniques of biopsy. Several studies have demonstrated that more than 70% of lung carcinomas are visible to bronchoscopy and combining bronchial biopsy, bronchial brushing, and bronchial washing results in an excellent diagnostic yield (Govert JA et al., 1998) and (Herth FJF, 2011).

The false-negative results of bronchoscopy found in the current study (16.2%) are due to the presence of peripheral lesions, particularly the smaller ones, because of the poor role played by bronchoscopy in these cases. Some published studies indicate that the sensitivity of bronchoscopy is poor for peripheral lesions that are < 2 cm in diameter (Chechani V, 1996), (Popovich J Jr et al., 1982) and (Schreiber G et al., 2003).

In the present investigation the authors obtained a sensitivity of 81.1% for CT, corroborating reports in the literature demonstrating that as lung cancer is detected by radiological methods, ¾ of the natural history of the pathology were already completed (Scagliotti G, 2001).

Radiology has traditionally played a crucial role in the evaluation and follow-up of patients with lung cancer. That role has changed with time, particularly with advances in surgical treatment and the introduction of new, less invasive techniques, such as video-assisted thoracoscopy and different imaging modalities have been used in the diagnosis and staging of lung cancer; reports refer that CT plays an important role in the diagnosis of lung cancer, however has been limited by uncertain detection rate for early stage of NSCLC, particularly central tumors (Jiang F et al., 2009) and (Shaffer K, 1997). CT scanning is required for a better delineation of the abnormality detected on plain radiographs.

Some studies in the literature mention that imaging plays an essential role in diagnosing, staging, and following patients with lung cancer (Patz EF Jr, 1999) and (Sarinas PS et al., 1996).

The specificity of CT in this investigation is a result of the number of false-positive results (36.4%) and this situation is due to the fact that radiological findings suggestive of lung cancer (that lead to the rate of a CT study as positive) such as parenchymal mass with speculated margins, thickwalled cavities, microlobulations, cavitary nodules and chest wall invasion may be observed in other diseases such as infections, pulmonary inflammatory processes, infarction and lung abscesses (George CJ et al., 2004), (Madhusudhan KS et al., 2007) and (Runciman DM et al., 1993).

Several studies indicate that the high proportion of false-positive CT findings may reach 70% and thus, histological confirmation is essential for diagnosis (Makris D et al., 2007) and (Swensen SJ et al., 2005).

5. Conclusion

Lung cancer is a common pathology that has a poor prognosis and survival is inversely proportional to the stage, with early detection and diagnosis being the key to achieving surgical cure.

Despite medical advances lung cancer remains the leading cause of cancer deaths (Serke M & Schönfeld N, 2007).

The diagnosis of lung cancer is essentially achieved by CT and bronchoscopic techniques. During these years numerous improvements of these diagnostic tools have been made available, which aspire to reduce the time to diagnosis and to simplify the initial staging approach.

The modality selected to diagnose a suspected lung cancer is based on the size and location of the primary tumor in the lung, the presence of potential metastatic spread, and the anticipated treatment plan (Schreiber G et al., 2003).

The main goals in selecting a specific diagnostic modality are to maximize the yield of the selected procedure for both diagnosis and staging and to avoid unnecessary invasive tests. The selection of the most appropriate test is done in a multidisciplinary way with contribution from a pulmonologist, radiologist and thoracic surgeon (Rivera MP et al., 2003).

The radiological diagnosis has become a key element in the evaluation and management of the patients with lung cancer and, in some instances, accurate staging and determination of appropriate treatment can be done noninvasively, with only imaging modalities, although in numerous situations surgical staging is also necessary.

Flexible Bronchoscopy with its attendant procedures is a valuable diagnostic tool in the workup of a patient who is suspected of having lung cancer. In the last decade, major advances have been made in interventional bronchoscopy.

Bronchoscopy results in this study corroborated the relevance of this method in the diagnosis of this malignant pathology, considering its dependence on the anatomopathological study of tissue or cells obtained through different biopsy techniques.

CT is today one of the cornerstones of imaging techniques and with the improved technical quality of CT scans, more small lesions are now detectable in the lungs.

The specificity of CT is limited and a histologic diagnosis or follow-up evaluation is, usually, necessary. The potential benefits of introducing CT screening for lung cancer detection may be its ability to detect more early stage tumors and decrease the numbers of later stage disease. And CT can best be thought of as a imaging tool that can provide a roadmap for more accurate surgical staging.

It is important to emphasize that in the detection and diagnosis of lung cancer should be carried out complementary exams that include CT and Bronchoscopy.

6. Definitions

False positive - is the proportion of absent events that yield positive test outcomes, i.e., the conditional probability of a positive test result given an absent event.

False – Negative – is the proportion of events that are being tested for which yield negative test outcomes with the test, i.e., the conditional probability of a negative test result given that the event being looked for has taken place.

Sensitivity - measures the proportion of actual positives which are correctly identified as such (e.g. the percentage of sick people who are correctly identified as having the condition).

Specificity - measures the proportion of negatives which are correctly identified (e.g. the percentage of healthy people who are correctly identified as not having the condition).

Positive predictive value - is the proportion of subjects with positive test results who are correctly diagnosed. It is a critical measure of the performance of a diagnostic method, as it reflects the probability that a positive test reflects the underlying condition being tested for.

Negative predictive value - is a summary statistic used to describe the performance of a diagnostic testing procedure. It is defined as the proportion of subjects with a negative test result who are correctly diagnosed. A high NPV means that when the test yields a negative result, it is uncommon that the result should have been positive

7. References

Agarwal, A., Ghotekar, L. H., Garbyal, R. S., Mital, V. P. & Chokhani, R. (2003). Evaluation of pulmonary malignancies in Kathmandu Valley and role of bronchoscopic techniques in diagnosis of such cases, *JIACM* 4:127–33.

Al Jahdali, H. (2008). Evaluation of the patient with lung cancer, *Ann Thorac Med* 3:74-8

Argiris, A. & Murren, J. R. (2001). Staging and clinical prognostic factors for small-cell lung cancer, *Cancer J* 7(5):437-47

Aristizabal, J. F., Young, K. R. & Nath, H. (1998). Can Chest CT decrease the use of evaluation of suspected bronchogenic preoperative bronchoscopy in the carcinoma?, *Chest* 113;1244-1249

Baughman, R. P. & Pina, E. M. (1999). Role of bronchoscopy in lung cancer research, *Clin Chest Med* 20(1):191-9

Beadsmoore, C. J. & Screaton, N. J. (2003). Classification, staging and prognosis of lung cancer, *Eur J Radiol* 45(1):8-17

Beckles, M.A., Spiro, S.G., Colice, G.L & Rudd, R. M. (2003). Initial evaluation of the patient with lung cancer: symptoms, signs, laboratory tests and paraneoplastic syndromes, *Chest* 123(1 Suppl);97S– 104S.

Bekett, W.S. (1993). Epidemiology and etiology of lung cancer, *Clin Chest Med* 14:1-15

Bilello, K.S., Murin, S. & Matthay, R.A. (2002). Epidemiology, etiology and prevention of lung cancer, *Clin Chest Med* 23(1):1-25

Brundage, M. D., Davies, D. & Mackillop, W. J. (2002). Prognostic Factors in Non-small Cell Lung Cancer* - A Decade of Progress, *Chest* 122:1037-1057

Bungay, H. K., Pal, C. R., Davies, C. W., Davies, C. W., Davies, R. J. & Gleeson, F. V. (2000). An evaluation of computed tomography as an aid to diagnosis in patients undergoing bronchoscopy for suspected bronchial carcinoma, *Clin Radiol* 55(7).554-60

Chang, J. W., Yi, C. A., Son, D. S., Choi, N., Lee, J., Kim, H. K., Choi, Y. S., Lee, K. S. & Kim, J. (2008). Prediction of lymph node metastasis using the combined criteria of helical CT and mRNA expression profiling for non-small cell lung cancer, *Lung Cancer* 60(2):264-70

Chechani, V. (1996). Bronchoscopic diagnosis of solitary pulmonary nodules and lung masses in the abscence of endobronchial abnormality, *Chest* 109(3):620-5

Chen, Y. M., Shih, J. F., Tsaim, C. M., Lee, Y. C., Perng, R. P. & Whang-Peng, J. (2009). Revisiting Squamous Cell Carcinoma of the Lungs – A Disease Given Less Attention, *J Chinese Oncol Soc* 25(6):393-402

Colice, G. L. (1994). Chest CT for known or suspected lung cancer, *Chest* 106(5):1538-50

Cook, R. M. & Miller, Y. E. (1995). Flexible fiberoptic bronchoscopy in the diagnosis and staging of lung cancer, *in* Johnson EB, Johnson HD, editors. Lung cancer. New York, NY: Wiley-Lyss, p. 123- 44.

Cordeiro, A. J. A. Robalo (1995). Pneumologia fundamental. Lisboa: Fundação Calouste Gulbenkian, p. 349-73.

Devbhandari, M. P., Quennell, P., Krysiak, P., Shah, R. & Jones, M. T. (2008). Implications of a negative bronchoscopy on waiting times to treatment for lung cancer patients: results of a prospective tracking study, *Eur J Cardiothorac Surg* 34(3):479-83

El-Bayoumi, E. & Silvestri, G. A. (2008). Bronchoscopy for the diagnosis and staging of lung cancer, *Semin Respir Crit Care Med* 29:261-70.

Figueiredo, L. & Bento, M. T. (1999). Neoplasia do pulmão, *in* Pisco JM & Sousa LA. Noções fundamentais de imagiologia. Lisboa: Lidel-Edições Técnicas, p. 195-209.

Gazdar, A. F. (2010). Should we continue to use the term non-small-cell lung cancer, *Ann Oncol* 21 Suppl 7:vii225-9

George, C. J., Tazelaar, H. D., Swensen, S. J. & Ryu, J. H. (2004). Clinicoradiological features of pulmonary infarctions mimicking lung cancer, *Mayo Clin Proc* 79(7):895-8.

Govert, J. A., Dodd, L. G., Kussin, P. S. & Samuleson, W. M. (1999). A prospective comparison of fiberoptic transbronchial needle aspiration and bronchial biopsy for bronchoscopically visible lung carcinoma, *Cancer* 87(3):129-34

Hansell, D. M., Boiselle, P. M., Goldin, J., Kauczor, H. U., Lynch, D. A., Mayo, J. R. & Patz, E. F. Jr. (2010). Thoracic Imaging, *Respirology* 15:393-400

Harewood, G. C., Wiersema, M. J., Edell, E. S. & Liebow, M. (2002). Cost-Minimization Analysis of Alternative Diagnostic Approaches in a Modeled Patient with Non-Small Cell Lung Cancer and Subcarinal Lymphadenopathy, *Mayo Clin Proc* 77:155-164

Henschke, C. I., Yankelevitz, D. F. & Altorki, N. K. (2007). The role of CT screening for lung cancer, *Thorac Surg Clin* 17(2):137-42

Henschke, C. I. & I-ELCAP Investigators. (2005). CT screening for lung cancer: update 2005, *Surg Oncol Clin N Am* 14(4):761-76

Herth, F. J. F. (2011). Bronchoscopic techniques in diagnosis and staging of lung cancer, *Breath* 7(4):325-337

Herth, F. J. & Eberhardt, R. (2010). Flexible bronchoscopy and its role in the staging of non-small cell lung cancer, *Clin Chest Med* 31(1):87-100.

Herth, F. J., Eberhardt, R. & Ernst, A. (2006). The future of bronchoscopy in diagnosing, staging and treatment of lung cancer, *Respiration* 73:399- 409.

Hicks, R. J., Lau, E., Alam, N. Z. & Chen, R. Y. (2007). Imaging in the diagnosis and treatment of non-small cell lung cancer, *Respirology* 12(2):165-72

Hollings, N. & Shaw, P. (2002). Diagnostic imaging of lung cancer, *Eur Respir J* 19:722-742

Jamnik, S., Santoro, I. L. & Uehara, C. (2002). Comparative study of prognostic factors among longer and shorter survival patients with bronchogenic carcinoma, *J. Pneumologia* 28(5): 245 - 249.

Jiang, F., Todd, N. W., Liu, Z., Katz, R. L. & Stass, S. A. (2009). Combined genetic analysis of sputum and computed tomography for noninvasive diagnosis of non-small-cell lung cancer, *Lung Cancer* 66(1):58-63

Jin, F., Um, D., Chu, D., Fu, E., Xie, Y. & Liu T. (2008). Severe complications of bronchoscopy, *Respiration* 76(4):429-33

Kamath, A. V. & Chhajed, P. N. (2006). Role of bronchoscopy in early diagnosis of lung cancer, *Indian J Chest Dis Allied Sci* 48(4):265-9

Landreneau, R. J., Hazelrigg, S. R., *et al.* (1996). Video-Assisted Thoracic Surgery, In Aisner J, Arriagada R, *et al*, editors. *Comprehensive Textbook of Thoracic Oncology*. Baltimore : Williams & Wilkins, p. 965-979

Laurent, F., Montaudon, M. & Corneloup, O. (2006). CT and MRI of lung cancer, *Respiration* 73:133–142.

Madhusudhan, K. S., Gamanagatti. S., Seith, A. & Hari, S. (2007). Pulmonary infections mimicking cancer: report of four cases, *Singapore Med J* 48:e327- 31.

Makris, D., Scherpereel, A., Leroy, S., Bouchindhomme, B., Faivre, J. B., Remy, J., Ramon, P. & Marquette, C. H. (2007). Electomagnetic navigation diagnostic bronchoscopy for small peripheral lung lesions, *Eur Resp J* 29:1187-1192

McLoud, T. C. (2006). "A System for the Clinical Staging of Lung Cancer" - A Commentary, *AJR* 187:269-270

Oliveira, C. & Saraiva, A. (2010). Comparative study between computed tomography and bronchoscopy in the diagnosis of lung cancer, *Radiol Bras* 43(4):229–235

Patz, E. F. Jr. (2000). Imaging Bronchogenic Carcinoma, *Chest* 117:90S-95S

Patz, E. F. Jr. (1999). Imaging lung cancer, *Semin Oncol* 26(5 Suppl 15):21-6

Plekker, D., Koegelenberg, C. F. N. & Bolliger, C. T. (2010). Different techniques of bronchoscopy, *Eur Respir Mon* 48:1-17

Popovich, J. Jr., Kvale, P. A., Eichenhorn, M. S., Radke, J. R., Ohorodnik, J. M. & Fine, G. (1982). Diagnostic accuracy of multiple biopsies from flexible fiberoptic bronchoscopy. A comparison of central versus peripheral carcinoma, *Am Rev Respir Dis* 125(5):521-3

Read, C., Janes, S., George, J. & Spiro, S. (2006). Early Lung Cancer: screening and detection, *Prim Care Respir J* 15 (6), 332-336.

Rivera, M. P., Detterbeck, F., Mehta, A. C. & American College of Chest Physicians. (2003). Diagnosis of lung cancer: the guidelines, *Chest* 123(1 Suppl 1):129S–36S.

Roberts, J. R., Blum, M. G., Arildsen, R., Drinkwater, D. C. Jr., Christian, K. R., Powers, T. A. & Merrill, W. H. (1999). Prospective comparison of radiologic, thoracoscopic, and pathologic staging in patients with early non-small cell lung cancer, *Ann Thorac Surg* 68(4):1154-8

Runciman, D. M., Shepherd, M. C. & Gaze, M. N. (1993). Lung abscesses mimicking multiple pulmonary metastases, *Clin Oncol (R Coll Radiol)* 5(5):317-8

Sarinas, P. S., Chitkara, R. K., Rizk, N. W., Segall, G. M. & Stark, P. (1996). Imaging in lung cancer, *Curr Opin Pulm Med* 2(4):263-70

Scagliotti, G. V., Ceppi, P., Novello, S. & Papotti, M. (2009). Chemotherapy Treatment Decisions in Advanced Non-small Cell Lung Cancer Based on Histology, *Am Soc Clin Oncol* 27:431-435

Scagliotti, G. (2001). Symptoms, signs and staging of lung cancer, *Eur Respir Mon* 17:86–119.

Schreiber, G. & McCrory, D. C. (2003). Performance Characteristics of Different Modalities for Diagnosis of Suspected Lung Cancer: Summary of Published Evidence, *Chest* 123:115S-128S

Serke, M. & Schönfeld, N. (2007). Diagnosis and staging of lung cancer, *Dtsch Med Wochenschr* 132(21):1165-9

Shaffer, K. (1997). Radiologic Evaluation in Lung Cancer: Diagnosis and Staging, *Chest* 112:235S-238S

Shah, P. L. (2008). Flexible bronchoscopy, *Medicine* 36(39:151-154

Shure, D. (1996). Tissue Procurement: Bronchoscopic Techniques for Lung Cancer, *in*: Pass HI, Mitchell JB, Johnson DH, editors, *Lung Cancer, Principles and Practice*. New York: Lippincott Williams and Wilkins, p. 471-477

Silva, A. C, Paiva, A. C., Nunes, R. A. & Gattass, M. (2011). Informatics and Computerized Tomogarphy Aiding Detection and Diagnosis of Solitary Lung Cancer. *in*, Homma N, editor. *Theory and Applications of CT Imaging and analysis*. Rijeka: In-Tech, p. 15 - 36

Silvestri, G. A., Gould, M. K., Margolis, M. L., Tanoue, L. T., McCrory, D., Toloza, E. & Detterbeck F (2007). Noninvasive Staging of Non-small Cell Lung Cancer*: ACCP Evidenced-Based Clinical Practice Guidelines (2nd Edition), *Chest* 132:178S-201S

Simon, M. & Simon, I. (2010). Update in bronchoscopic techniques, *Pneumologia* 59:53–6.

Spiro, S. G., Tanner, N. T., Silvestri, G. A., Janes, S. M., Lim, E., Vansteenkiste, J. F. & Pirker, R. (2010). Lung cancer: progress in diagnosis, staging and therapy, *Respirology* 15(1):44-50

Stinchcombe, T. E. & Socinski, M. A. (2009). Current treatments for advanced stage non-small cell lung cancer, *Proc Am Thorac Soc* 6:233–41.

Suleman, A., Ikramullah, Q., Ahmed, F. & Khan, M. Y. (2008). Indications and Complications of Bronchoscopy. An experience of 100 cases in a tertiary care hospital, *JMPI* 22(3):210-214

Swensen, S. J., Jett, J. R., Hartman, T. E., Midthun, D. E., Mandrekar, S. J., Hillman, S. L., Skyes, A. M., Aughenbaugh, G. L., Tatjana, Z. & Busayarat, S. (2011). Computer-aided Analyses and Interpretation of HRCT Images of the Lung, *in* Homma N, editor, *Theory and Applications of CT Imaging and analysis*. Rijeka: In-Tech, p. 37-62

Thomas, P.A. (2009). Standards of surgery in lung cancer., *Rev Prat* 59(7):934-8

Udaya, B. & Prakash, S. (1999). Advances in Bronchoscopic Procedures, *Chest* 116.1403-1408

Yasufuku, K. (2010). Early diagnosis of lung cancer, *Clin Chest Med* 31(1):39-47

Xiuhua, G., Tao, S., Huan, W. & Zhigang L. (2011). Prediction Models for Malignant Pulmonary Nodules Based-on Texture Features of CT Image, *in* Homma N, editor. *Theory and Applications of CT Imaging and Analysis*. Rijeka:In-Tech; 2011.p. 63-76

Xu, Y., Van Beek, E. J., Hwanio, Y., Guo, J., McLennan, G. & Hoffman, E. A. (2006). Computer-aided classification of interstitial lung diseases via MDCT: 3D adaptive multiple feature method (3D AMFM), *Acad Radiol* 13(8):969-78

Wang, T., Nelson, R. A., Bogardus, A. & Grannis, F. W. Jr. (2010). Five-year lung cancer survival: which advanced stage nonsmall cell lung cancer patients attain long-term survival, *Cancer* 116(6):1518-25

Westeel, V. (2003). Diagnosis of lung cancer, *Rev Prat* 53:727–34.
Witschi, H. (2001). A Short Story of Lung Cancer, *Toxicol Sci* 64(1):4-6
Wynants, J., Stroobants, S., Dooms, C. & Vansteenkiste, J. (2007). Staging of lung cancer, *Radiol Clin North Am* 45:609–25

Section 3

Bronchoscopy in Special Situations

5

Bronchoscopy in Mechanically Ventilated Patients

Angel Estella
Intensive Care Unit Hospital of Jerez
Spain

1. Introduction

The origins of bronchoscopy date back to 1897 when Gustav Killian, considered "the father of bronchoscopy", performed the first airway examination with a rigid esophagoscope to a farmer extracting a piece of bone that had lodged in the main stem bronchus. Shigeto Ikeda in 1964 revolutionized the field of bronchoscopy with the introduction of a flexible instrument that could be introduced to sub-segmental bronchi and allowed the extraction of samples for cytological examination. Endoscopy Machida Company Ltd and Olympus Optical Company Ltd in 1966 built the first prototype of a fiberoptic bronchoscope. Since its introduction in routine clinical practice in the decade of 60 has been improved, increasing its indications. 30 years ago, rigid bronchoscope was the main instrument for the direct examination of the tracheobronchial tree; and even today is considered the choice procedure in two emergencies, haemoptysis and removal of foreign bodies.

Currently, flexible fiberoptic bronchoscopy is an invasive procedure widely applied in pneumology, intensive care and thoracic surgery. It has become the procedure of choice in most examinations of the tracheobronchial tree and it is of significant help in the diagnosis and treatment of pulmonary pathology in critically ill patients. It is increasingly being used in intensive care units (ICU) because it is easy to perform at the bedside, thus avoiding potentially dangerous transfers out of the ICU, and few complications have been described with its use. The procedure revolutionized the management of respiratory diseases and in the critically ill patients is considered a safe procedure. In view of this, it is currently considered to be an essential piece of ICU equipment.

Although, by definition, critically ill patients are a priori more susceptible to developing complications during the procedure, mechanically ventilated patients, because their airway is secured, are paradoxically less at risk than when the procedure is performed on patients breathing spontaneously.

Actually flexible fiberoptic bronchoscopy is a common diagnostic and therapeutic tool for patients admitted in ICU. In the literature flexible fiberoptic bronchoscopy has been scarcely documented in critically ill patients. This chapter summarizes main indications, complications and requirements necessary to perform a bronchoscopy in mechanically ventilated patients.

2. Procedure in mechanically ventilated patients

In mechanically ventilated patients bronchoscopy is performed through the endotracheal or tracheotomy tube by means of a specially adapted valve that facilitates the introduction of the bronchoscope into the airway without disconnection of mechanical ventilation. The adapter connects the endotracheal tube with the ventilator circuit and has a side port to allow entry of the bronchoscope into the endotracheal tube without disrupting the ongoing mechanical ventilation (figure 1).This valve allows continued ventilation and maintenance of PEEP during the technique.This is especially important in patients with adult respiratory distress syndrome.

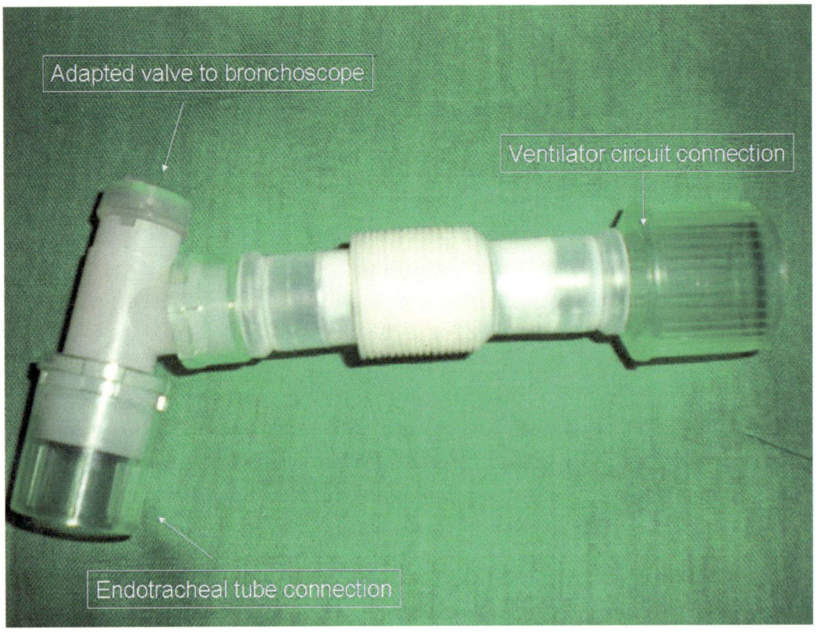

Fig. 1. Adapted valve to perform bronchoscopy in mechanically ventilated patients.

It has been studied that bronchoscope diameter plays an important role in airway flow obstruction in intubated patients.Without the orotracheal tube the bronchoscope only occupies 10% of the trachea. The internal diameter of the endotracheal tube influences the size of the bronchoscope.

In order to maintain the adequate minute volume and to minimize barotrauma it is recommended to use an endotracheal tube with a probe diameter of at least 2 mm larger than the bronchoscope diameter. An adult bronchoscope of 5.7 mm occupies 40% of the orotracheal lumen in a 9 mm endotracheal tube, which equals 51% and 66% of the lumen for 8 and 7 mm respectively. Use of a narrow bronchoscope may avoid the risk of barotrauma but has the disadvantage of less suction capacity through the bronchoscope channel.

Despite all these factors fiberoptic bronchoscopy is considered a safe procedure; patients admitted in the Intensive Care Unit should be considered at high risk from complications when undergoing fiberoptic bronchoscopy.Several recommendations must to be applied to guarantee the security of the technique and improve patient safety.

In mechanically ventilated patients several considerations (table 1) are recommended during the peribronchoscopy period to ensure the maintenance of adequate ventilation and oxygenation while minimizing the risk of barotrauma. Continuous physiological monitoring must be continued during and after the procedure. During the bronchoscopy exhaustive ventilator parameter monitoring is required to take care to maintain tidal volume and to control airway pressures. Continuous haemodynamic monitoring with heart rate, arterial pressure and oximetry is mandatory.

- Internal diameter of endotracheal tube at least 2 mm larger than bronchoscope diameter.
- Specially adapted valve, allowing minimal loss of tidal volume.
- Lubricate bronchoscope.
- Inspired fraction of oxygen of 1 prior to and during bronchoscopy.
- Short suction periods.
- Continuous haemodynamic monitoring: heart rate, blood pressure, respiratory rate.
- Continuous pulse oximeter during the procedure.
- Ventilator parameters monitoring: tidal volume, airway pressure.
- Sedation and sometimes muscle relaxation must to be considered.
- To interrupt enteral nutrition during procedure.
- Verbal and written consent form.

Table 1. Recommendations to perform bronchoscopy in mechanically ventilated patients.

Prior to and during fiberoptic bronchoscopy inspired fraction of oxygen (FiO_2) must be increased to 1 and following the procedure the FiO_2 will be adjusted according to the clinical situation of the patient. Pressure-control mode has demonstrated to deliver a greater baseline volume than volume- control mode in a lung model; careful readjustment of the inspiratory pressure level is necessary in Pressure-control mode to maximize exhaled tidal volume. Finally inspiratory pressure level must be reduced to pre-procedure values when the bronchoscope is removed. Effects of fiberoptic bronchoscopy on the respiratory function have been amply analyzed in patients with spontaneous breathing but in mechanically ventilated patients has been scarcely studied. Recently it was documented in a study to analyze the effects on respiratory mechanics of flexible bronchoscopy in mechanically ventilated patients. A transitory deterioration of pulmonary mechanics with a decrease of respiratory system compliance and an increase in airway resistance was observed in fifty mechanically ventilated patients after bronchoscopy with bronchoalveolar lavage (Estella,2010).

Sedation and muscle relaxation may be necessary during the procedure to prevent barotrauma caused by airway irritation reflex and cough; although critically ill patients may be heavily sedated we recommend short-acting benzodiazepines.

Flexible bronchoscopy is an invasive procedure and therefore needs documented informed consent from the patient or legal representative if the patient lacks medical decision-making capacity.

3. Fiberoptic bronchoscopy indications in an Intensive Care Unit

Flexible fiberoptic bronchoscopy is an essential diagnostic and therapeutic tool for management of critically ill patients. The present chapter summarizes the indications of these procedures in the Intensive Care Unit; many indications require both diagnostic and therapeutic objectives simultaneously. It is currently a usual procedure in mechanically ventilated patients. Table 2 summarizes the indications of flexible bronchoscopy in this group of patients.

- Pneumonia diagnosis, mainly ventilator associated pneumonia or immunocompromised patients. - Atelectasis, mainly caused by a central mucous plug. - Haemoptysis. - Bronchorrhea. - Difficult airway management. - Percutaneous tracheostomy control. - Foreign bodies. - Chest/airway trauma. - Diffuse lung diseases. - Acute inhalational injury. - Others: assessment of glottic damage, insertion of double-lumen endotracheal tube.

Table 2. Indications for bronchoscopy in mechanically ventilated patients.

3.1 Pneumonia diagnosis in mechanically ventilated patients

The most frequent diagnostic indication of flexible bronchoscopy in mechanically ventilated patients is to collect samples for microbiological analysis in patients with suspected pneumonia.

Pneumonia is the most frequent nosocomial infection occurring in critically ill patients in the Intensive Care Unit and is associated with a high mortality rate, prolonged mechanical ventilation and intensive care unit stay. It is associated with a high cost due to extended hospital stay and a greater consumption of antimicrobial agents. It is necessary to distinguish three kinds of pneumonia in mechanically ventilated patients to analyze the role of flexible bronchoscopy: community acquired pneumonia, ventilator associated pneumonia and pneumonia in immunocompromised patients.

In Europe, only in half of patients with community acquired pneumonia requiring hospitalization etiological diagnosis is finally known (Woodhead M, 2002). Streptococcus pneumoniae is the most frequent etiologic cause. In community acquired pneumonia invasive techniques are not usually indicated. It is recommended in cases with fulminant evolution or cases without adequate response to empirical antibiotics. In an analysis of the role of bronchoalveolar lavage in 96 mechanically ventilated patients the group with community acquired pneumonia had the lower diagnostic yield compared with ventilator associated pneumonia and immunocompromised patients (Estella, 2008). Our hypothesis is that recent introduction of antibiotics reduce the diagnostic yield of respiratory samples and empiric treatment is usually administered in a previous admission in the Intensive Care Unit.

Despite prior antibiotic therapy bronchoalveolar lavage is a useful diagnostic tool in immunocompromised patients. In ventilator associated pneumonia, in spite of the number of studies carried out, the diagnosis of pneumonia during mechanical ventilation is still disputed. Actually there are two diagnostic strategies: the "non-invasive" strategy, based on clinical criteria and a culture of secretions from upper airways (Heyland, 2006), and the "invasive" strategy, based on the use of flexible bronchoscopy for microbiological diagnosis using quantitative cultures from samples obtained selectively from the affected area (Fagon,2000). This particular strategy is recommended in the clinical guidelines of leading scientific societies for diagnosing ventilator-associated pneumonia like the American Thoracic Society, yet is one of the diagnostic methods least used in Europe, the tracheal aspirate was the most frequent diagnostic sample used in twenty-seven intensive care units of nine european countries (Koulenti,2009).

The strengths and weaknesses of the use of bronchoscopy comparing with the clinical strategy based in tracheal aspirate samples are shown in Table 3. The explanations for the low use of fiberoptic bronchoscopy in Intensive Care Unit for pneumonia diagnosis are probably the lack of experienced personnel , procedure time spent compared with other samples like tracheal aspirate and the lack of a definitive well designed study that definitively define a gold standard for the diagnosis of pneumonia.

Advantages - Lower respiratory tract - Guided sample obtained. - High specificity. - Distinguish between infection and colonization.
Disadvantages - Staff need training in bronchoscope use. - Complications. - Relative contraindications.

Table 3. Strengths and weaknesses of bronchoscopy for pneumonia diagnosis.

The year 2009 was characterized in worldwide Intensive Care Units by the Influenza A (H1N1)v pandemic. Initially bronchoscopy was not routinely recommended to obtain respiratory samples for the Influenza A (H1N1)v pneumonia due to critically ill patients presenting with severe hypoxemia and for the risk of generating aerosol. Interestingly bronchoalveolar lavage was described in a short series of patients as a useful diagnostic method in patients with false negatives obtained by upper airway respiratory samples (ANZIC influenza investigators,2009). Future studies are necessary for determining the role of bronchoscopy in the diagnosis of Influenza A (H1N1)v pneumonia. We proposed a diagnostic algorithm with the recommendation to perform bronchoscopic bronchoalveolar lavage in cases with a high clinical suspicion and negative microbiologic results of samples obtained from upper respiratory airway (Estella, 2010).

3.2 Atelectasis

Atelectasis and retention of secretions are common complications in critically ill patients. They usually present with excess airway secretions or inability to generate a cough. Frequently it is due to postoperative state, prolonged mechanical ventilation or sedation. Atelectasis is one of the most frequent therapeutic indications for flexible fiberoptic bronchoscopy in the Intensive Care Unit. For this use the size of the bronchoscope is important as efficient suctioning requires a large bronchoscope with a wide suction channel. In adult mechanically ventilated patients paediatric bronchoscopes are not recommended for this indication.

But the effectiveness of bronchoscopy to resolve it is the subject of controversy. A systematic review of several publications (Kreider, 2003) finding important differences in the effectiveness of flexible bronchoscopy: from 19% to 89%, with the best results found in lobar atelectasis caused by a central mucous plug, and the worst in subsegmental atelectasis. Figure 2 shows the sequence of endoscopic images of a central mucous plug located in the right main stem (1,2,3) and its resolution with the aspiration through the suction channel (4,5,6). Marini et al compared the use of flexible bronchoscopy with intense respiratory physiotherapy for treating atelectasis and found no differences in either group, attributing, in this study, delayed resolution to the presence of air bronchograms in the chest x-ray (Marini, 1979).

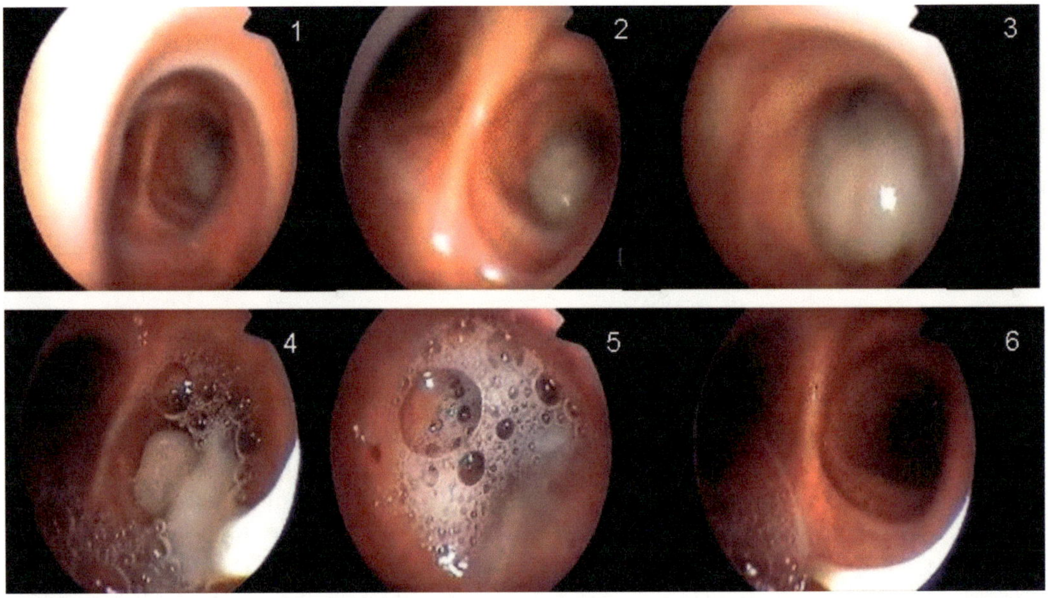

Fig. 2. Endoscopic image of a central mucous plug located in the right main stem and its resolution.

3.3 Hemoptysis

Rigid bronchoscopy is the procedure of choice for acute life-threatening haemoptysis, defined as the expectoration of more that 600 ml of blood over a 48 hour period, or of 400 ml in 24 hours in an isolated episode. In patients with haemoptysis, flexible bronchoscopy is a useful tool for locating the point of bleeding and also for administering through the bronchoscopic channel cold saline solution and adrenaline 1:10000 to control haemorrhaging. Haemoptysis is one of the commonest situations for which emergency bronchoscopy is indicated.

In cases of life-threatening haemoptysis in intubated patients and in distal locations, flexible bronchoscopy has been shown to be useful, with reports of cases of unrelenting haemorrhage where the source of bleeding has been plugged using a Fogarty catheter placed through the aspiration channel of the endoscope (Gottlieb LS,1975). Likewise, cases have been documented in which plugging was performed using the same technique described, but with a Swan-Ganz catheter. Flexible bronchoscopy can help position double-lumen endotracheal tubes for pulmonary isolation and selective ventilation in cases of massive unilateral haemoptysis. Recently a new way of administration of drugs has been described where a good response to intrapulmonary treatment with activated recombinant factor VII instilled through the channel of the bronchoscope in cases of diffuse alveolar haemorrhage has been documented (Heslet, 2006; Estella,2008).

3.4 Chest trauma

Patients with chest trauma present potential risk of lesions of the bronchial tree. Sometimes several lesions are not clinically evident and flexible bronchoscopy may be indicated to explore the airway and respiratory tract. It can be useful in diagnosis by enabling direct endoscopic visualisation of tracheal lacerations, bronchial transection or lacerations at any point of the bronchial tree, haemorrhage, contusions of the mucous membrane or aspirated material.

3.5 Percutaneous tracheostomy control

Percutaneous tracheostomy is a simple bedside procedure frequently used in Intensive Care Units, it is considered as the airway management of choice for patients with prolonged mechanical ventilation requirements. The procedure is associated with a low complication rate. It does have a few, but potentially life-threatening, complications like creation of a false airway, pneumothorax, subcutaneous emphysema, tracheoesophageal fistula. These complications are mainly associated with failure to visualise the area during the technique.

Bronchoscopic control with direct visualization minimises the complications associated with the procedure.It is recommended particularly in patients with anatomically difficult necks.

Figure 3 shows the different steps of the percutaneous tracheostomy technique and their endoscopic visualization. 1: advancement of the needle until free withdrawal of air into the fluid filled syringe and bronchoscopic visualization confirming the entry of the needle and cannula into the trachea; 2: a) introduction of the guide-wire, b) predilation, passing of the pre-dilator over the guide wire penetrating soft tissues and tracheal wall; 3: tracheal dilation, advancing the guide wire dilating forceps over the guide wire and opening of the forceps to dilate tracheal wall in order to accept the tracheotomy tube; 4: tube insertion, endoscopic image of the advancement of the tracheotomy tube into the trachea.

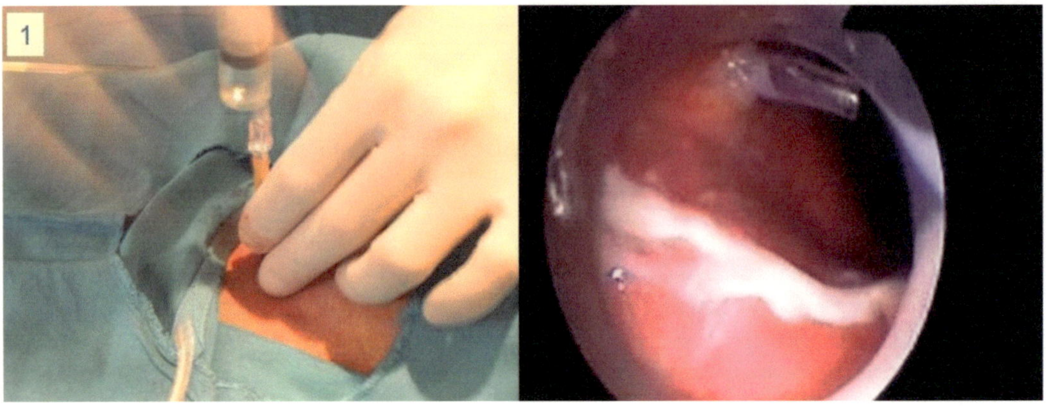
1

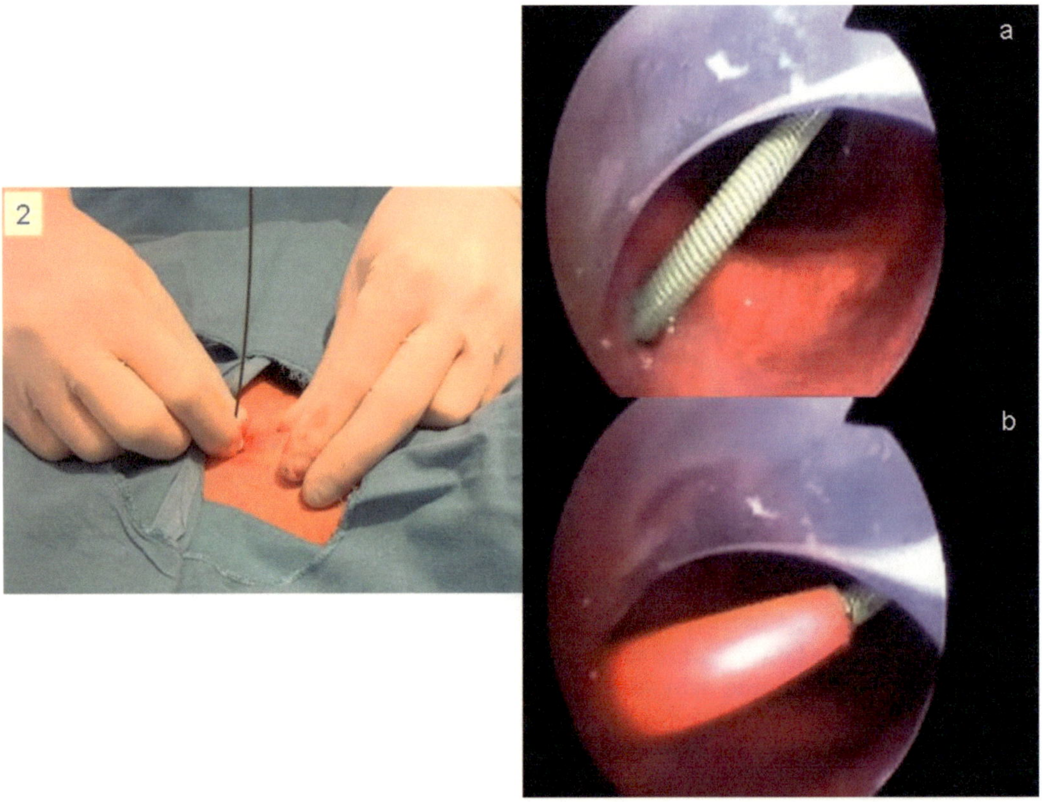
2
a
b

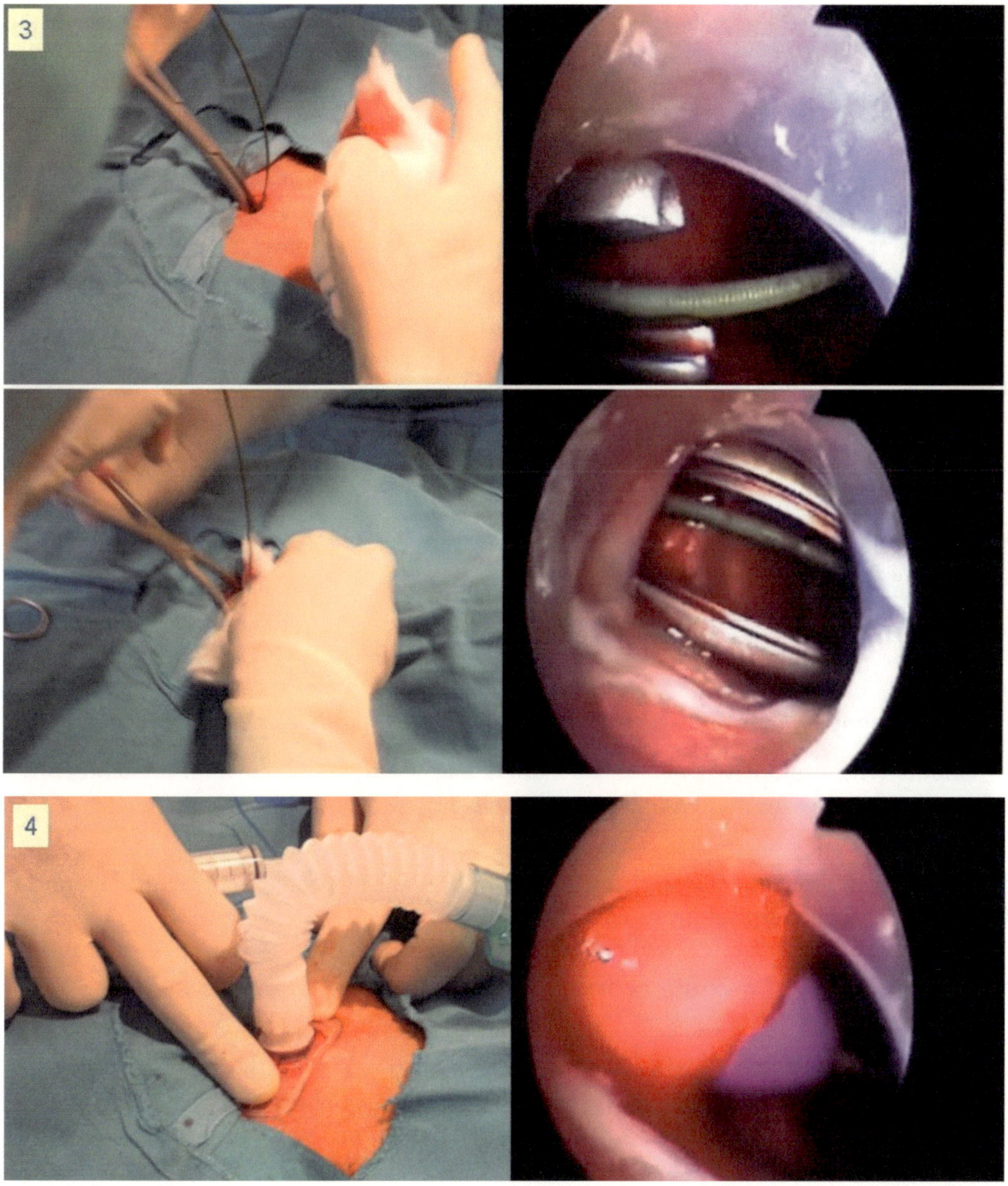

Fig. 3. Bronchoscopic images of different steps of percutaneous tracheostomy technique.

3.6 Management of difficult airway

The availability of flexible bronchoscopy in the Intensive Care Unit is essential for management of so called "difficult airways", although the indication is seen in fewer than 1% of all bronchoscopies performed in critically ill patients. This low percentage may be due to the fact that experience is required to perform the procedure and to the emergence of more easily managed devices for treatment of difficult airways, such as the Combitube, the laryngeal mask and Fastrack mask, which are increasingly used. Really, flexible bronchoscopy is a very useful tool for management of difficult intubation, usually caused by upper airway obstruction, anatomic disorders that reduce visibility of vocal cords and/or mobility of the head and neck like short neck, protruding incisor teeth or long high arched palate. Moreover in severe bleeding which makes laryngoscope intubation more risky, bronchoscopy is recommended. Finally it should be noted that bronchoscopyic endotracheal intubation is contraindicated in apnoeic patients. The oral route is preferred than nasal because of avoiding damage to the nasal mucosa and further nosocomial sinusitis. Moreover it allows intubation with an endotracheal tube with a larger diameter.

Other indication is for changing the endotracheal tube in patients with an expected difficult intubation. The new endotracheal tube is inserted over the bronchoscope and it is passed into the trachea by going outside parallel to the old endotracheal tube after deflation of the old endotracheal tube cuff.

3.7 Extracting foreign body

For extracting foreign bodies, the procedure of choice is the rigid bronchoscope, although flexible bronchoscopy using specialised instruments like hooks, Dormia baskets or biopsy forceps is also possible.

3.8 Other indications

A further use of flexible bronchoscopy is to correctly place double-lumen endotracheal tubes for selective ventilation in cases of massive haemoptysis or bronchopleural fistulas.

In patients who present with acute inhalation injury and burns flexible bronchoscopy is indicated to identify the anatomic level of the injury.

Assessment of glottis damage may be necessary in patients with prolonged mechanical ventilation.Flexible bronchoscopy is indicated to evaluate suspected neoplastic mass and for initiation of independent lung ventilation.

4. Complications of flexible bronchoscopy in mechanically ventilated patients

Taking into account recommendations commented in table 1 flexible bronchoscopy is an extremely safe procedure, if it is performed by a trained specialist.In mechanically ventilated patients it is easier to perform than in spontaneous breathing, as there is no upper airway to traverse. The risk of major complications in Intensive Care Unit is less than 1% and mortality related with the procedure is less than a 1%. Minor complications (table 4) have been associated with the procedure and occur in the first 24 hours within the procedure.

Cardiac arrhythmias, mainly supraventricular tachycardia are more like to occur in critically ill patients.Hypoxemia and insufficient sedation are associated with this complication and patients with cardiovascular disease are at highest risk for this complication.

Hypoxemia is common in mechanically ventilated patients undergoing flexible bronchoscopy, especially in patients with acute respiratory distress syndrome (ARDS).Continuous pulse oximeter during the procedure is recommended, and if a relevant decrease of oxygen saturation is observed the procedure must to be stopped.

Hypercapnia may be due to hypoventilation during the procedure and the monitoring of the tidal volume is necessary to ensure the maintenance of adequate ventilation; sedation and supplemental oxygen must be used with caution.

Bleeding of the mucous membrane occurs uncommonly during flexible bronchoscopy and is rarely harmful and usually transitory with spontaneous resolution.Patients with coagulation disorders or thrombocytopenia have high risk for bleeding. Transbronchial biopsy or brushing has more risk than bronchoalveolar lavage for bleeding with these conditions.

Pneumothorax has been documented especially when a biopsy or brush is performed while with other procedures like bronchoalveolar lavage the incidence is less than 1% (Hertz MI, 1991).

Laryngospasm and bronchospasm rarely occurs after flexible bronchoscopy in mechanically ventilated patients.

Recently we have documented the effects in respiratory mechanics with bronchoscopic bronchoalveolar lavage in mechanically ventilated patients; we conducted a study in mechanically ventilated patients observing a transitory deterioration of the respiratory mechanics with a decrease of respiratory compliance and an increase in airway resistance (Estella A, 2010).

- Anesthesia-related problems.
- Cardiac arrhythmias
- Hypoxemia
- Hypercapnia
- Hemorrhage
- Pneumothorax
- Laryngospasm
- Bronchospasm
- Pneumonia
- Fever
- Hypotension
- Decrease of respiratory system compliance.
- Increase in airway resistance.

Table 4. Complications of bronchoscopy in mechanically ventilated patients.

Post-bronchoscopy complications.

Until now we have commented on complications during flexible bronchoscopy. Complications developing in the hours after the procedure have been scarcely investigated in critically ill patients.

Post-bronchoscopy fever has not been much studied in mechanically ventilated patients, although its appearance has been reported in 16% of the patients (Shennib H, 1996). By contrast, in patients with spontaneous breathing this complication has been sufficiently documented as self-limited in 24 hours with an incidence between 6 to 19% of the cases. In a large series of 518 patients (Um SW,2004), 5% had post-bronchoscopy fever.It was not demonstrated to be related with bacteremia. A significant increase of leukocytes and neutrophils were observed. The combination of leukocytosis, fever and negative blood cultures supports the theory that fever is due to a systemic inflammatory response; a possible mechanism involves the activation of lung macrophages on contact with the liquid instilled with the bronchoalveolar lavage, which causes a release of proinflammatory mediators into the circulation and thereby triggers a systemic inflammatory response. In mechanically ventilated patients complications in the hours following the procedure has been scarcely investigated. A rise in temperature three hours after and a significant decrease of the arterial pressure five hours after flexible bronchoscopy was documented in patients with pneumonia in a series of 34 procedures in 25 intubated patients (Pugin J,1992). Only one study, (Bauer, 2001), has investigated the cytokine inflammatory response after bronchoalveolar lavage in 30 mechanically ventilated patients. They did not find differences in cytokine concentrations 12 and 24 hours after the procedure.

5. Contraindications to flexible bronchoscopy in mechanically ventilated patients

With adequate training and experienced operators flexible bronchoscopy has few if any absolute contraindications. It is mandatory to have careful patient selection, identifying the situations in which the clinical conditions and/or haemodynamic status do not guarantee the completion of the bronchoscopy safely.The inability to adequately oxygenate or ventilate increase the risk of bronchoscopy in mechanically ventilated patients.The clinical conditions in which the risk in performing a flexible bronchoscopy is increased are cited in the table 5.

Conditions cited in table 5 are relative contraindications because if they are normalized flexible bronchoscopy can be performed.

Even in paralyzed patients increase of intracranial pressure occurs. In patients with increased intracranial pressure it is mandatory to perform the procedure with deep sedation and paralysis with muscle relaxation and continous monitoring of cerebral hemodynamics.

Endotracheal tube with an internal diameter less than 8 mm with a standard adult bronchoscope (5.8mm).
Presence of pneumothorax on chest radiograph.
Oxygen saturation below 90% with FiO2 of 1.
Active bronchospasm.
Severe acidosis, Ph<7,2.
Haemodynamic instability, defined by systolic blood pressure <90 mmHg despite vasoactive drugs.
Unstable arrhythmia.
Coagulation disorders with indications for brush or biopsy.
Increased intracranial pressure.

Table 5. Conditions of increased risk of bronchoscopy in mechanically ventilated patients.

Although cardiac ischemia is supposed to increase the risk of flexible bronchoscopy there is no clear data in the literature supporting this consideration. In critically ill patients the risk for developing cardiac arrhythmias is increased.

6. Final considerations

Flexible bronchoscopy must be an essential piece of Intensive Care Unit equipment; it is a safe and useful procedure for the management of several pulmonary disorders in mechanically ventilated patients.

It is relatively easy to perform at the bedside and clinicians trained in its use are necessary in the Intensive Care Unit. This valuable procedure should be available to perform urgently for a wide range of therapeutic and diagnostic indications.

The following features attest to the increasing use of flexible bronchoscopy in mechanically ventilated patients: proven useful for a wide range of respiratory diseases in critically ill patients, easy to achieve at the bedside avoiding potentially dangerous transfers out of the Intensive Care Unit, relatively inexpensive clinical tool, demonstrated safely of the procedure described with careful preparation and close monitoring in selected patients and few relative contraindications.

7. References

Álvarez-Lerma F, Álvarez-Sánchez B, Barcenilla F. Protocolo diagnóstico y terapéutico de la neumonía asociada a ventilación mecánica. Guía de práctica clínica en medicina intensiva. Sociedad Española de Medicina Intensiva y Unidades Coronarias. Barcelona: Meditex, 1996; 1-8.

American Thoracic Society Documents. Guidelines for the management of adults with hospital-acquired, ventilator-associated, and health care-associated pneumonia. Am J Respir Crit Care Med 2005;171:388-416.

Barba CA, Angood PB, Kauder DR, Latenser B, Martin K, McGonigal MD, et al. Bronchoscopic guidance makes percutaneous tracheostomy a safe,cost-effective,and easy-to-teach procedure. Surgery 1995;118:879-83.

Bauer TT, Arosio C, Monton C, Filella X, Xaubet A, Torres A. Systemic inflammatory response after bronchoalveolar lavage in critically ill patients. Eur Respir J 2001;17:274-80.

British Thoracic Society Guidelines on diagnostic flexible bronchoscopy. Thorax 2001;56:(Supl 1):1-21.

Butler KH, Clyne B. Management of the difficult airway: alternative airway techniques and adjuncts. Emerg Med Clin North Am 2003;21:259.

Davis KA. Ventilator-Associated Pneumonia: a review. J Intensive Care Med 2006;21:211-26.

Dellinger RP, Bandi V. Fiberoptic bronchoscopy in the intensive care unit. Crit Care Clin 1992; 8:755-72.

Dupree HJ, Lewejohann JC, Gleiss J, Muhl E, Bruch HP. Fiberoptic bronchoscopy of intubated patients with life-threatening hemoptysis. World J Surg 2001;25:104-7.

Estella A, Jareño A, Pérez Bello Fontaiña L. Intrapulmonary administration of recombinant activated factor VII in diffuse alveolar haemorrhage: a report of two case stories. Case J. 2008 Sep 12;1(1):150.

Estella A, Monge MI, Pérez Fontaiña L et al. Bronchoalveolar lavage for diagnosing pneumonia in mechanically ventilated patients. Med Intensiva. 2008 Dec;32 (9): 419-423.

Estella A. Bronchoalveolar lavage for pandemic influenza A (H1N1)v pneumonia in critically ill patients. Intensive Care Med. 2010 Nov;36(11):1976-7.

Estella A. Effects on respiratory mechanics of bronchoalveolar lavage in mechanically ventilated patients. Journal of bronchology and interventional pulmonology 2010. 17(3);228-231.

Fagon JY, Chastre J, Wolff M, et al. Invasive and noninvasive strategies for management of suspected ventilator-associated pneumonia: a randomized trial. Ann Intern Med 2000;132:621-30.

Fagon JY, Chastre J, Wolff M, Gervais C, Parer-Aubas S, Stephan F, et al. Invasive and noninvasive strategies for management of suspected ventilator-associated pneumonia. A randomized trial. Ann Intern Med. 2000;132:621-30.

Fagon JY. Diagnosis and treatment of ventilator-associated pneumonia: fiberoptic bronchoscopy with bronchoalveolar lavage Is essential. Semin Respir Crit Care Med 2006;27:034-044.

Gottlieb LS, Hillberg R. Endobronchial tamponade therapy for intractable hemoptysis. Chest 1975;67:482-3.

Hara KS, Prakash UB. Fiberoptic bronchoscopy in the evaluation of acute chest and upper airway trauma. Chest 1989;96:627-30.

Heslet L, Nielsen JD, Levi M et al. Succesful pulmonary administration of activated recombinant factor VII in diffuse alveolar hemorrhage. Crit Care 2006; 10 (6):R177.

Jolliet Ph, Chevrolet JC. Bronchoscopy in the intensive care unit. Intensive Care Med 1992;18:160-9.

Kost KM. Percutaneous tracheostomy: comparison of Ciaglia and Griggs techniques. Critical Care Med 2000;4:143-6.

Koulenti D, Lisboa T, Brun-Buisson C, Krueger W, Macor A, Sole-Violan J, Diaz E, Topeli A, DeWaele J, Carneiro A, Martin-Loeches I, Armaganidis A, Rello J; EU-VAP/CAP Study Group. Spectrum of practice in the diagnosis of nosocomial pneumonia in patients requiring mechanical ventilation in European intensive care units. Crit Care Med. 2009 Aug;37(8):2360-8.

Kreider MD, Lipson DA. Bronchoscopy for atelectasis in the ICU. A case report and review of the literature. Chest 2003;124:344-350.

Lawson RW, Peters JI, Shelledy DC: Effects of fiberoptic bronchoscopy during mechanical ventilation in a lung model. Chest 2000, 118(3):824-831.

Liebler JM, Markin CJ. Fiberoptic bronchoscopy for diagnosis and treatment. Crit Care Clin 2000;16:83-100.

Lindholm CE, Ollman B, Snyder JV et al: Cardiorespiratory effects of flexible fiberoptic bronchoscopy in critically ill patients. Chest 1978, 74(4):362-368.

Marini JJ, Pierson DJ, Hudson LD. Acute lobar atelectasis: a prospective comparison of fiberoptic bronchoscopy and respiratory therapy. Am Rev Respir Dis 1979; 119:971-8.

Moine P, Vercken JB, Chevret S, Chastang C, Gagdos P. Severe community-acquired pneumonia: etiology, epidemiology, and prognosis factors. Chest1995; 107:1182-3.

Olaechea PM, Ulibarrena MA, Álvarez-Lerma F, Insausti J, Palomar M, de la Cal MA. Factors related to hospital stay among patients with nosocomial infection acquired in the intensive care unit. The ENVIN-UCI Study Group. Infect Control Hosp Epidemiol 2003;24:207-13.

Olopade CO, Prakash UB. Bronchoscopy in the critical care unit. Mayo Clin Proc 1989;64:1255-63.

Olopade CO, Prakash UB. Bronchoscopy in the critical care unit. Mayo Clin Proc 1989;64:1255-63.

Ovassapian A. The flexible bronchoscope. A tool for anesthesiologists (review). Clin Chest Med 2001; 22:281-99.

Pardon R, Ranic V, Rakaric-Poznanovic M. Bronchoscopy in the diagnosis and therapy of chest injuries. Acta Med Croatica 1997;51:29-36.

Poe RH, Israel RH, Marin MG, Ortiz CR, Dale RC, Wahl GW, et al. Utility of fiberoptic bronchoscopy in patients with hemoptysis and a nonlocalizing chest roentgenogram. Chest 1988; 93:70-5.

Polderman KH, Spijkstra JJ, de Bree R, Christiaans HM, Gelissen HP, Wester JP, et al. Percutaneous dilatational tracheostomy in the ICU: optimal organization, low complication rates, and description of a new complication. Chest 2003;123:1595-602.

Pugin J, Suter PM. Diagnostic bronchoalveolar lavage in patients with pneumonia produces sepsis-like systemic effects. Intensive Care Med 1992;18:6-10.

Rello J, Ollendorf DA, Oster G, Vera-Llonch M, Bellm L, Redman R et al. Epidemiology and outcomes of ventilator-associated pneumonia in a large US database. Chest 2002;122:2115-21.

Richards MJ, Edwards JR, Culver DII, et al. Nosocomial infections in combined medical-surgical intensive care units in the United States. Infect Control Hosp Epidemiol 2000;21:510-5.

Shennib H, Baslaim G. Bronchoscopy in the intensive care unit. Chest Surg Clin N Am 1996; 6: 349-61.

Shorr AF, Sherner JH, Jackson WL, Kollef MH. Invasive approaches to the diagnosis of ventilator-associated pneumonia: a meta-analysis. Crit Care Med 2005;33:46-53.

Snow.N, Lucas AE. Bronchoscopy in the critically ill surgical patient. Am Surg 1984;50:441-5.

Swanson KL, Udaya B, Prakash S, Midthun DE, Edell ES, Utz JP, et al. Flexible bronchoscopic management of airway foreign bodies in children. Chest 2002; 121:1695-1700.

The ANZIC Influenza Investigators. Critical care services and 2009 H1N1 influenza in Australia and New Zealand. N Engl J Med 2009;361:1925-34.

The Canadian Critical Care Trial Group. A randomized trial of diagnostic techniques for ventilator associated pneumonia. N Engl J Med. 2006;355:2619-30.

Timsit JF, Cheval C, Gachot B, Bruneel F, Wolff M, Carlet J, Regnier B. Usefulness of a strategy based on bronchoscopy with direct examination of bronchoalveolar lavage fluid in the initial antibiotic therapy of suspected ventilator-associated pneumonia. Intensive Care Med 2001;27:640-7.

Turner JS, Willcox PA, Hayhurst MD, Potgieter PD. Fiberoptic bronchoscopy in the intensive care unit. A prospective study of 147 procedures in 107 patients. Crit Care Med 1994; 22:259-64.

Um SW, Choi CM, Lee CT, Kim YW, Han SK, Shim YS, et al. Prospective analysis of clinical characteristics and risk factors of postbronchoscopy fever. Chest 2004;125:945-52.

Vincent JL, Bihari DJ, Suter PM, Bruining HA, White J, Nicolas-Chanion MH, et al. The prevalence of nosocomial infection in Intensive Care Units in Europe. Results of the European Prevalence of Infection in Intensive Care (EPIC) study. JAMA 1995; 274:639-44.

Woodhead M. Community-acquired pneumonia in Europe: causative pathogens and resistance patterns. Eur Respir J Suppl. 2002 Jul;36:20s-27s.

6

Bronchoscopy in Bronchiectasis and Cystic Fibrosis

Aditya Kasarabada, Mark E. Lund and Jeffrey B. Hoag
Cancer Treatment Centers of America,
Drexel University College of Medicine, Philadelphia, PA
USA

1. Introduction

Bronchiectasis is a constellation of diseases characterized by abnormally dilated bronchi with thickened bronchial walls due to repeated infection and inflammation. Bronchiectasis causes impairment of mucociliary clearance, airflow limitation, bronchorrhea, and predisposes to recurrent respiratory infections. It has a number of potential underlying causes. Laennec first described bronchiectasis as a distinct clinical entity in 1819 (Barker 2002, O'Donnell 1998). The diagnosis, investigation and particularly management of bronchiectasis has been largely empirical and unfortunately, the subject of relatively few controlled clinical trials. Cystic fibrosis causes about a third of all bronchiectasis in United States (O'Donnell 1998), and is common worldwide. Cystic fibrosis (CF) is a recessive genetic disease characterized by dehydration of the airway surface liquid and impaired mucociliary clearance caused by altered functioning of a chloride channel called the Cystic Fibrosis Transmembrane Conductance Regulator (CFTR). Impaired chloride conductance through the apical portion of airway cells leads to dehydration of airway secretions causing lung destruction through obstruction of the airways with thickened secretions. The resultant endobronchial infection and exaggerated inflammatory response leads to the development of bronchiectasis (destruction and widening of airways) and progressive obstructive airway disease. This chapter provides insight into the specific diagnostic and therapeutic roles of bronchoscopy in patients with bronchiectasis and Cystic Fibrosis.

2. Overview of bronchiectasis

Bronchiectasis is generally defined as an abnormal and permanent dilatation of the bronchi with thickening of the bronchial wall. In a retrospective cohort study of the insurance claims made in United States, Weycker et al. showed the prevalence of bronchiectasis ranged from 4.2 per 100,000 persons aged 18-34 years to 271.8 per 100,000 among those aged ≥75 years. Prevalence is higher among women than men at all ages (Weycker, D 2005). Bronchiectasis is being recognized with increasing frequency because of the widespread use of high-resolution chest computed tomography (HRCT) scanning (Cohen, M 1999). A bronchus is thought to be dilated if on the CT scan the broncho-arterial ratio with the adjacent accompanying artery exceeds 1. There are many causes of bronchiectasis that can be classified as due to anatomic, systemic diseases, congenital, post infectious, or idiopathic

(Barker, A.F. 2002, O'Donnell, A.E. 2008). Table 1. Based on the HRCT, bronchiectasis can be classified into 3 types cylindrical bronchiectasis, varicose bronchiectasis and saccular or cystic bronchiectasis. In cylindrical bronchiectasis the bronchi fail to taper as the bronchi progress peripherally. Varicose bronchiectasis has an irregular and beaded appearance and appears as "a string of pearls". Saccular or cystic bronchiectasis appears as a group of cysts without recognizable bronchial structures distal to the sacs (Webb, WR, High resolution CT chest of the Lung 2009).

Post-Infectious Lower Respiratory Tract Granulomatous Infections Nectrotizing Pneumonias Other Respiratory infections	**Inhalational and Obstruction** Severe Gastroesophageal Reflux Disease Chronic Aspiration Pneumonia Toxic or Thermal Inhalational Injury
Primary Immune Disorders Hypogammaglobulinemia Waldendstrom's Other Humoral / Cellular Disorders Neutrophil abnormalities	**Cystic Fibrosis** **Young's Syndrome** **Alpha$_1$-Antitrypsin Deficiency**
Heritable Structural Abnormalities Ciliated epithelium such as Primary Ciliary Diskinesia Cartilage or Connective Tissue (Tracheobronchiomegaly; Williams-Campbell) Sequestration, agenesis, hypoplasia	**Allergic Bronchopulmonary Aspergillosis** Or Other Mycosis **Post-obstruction** Foreign body Tumor (benign and malignant)
Idiopathic Inflammatory Disorders Sarcoidosis Rheumatoid Arthritis Systemic Lupus Erythematosis Sjogren's Syndrome Inflammatory Bowel Disease Relapsing polychondritis	**Miscellaneous** HIV infection / AIDS Yellow Nail Syndrome Radiation Injury

Table 1. Differential Diagnosis of Known Etiologies of Bronchiectasis

Patients with bronchiectasis typically present with chronic cough recurrent infections and sputum production (Morrissey 2007). Recurrent infections lead to further airway inflammation and damage which worsens the condition. Other presentations include hemoptysis, chronic airflow obstruction, and slow progressive shortness of breath or dyspnea. Physical examination is variable based on the etiology. Bronchography was used in the past for visualization of bronchiectatic airways. This involved coating the airways with a radiopaque dye instilled through a catheter or a bronchoscope. However, with the advent of HRCT this procedure is rarely being utilized. Pulmonary function tests may show airflow obstruction.

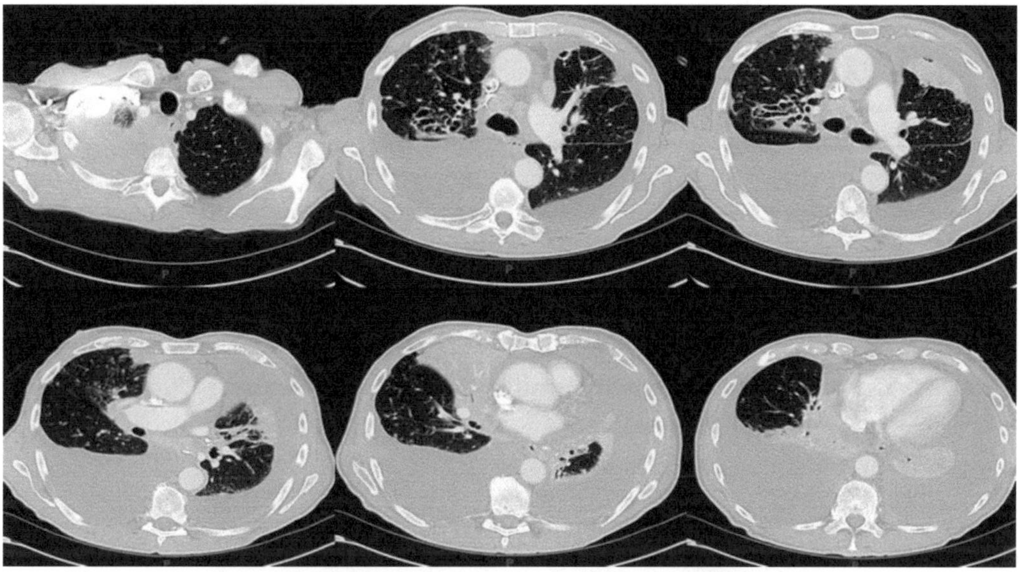

Fig. 1. CT images of a patient with Yellow Nail Syndrome with pleural effusion. Yellow Nail Syndrome is characterized by slow growing curved thickened yellow nails with lymphedema, pleural effusion and bronchiectasis on Computed Tomography. Note the bronchiectatic airways in the right middle lobe.

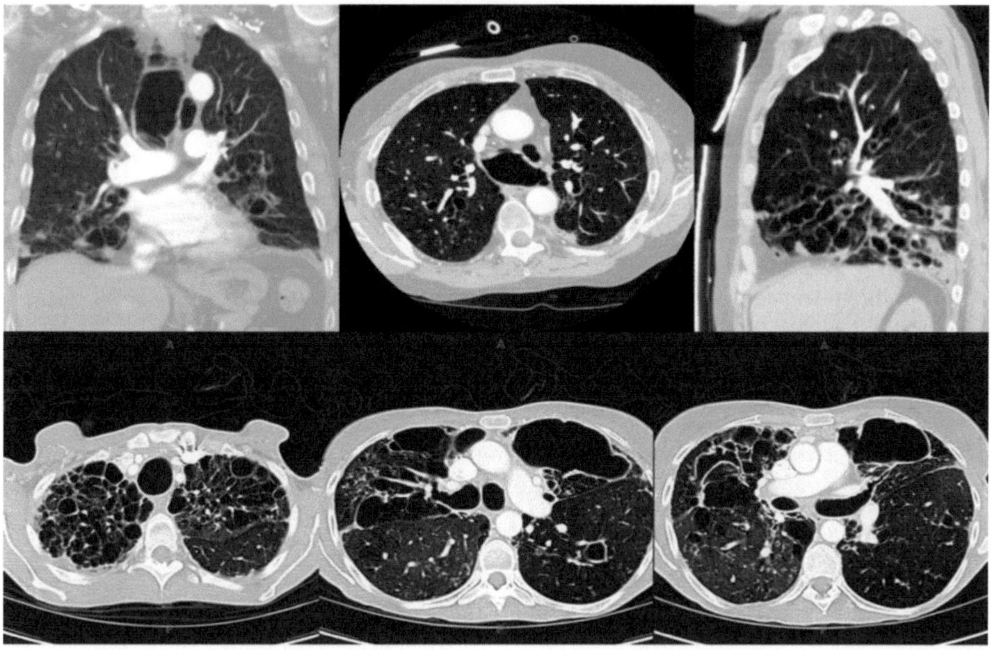

Fig. 2. Tracheobroncheomegaly or Mounier-Kuhn Syndrome. Images show marked dilatation of the trachea and the main stem bronchi. It is characterized by tracheal diameter greater than 3 cm that is measured 2 cm above the aortic arch. The right main bronchus should be greater than 2.4 cm and the left main bronchus greater than 2.3 cm.

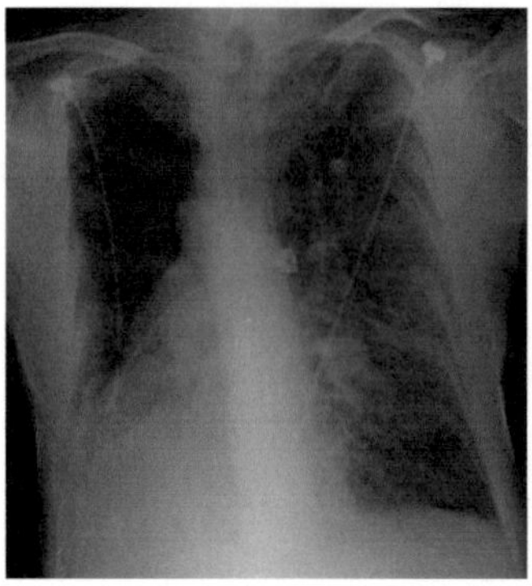

Fig. 3. Plain radiograph of Kartagener's Syndrome, characterized by situs inversus, azospermia, and bronchiectasis.

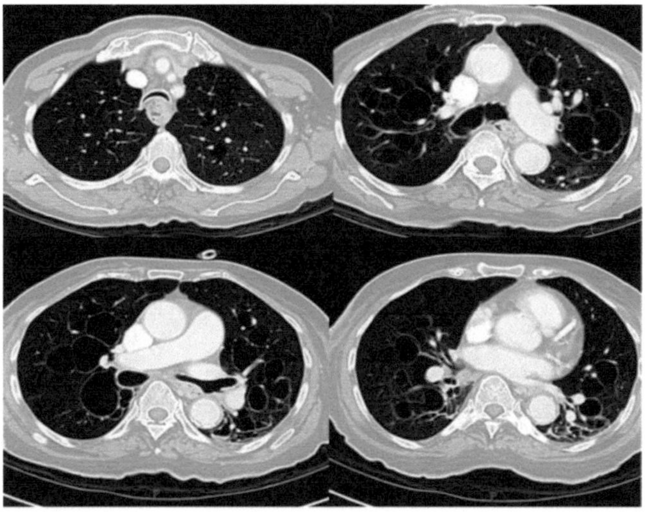

Fig. 4. CT cross sections of a patient with Williams-Campbell syndrome which show bilateral cystic bronchiectasis distal to the third-generation bronchi with abnormal distal lucency probably due to air trapping hyperinflation of lung or bronchiolitis

3. Overview of Cystic Fibrosis

Cystic Fibrosis is the most common life-shortening genetic disease of Caucasians affecting more than 25,000 individuals in the United States. Cystic Fibrosis is an autosomal recessive disease due to alteration in the function of a chloride channel; the Cystic Fibrosis Transmembrane Conductance Regulator (CFTR) (Rowe S. M. 2005). In the setting of CFTR dysfunction, an inability of chloride to pass through the channel in the apical membrane of epithelial cells leads to less hydrated secretions from exocrine glands. In the lungs, this causes airway secretions to be thick and difficult to clear. In this milieu, inflammatory cells and colonizing bacteria clogging the airways leads to destruction and dilation with subsequent development of bronchiectasis. The bronchiectasis in patients with Cystic Fibrosis is classically an upper lobe process. However, over time, the destruction becomes widespread involving all lobes.

In addition to the development of bronchiectasis in individuals with Cystic Fibrosis through the pathophysiology of CFTR dysfunction, coincident bacterial and fungal colonization and infection propagate the airway dilation. Patients with Cystic Fibrosis are often colonized with atypical Mycobacterium (Whittaker, L. A 2009). *Mycobacterium avium intracellulare* is the most common such infection which leads to bronchiectasis in middle lobe and lingular segments. Moreover, Allergic Bronchopulmonary Aspergillosis affects up to 10% of CF patients leading to worsening central bronchiectasis (Laufer, P 1984, Knutsen A. P. 2011). The role of bronchoscopy in Cystic Fibrosis will be discussed herein.

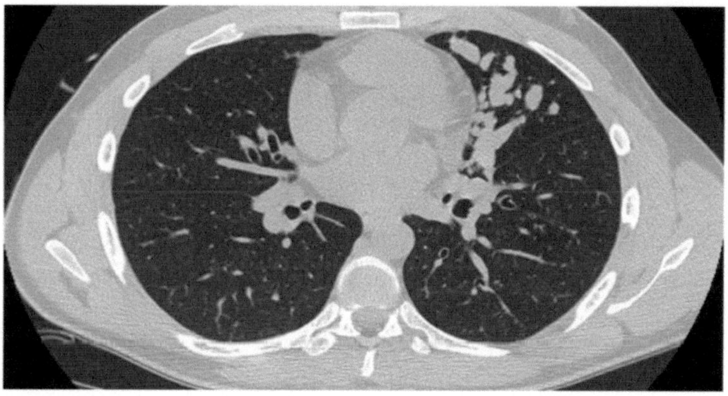

Fig. 5. CT image of right middle lobe involvement of Allergic Bronchopulmonary Aspergillosis with mucus impaction in a patient with Cystic Fibrosis.

4. Role of bronchoscopy

4.1 Role of diagnostic bronchoscopy in bronchiectasis

Bronchoscopy is not routinely indicated for the diagnosis of bronchiectasis. With the increasing resolution and availability of high-resolution computed tomography (HRCT) scanning, the utility of bronchoscopy in patients with bronchiectasis is not clear, although there exist certain situations in which bronchoscopy provides vital information.

Bronchoscopy for localized bronchiectasis is indicated to evaluate for the presence of an obstructing lesion causing distally located bronchiectasis when lobar or segmental bronchiectasis is apparant on CT imaging. For example, Middle Lobe Syndrome refers to the chronic collapse of the middle lobe which is often associated with distal middle lobe bronchiectasis. The etiology of Middle Lobe Syndrome has both infectious and non infectious causes. It can be divided into obstructive and non obstructive types (Albo, R.J. 1966, Wagner RB 1983, Einarsson, J.T. 2009,). Bronchoscopy is indicated in all patients with Middle Lobe Syndrome to evaluate for a compressing or obstructing lesion as malignancy is a common cause. (Albo, R.J. 1966, Wagner R.B. 1982, Priftis, K.N. 2005,). Foriegn body may not be apparant on HRCT. Dikensoy et al in their review of foreign body aspiration reported cases of foreign body seen at bronchoscopy which was not evident on CT of the chest (Dikensoy, O. 2002). Cytological examination of bronchoscopic specimens can provide evidence supporting gastric aspiration as a cause of bronchiectasis in dependent lung segments(Pasteur, M.C. 2010). Li et al showed 3/4 cases of bronchiectasis thought to be due to aspiration had lipid-laden macrophages on cytology (Li, A.M. 2005)

The British Thoracic Society published guidelines related to the utility of bronchoscopy in non-Cystic Fibrosis Bronchiectasis in 2010, which lists several indications for diagnostic bronchoscopy (Pasteur, M.C. 2010). Table 2.

Pasteur et al identified a study by Fernald at el in 1978 in stable state in which bronchoscopy did not show any advantage over sputum culture at identifying lower respiratory tract pathogens (Pasteur, M.C. 2010 Fernald G.W., 1978). Shiekh et al retrospectively evaluated the occurence of bronchiectasis in children with HIV pneumopathy (Shiekh, S. 1997). They found that bronchoalveolar lavage (BAL) had a high yield of clinically relevant information that required specific treatment. 22/57 (38.6%) were positive of Pneumocystis carinii, 14/27 (24.5%) had CMV and 12/27 (21%) were positive for MAI.

1. Bronchiectasis in a single lobe to exclude a foreign body obstruction especially in children;
2. In adults with localized disease, bronchoscopy may be indicated to exclude proximal obstruction;
3. Bronchoscopy is useful for obtaining microbiological results in patients who are acutely ill;
4. Bronchoscopic sampling of lower respiratory tract secretions may be indicated in patients with bronchiectasis in whom serial sputum testing is not yielding results and who are worsening;
5. Bronchoscopy can be used to obtain endobronchial biopsy of airway cilia to investigate causes of bronchiectasis
6. Bronchoscopy can be used to localize the site of bleeding in patients with bronchiectasis and hemoptysis which can guide further interventional therapies.

Table 2. British Thoracic Society Guidelines on non-Cystic Fibrosis Bronchiectasis

Pang et al while evaluating the bacteriology of bronchiectasis in Hong Kong, concluded that BAL and protected specimen brush are comparably sensitive in detecting lower respiratory tract organisms (Pang, J.A. 1989). Cabello et al looked at distal airway flora of healthy subjects with chronic lung disease including those with bronchiectasis and found that 88% of patients had bacterial colonization (Cabello, H. 1997). They also found comparable sensitivities between both BAL and protected specimen brush. Tanaka et al found that bronchial washings was twice as sensitive as expectorated sputum for isolation of Mycobacterium avium complex (Tanaka, E. 1997). They also went on to show that granuloma formation as seen on lung biopsy would suggest infection rather than colonization.

Bronchoscopy in the setting of Tuberculosis is a vast topic and is beyond the scope of this chapter, however, a brief review is warranted. In endemic areas, a positive sputum acid-fast bacilli (AFB) smear is frequently regarded as diagnostic of pulmonary tuberculosis. Negative AFB smears often poses a diagnostic challenge. Tan et al examined the clinical utility of rapid Mycobacterium tuberculosis (MTB) detection in bronchoalveolar lavage (BAL) samples by polymerase chain reaction (PCR). BAL PCR had sensitivity, specificity, positive and negative predictive values of 66.7%, 100%, 100% and 88%, respectively, for the group with upper lobe infiltrates (Tan YK 1999). Ismail and coworkers reviewed 232 cases of pulmonary tuberculosis and found that 22.8 % of patients had smear positive acid fast bacilli, 11.2 % of patients were diagnosed with tuberculosis based on this. In the setting of negative sputum testing in patients with typical clinical and chest radiographic presentations, the diagnostic accuracy was improved to 49.1% with bronchoscopic washings. Twenty-four percent of these demonstrated smear positivity and the other 25% were culture positive (Ismail Y 2004). Watanuki et al. examined 14 subjects with abnormal chest radiographs in which no definite diagnosis could be obtained through sputum analysis including smears and cultures. Bronchoscopic washings were positive for Mycobacterium in 7 patients on smear while cultures were positive in 8 patients. Mycobacterium avium complex (MAC) was identified in 13 patients; however, only 36% of those tested by specific polymerase chain reaction probes were MAC-positive. In patients undergoing transbronchial lung biopsy (n=11), histological review showed granuloma formation in four and caseation in another three patients (Watanuki Y 1999). Watanabe described 19 cases of bronchial stricture or obliteration due to endobronchial tuberculous lesions. Based on their findings, these authors recommended bronchoscopy and computed tomography as methods of choice for accurate diagnosis of tuberculous bronchial involvement (Watanabe Y 1997). Moreover, these modalities may aid in the assessment for surgery. Based on review of the available literature focusing on Tuberculosis or other Mycobacterial infections in the setting of bronchiectasis, bronchoscopy should be considered when diagnosis is uncertain in high-risk patients or when assessment of intervention is necessary.

4.2 Role of bronchoscopy in Cystic Fibrosis

Most of the current literature about the use of bronchoscopy in Cystic Fibrosis comes from pediatric experience. In infants with asymptomatic CF and those diagnosed through newborn screening, bronchoscopy is useful in defining bacterial colonization and inflammation in the airways not obtainable through less invasive means (Rosenfeld, M. 2001). The high yield of microbiology, cytology, and pH probe investigations in newborn infants with CF suggests that invasive surveillance fiber optic bronchoscopy (FOB) should be considered (Stafler, P. 2001). Bronchoscopy has been used for studying inflammatory markers such as Interleukin -8 and nitrite in the lower airway of patients with Cystic Fibrosis (Noah, T.L. 2003, Cetin, I. 2004, Davis, S.D. 2007, Cobanoglu, N. 2010). Bronchoscopy has similarly been used for identification of atypical airway infections. Semi quantitative culture of bronchoalveolar lavage (BAL) fluid was a useful diagnostic tool in CF patients in whom empiric therapy failed (Baughman, R.P. 1997). Dahm et al. showed fiberoptic bronchoscopy to be a superior technique for obtaining BAL samples as compared to rigid bronchoscopy or bronchial washout (Dahm, L.S. 1977). Davis et al. showed that the BAL fluid inflammation as indicated by the percent of recovered neutrophils and Interleukin -8 levels was significantly higher in the area identified as having the greatest disease on a high resolution chest CT (Davis, S.D. 2007). This highlights the potential importance of performing BAL in more than one area in patients with CF. In a retrospective study, Gilchrist et al showed that single-lobe bronchoalveolar lavage is not sufficient in assessing patients with cystic fibrosis for lower airway infection (Gilchrist, F.J. 2011). Studies have also compared sputum versus BAL in CF (Aaron, S.D. 2004). Bronchoscopy has been used to localize the site of bleeding in patients with CF-related hemoptysis, although there is little evidence for its benefit (Flume, P.A. 2010).

4.2.1 Role of Bronchoalveolar Lavage (BAL) in bronchiectasis and CF

There is evidence of early functional structural and pathological changes including bronchiectasis in babies with CF (Linnane, B.M. 2008, Linnane, B.M., Hall G.L.2008). Hillard et al in UK showed that 44% of asymptomatic children investigated with Bronchoscopy and BAL had a positive culture prior to newborn screening (Hillard, T.N. 2007). While looking at the patient's after newborn screening they found 27% of asymptomatic patient's had positive BAL cultures. There was evidence of airway inflammation as well. Whether early identification and aggressive treatment of asymptomatic pulmonary infections delays the decline in lung function is a matter of debate and at the present time there are no longitudinal studies. In a retrospective review of bronchoscopies performed in pediatric cystic fibrosis patient's Boogarard et al showed that 28/66 (42%) of the BAL provided information that had therapeutic consequences (Boogaard, R. 2008). The European Respiratory Society guidelines in 2000 recommended taking one BAL specimen from the most effected lobe or the right middle lobe (de Blic J 2000). This was later changed to two BALs specimens in 2007 (Brennan, S. 2008). In a retrospective review Gilchrist et al found that if they have used the 2000 ERS guidelines of only sampling a lobe they could have missed 26 positive cultures, while if they used the most current or 2007 guidelines for BAL sampling with 2 BALS at 2 different lobes then they would have missed only 12 positive cultures out of 39 (Gilchrist, F.J. 2011).

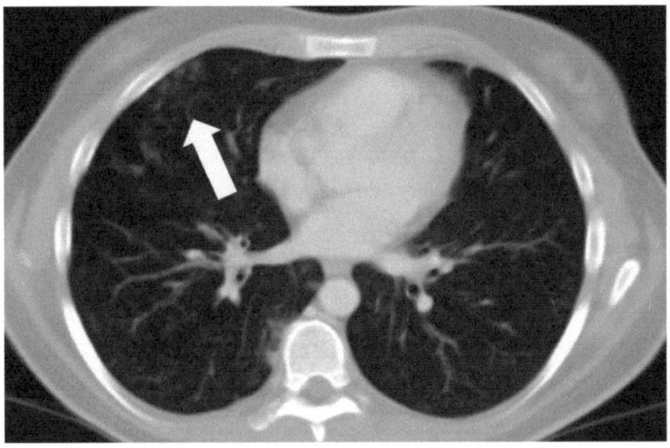

Fig. 6. CT image of a 24-year-old female with Cystic Fibrosis. The patient had frequent pulmonary exacerbations of Cystic Fibrosis and progressive decline in lung function in spite of aggressive appropriate antibiotic therapy guided by expectorated sputum cultures. She subsequently underwent a directed bronchoscopy with BAL in the right middle lobe (arrow) which grew *Mycobacterium abscessus*. Treatment of this infection broke the cycle of recurrent pulmonary exacerbations.

BAL has also been compared to oropharyngeal swabs to determine the pathogen causing sinus infection by Muhlebach et al. Sinusitis can cause CF exacerbations. The diagnostic accuracy of BAL and oropharyngeal swabs cultures was low in predicting sinus infections especially at younger ages. The positive predictive value of BAL sample for *Pseudomonas aeruginosa* infection was 65% while the negative predictive value was 67%. These were similar to oropharyngeal swab cultures. The positive predictive value for *Staphylococcus aureus* was 76% and a negative predictive value was 63% for the BAL fluid. Based on this study both BAL and oropharyngeal swabs are poor predictors of the organisms present in the sinus (Muhlebach, M.S. 2006). In the Australasian Cystic Fibrosis Bronchoalveolar Lavage randomized controlled trial cystic fibrosis patients identified through newborn screening were randomly assigned to BAL directed therapy versus standard therapy (Wainwright, C.E. 2011). They reported similar prevalence of Pseudomonas and other organisms amongst the two groups. There were no significant differences in the secondary outcomes such as FEV1, weight or BMI amongst the two groups. BAL fluid in cystic fibrosis patients has also been used to quantify and assess BAL fluid nitrite levels as this may reflect adequate the degree of inflammation in the respiratory tract and could potentially be a useful indicator of airway inflammation for patients with CF (Cetin, I 2004).

Cobanoglu et al studied the levels of ANCA in serum and BAL fluid to identify any relationship with infection (Cobanoglu, N 2010). MacGregor et al analyzed the BAL fluid obtained from CF patients using mass-spectrometry techniques (MacGregor, G 2008).

4.2.2 Role of protected brushing in bronchiectasis and CF

Bronchoscopy with protected Brush has been used to collect uncontaminated airway specimen for culture from the lower airways. As the brush is used to directly obtain secretions and bacteria from the airway lumen and then retracted into a sterile sheath, it is thought to have minimal contamination from other airway secretions. Aaron et al (2004) tried to see if bronchoscopy with protected brush would sample biofilm-forming bacteria on the airway wall as opposed to traditional sputum collection techniques. A total of 12 patients were evaluated with protected brush bronchoalveolar lavage and expectorated sputum collection. They showed that 10 patients (83%) had the same strain of *Pseudomonas aeruginosa* found using all 3 techniques. They concluded that sputum collection provided as much information for characterization and antibiotic susceptibility testing of *Pseudomonas aeruginosa* infection as bronchoscopy with protected brush (Aaron, S.D. 2004). As mentioned in previous sections Pang et al as well as Cabello et al showed that protected brush specimen was comparably sensitive to bronchoalveolar lavage in detecting lower respiratory tract organisms in patients with bronchiectasis (Pang, J.A. 1989, Cabello, H. 1997).

4.2.3 Role of endobronchial and transbronchial biopsy in bronchiectasis and CF

Endobronchial biopsy during bronchoscopy is a minimally used technique in the diagnostic evaluation of patient's with cystic fibrosis. There is a theoretical concern of bleeding with endobronchial biopsy in these patients due to increased blood flow. Endobronchial biopsy has been used safely in adults with cystic fibrosis during research protocols. Molina-Teran et al retrospectively looked at 45 bronchoscopies with endobronchial biopsies in children with cystic fibrosis at their Institute and matched them to control. They noted 6/45 (13%) had complications during the procedure of which 4 had significant coughing, 1 had > 10 % drop in oxygen saturation which improved with oxygen and 1 had dental loss. During the 12 hours after the procedure there was no significant complications in both patients with cystic fibrosis and the controls. They did not note any significant bleeding (Molina-Teran, A. 2006). One of the drawback of this study is that they is did not quantify the bleeding. Patients with severe CF were excluded from the study. In 2007 Regamey et al prospectively assessed the quality of the biopsy specimen obtained from children with cystic fibrosis using non-CF patients as control. They concluded that adequate biopsy specimens could be obtained to study the airway of patients with cystic fibrosis (Regamey, N. 2007). They did suggest taking at least 2 biopsies and the use of large forceps during the biopsy procedure. As mentioned earlier, in patients with bronchiectasis with suggestion of MAC on HRCT Tanaka et al found that 10/26 who underwent transbronchial lung biopsy had granuloma formation, 8 of whom were positive for MAC and 2 were positive for M. *abscessus* and M. *fortuitum*. They showed that this was present with infection and not with colonization (Tanaka, E. 1997).

We can conclude that in the bronchial biopsy can be used safely as a diagnostic tool in the evaluation and management of patient's with Cystic Fibrosis and bronchiectasis. In the setting of uncertainty in CF, it can yield important information leading to therapeutic guidance.

4.3 Role of bronchoscopy for therapeutics

Despite the paucity of literature in bronchoscopy for patients with cystic fibrosis and bronchiectasis there are reports of its therapeutic use. Lobar atelectasis is a common complication in patients with cystic fibrosis. Morbidity and mortality of patient's with cystic fibrosis has been linked to their FEV1. As such the consequences of persistent atelectasis in these patients can be serious (Stern, R.C. 1978). Whitaker et al reported a case series of CF patients with Allergic Bronchopulmonary Aspergillosis (ABPA) who successfully underwent sequential bronchoscopy with installation of recombinant human DNase to achieve re-expansion of the lung after they had failed standard medical therapy (Whitaker, P. 2011). McLaughlin et al. successfully treated lobar atelectasis in CF patients with ABPA, which was resistant to conventional therapy with antibiotics and chest physiotherapy, with bronchoscopic instillation of recombinant human deoxyribonuclease (rhDNase) (McLaughlin, A.M. 2008). Slattery et al also showed similar results in another retrospective study. They showed therapeutic bronchoscopy with rhDNase lavage was shown to be safe and associated with improved chest radiographs in pediatric CF patients with persistent atelectasis (Slattery, D.M. 2001).

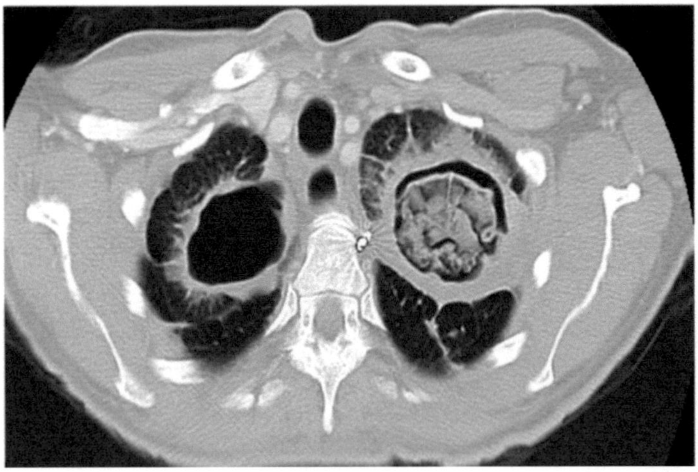

Fig. 7. CT image of a 42-year-old woman with Cystic Fibrosis with recurrent massive hemoptysis. Initially based on imaging, a left-sided source was assumed and she underwent bronchial artery embolization (BAE). As hemoptysis was unremitting, bronchoscopy was performed to localize the source, which was identified and successfully treated with BAE of the right upper lobe vessels.

Bronchomalacia or collapse of the large airway is only rarely reported as a complication of CF. Herlitz et al. were the first to report the successful deployment of an expandable silicone stent to treat bronchomalcia in a 15 year old with CF (Herlitz, G.N. 2006). This led to clinical improvement as well as improvement in the pulmonary function test obviating the immediate need for lung transplant. Bronchoscopy and transbronchial stenting have been used to treat complications arising from lung transplantation or surgery in patients with cystic fibrosis. Wood at al reported a case of a 20-year-old with cystic fibrosis who came with recurrent massive hemoptysis that was due to bronchopleural fistula at the stump site. They used superglue (butyl or Methy methacrylate) passed through a Teflon catheter through the working channel of the bronchoscope to seal the stump (Wood, R.E. 1992). Bronchoscopy has been used in management of hemoptysis in patients with CF and bronchiectasis. Joseph at al used bronchoscopic techniques for gene transfer to airway epithelium using adenoviruses for cystic fibrosis (Joseph, P.M. 2001, Perricone, M.A. 2001).

5. Safety of bronchoscopy in Cystic Fibrosis

Adverse events are common with BAL in young CF children, but are usually transient and well tolerated (Wainwright, C.E. 2008). Wainwright at al conducted a prospective multi-center study to systematically evaluate safety and adverse events associated with BAL in pediatric CF patients. They looked at pediatric patients undergoing BAL between September 1999 and December 2005. Twenty-nine of 333 (8.7%) of the BALs were followed by fever; 10 (3%) had clinically significant deterioration of which five required assisted ventilation during the procedure due to desaturation; one had a ventricular tachyarrhythmia after the use of an anesthetic agent; and one was hospitalized for stridor and respiratory distress. The rates of patients with fever in this study were no different than the rates reported in other studies in children without CF. Transient fever after BAL is thought to be associated with elevated serum pro inflammatory markers and can develop without bacteremia. They did find that focal bronchitis was associated with clinically significant deterioration during or after the BAL procedure, the reason for which were not entirely clear. Another strong association noted was between *Streptococcus pneumonia* in BAL fluid and fever afterwards. Worsening of cough was the most frequently reported minor event. It did not result in any increase in hospitalization. As mentioned previously, in a retrospective review Molina-Teran et al. showed that endobronchial biopsy performed under general anesthesia can be done safely in children with CF (Molina-Teran, A. 2006). They noted 6/45 (13%) had complications during the procedure of which 4 had significant coughing, 1 had > 10 % drop in oxygen saturation which improved with oxygen and 1 had dental loss. During the 12 hours after the procedure there was no significant complications in both patients with cystic fibrosis and the controls. They did not note any significant bleeding. The major drawback of this study was that it did not quantify the bleeding or include patients with severe disease. Endobronchial biopsy has been performed safely in adult CF patients for the purpose of research.

6. Role of anaesthesia and sedation

As with all procedures, the safety of the patient is paramount. Decisions regarding the best approach for patient control and comfort surround multiple patient factors as well as consideration for the duration and technical aspects of the procedure. Conscious sedation is performed by many providers performing bronchoscopies on patients with bronchiectasis and cystic fibrosis. However, due to profound bronchoscopasm often experienced with airway manipulation, consideration for the utilization of anesthesia support should strongly be considered in patients with bronchiectasis and cystic fibrosis.

Little was known initially about the role of general anesthesia in patients with Cystic Fibrosis. Price showed that a marked deterioration in lung function took place after a brief anesthetic for a relatively minor surgical procedure (Price, J.F. 1986). In a retrospective review, Chhajed et al showed that the sedative drug requirements during bronchoscopy were higher in patients with CF, especially after lung transplantation (Chhajed, P.N. 2005). Few authors reviewed the preoperative assessment, intraoperative and postoperative management of patients with CF (Huffmyer, J.L. 2009, Della Rocca, G. 2002, Walsh, T.S. 1995). An anesthetic plan for patients with CF undergoing procedures was described by Karlet et al (Karlet, M.C. 2000).

The respiratory dysfunction associated with cystic fibrosis should be the major focus of preoperative evaluation by the anesthesiologist. The anesthesiologist should quantify the level of pulmonary function and extent of cardiopulmonary limitation preoperatively and attempts must be made to optimize it prior to the procedure. Historically, the amounts of sputum production, decreased exercise tolerance, decreasing weight are important features. If patients report an increased cough, wheezing, increased sputum production, decreased activity level, infection or other symptoms to suggest CF exacerbation, admission to the hospital for optimization of lung function should be considered. Hypercarbia typically develops late in cystic fibrosis.

All cases should receive chest radiograph, pulmonary function testing, serum electrolyte levels including blood glucose levels, complete blood cell count and liver function tests (Della Rocca, G. 2002). Depending on the type of bronchoscopy being performed and the patient's history of liver involvement, further coagulation testing may be ordered. Moreover, arterial blood gas measurements, electrocardiogram, and echocardiogram may also be performed prior to the procedure if warranted by the patient's history.

Patient's routine medications including bronchodilators and corticosteroids should be continued into the perioperative period. Sedatives and analgesics should be used cautiously in the preoperative period as they can depress the respiratory drive and patient's inability to clear secretions (Huffmyer, J.L. 2009). Premedication with an antacid such as H2 blocker should be considered as there is a higher incidence of gastroesophageal reflux (Weeks, A.M. 1995).

Procedural monitoring should include continuous electrocardiography, respiratory rate, oximetry, and blood pressure. Capnography may be beneficial in patients requiring significant sedation or in those with moderate to severe lung disease. Arterial blood gas monitoring should be performed for patients with severe disease. Frequent intraoperative and postoperative management of blood sugars is indicated for prolonged procedures. Ventilating pressures should be monitored carefully as patients with CF are at risk for rupture of emphysematous bullae resulting in a pneumothorax (Karlet, M.C. 2000) in the setting of air trapping.

Preoxygenation to achieve higher oxygen saturation before induction is important. History of significant gastroesophageal reflux would require a rapid sequence induction. The short life of

Propofol makes it an ideal choice. Ketamine is relatively contraindicated due to increased bronchial secretions. The advantage of volatile inhalational agents used in general anesthesia is that they cause bronchodilation, decrease muscle relaxant dosage, and reduced airway hyperreactivity. Although Desflurane has an undesired pungent odor and respiratory tract irritability which makes it a poor choice of agent. Systemic hydration and humidification of inspired gasses are important for maintaining secretions in a less viscous state. If muscle relaxants are used short-acting nondepolarizing agents may be more appropriate. They should be administered in minimum possible doses. It should be noted that the aminoglycoside antibiotics use to treat infections might prolong the neuromuscular blocking affect. Extubation should be delayed until the effect of muscle relaxants has worn off.

Anesthesia should be tailored towards rapid postoperative recovery of the ability to cough and take deep breaths to actively clear secretions. Post procedure aggressive suctioning, chest physiotherapy and oxygen supplementation should be continued till the effect of the anesthetic agent has worn off and patient is back to his/her previous state of health.

Suggested tests	**Further testing**
Serum electrolytes	Coagulation tests
Complete blood count	Arterial blood gas
Liver function tests	Echocardiogram
Chest X ray	
Pulmonary function tests	
Blood glucose levels	
Electrocardiogram	

Adapted from Karlet, 2002

Table 3. Preoperative test for Anesthesia

7. Approach to performing bronchoscopy in bronchiectasis and CF

Preparation for bronchoscopy in patients with cystic fibrosis or chronic suppurative bronchiectasis is similar to the initial evaluation for anaesthesia. Important aspects include a clear understanding of the indication for bronchoscopy. As the pulmonologist understanding the current and usual steady state of the patients' respiratory function is critical. While there are no clear guidelines to support peri-operative antibiotics these patients may have a higher likelihood of transient bacteraemia or post bronchoscopic febrile episodes. Judicious clinical judgement of the patients overall condition should be followed in determining which patients may benefit from peri-operative antibiotics.

Having a clear understanding of the indications for the procedure in these patients is not only important in weighing risk and benefit but in allowing an expeditious procedure. Patients with advanced obstructive lung disease may have difficulty with hypoxemia and other complications. A well planned procedure will shorten the duration and attempt to mitigate risk.

If the indication is for airway sampling for culture, care must be taken to avoid contamination of the cultures by suctioning in the upper airway. This may be difficult due to the tenacious sputum and upper airway secretions in patients with cystic fibrosis. This is usually less of an issue in those with suppurative bronchiectasis. Strong consideration should be given to protected brush specimen retrieval in all these patients. Ensuring rapid and appropriate transport to the laboratory and rapid plating will significantly aid in obtaining viable culture specimens.

Patients with chronic suppuration coincident with bronchiectasis may have mucosa that is particularly friable. Having a seasoned bronchoscopist is the best choice to avoid mucosal injury and provide the shortest procedural time. These patients are likely not the best candidates for early trainees in bronchoscopy or those who rarely perform bronchoscopy. When these patients present with haemoptysis localization may be critical to guiding bronchial or intercostals arterial embolization. In addition, visualization of a more proximal bleed can occasionally occur. In these cases endobronchial therapies are warranted. The authors would recommend non contact therapies such as argon plasma coagulation or very low wattage Nd:YAG laser. If the indication for the bronchoscopy is mucosal sampling for ciliary dyskinesias a critical step is ensuring the correct specimen handling procedures are known and strictly followed. Most laboratories do not routinely process specimen's electron micrography. Ensuring good pre-procedural communication cannot be understated.

With the advancing population age of cystic fibrosis patients and the presence of bronchiectasis in middle age or older individuals the potential of central airway obstruction must be considered. Both primary bronchogenic carcinoma and metastatic airway disease may occur. Therapeutic bronchoscopy should be considered for these patients if central airway obstruction is due to endobronchial tumor. Therapeutic decision-making, such as risk to benefit of placing a endobronchial foreign body in a suppurative airway makes these cases extremely challenging. The authors would recommend referral to an interventional pulmonologist in a "center of excellence" to provide the best care for these complicated patients. Endoluminal ablative therapies are not contraindicated in these patients but experience is fairly limited. A center with a high volume of therapeutic bronchoscopy is likely the best choice.

8. Conclusions

Bronchoscopy provides useful diagnostic information in patients with bronchiectasis and Cystic Fibrosis. The use of these techniques aids the clinician in preventing the considerable morbidity associated with these conditions, and a proper understanding of the intricices of bronchoscopic procedures in these patients is paramount to success.

9. References

Aaron, S. D., D. Kottachchi, et al. (2004). "Sputum versus bronchoscopy for diagnosis of Pseudomonas aeruginosa biofilms in cystic fibrosis." *Eur Respir J* 24(4): 631-637.

Albo, R. J. and O. F. Grimes (1966). "The middle lobe syndrome: a clinical study." *Dis Chest* 50(5): 509-518.

Barker, A. F. (2002). "Bronchiectasis." *N Engl J Med* 346(18): 1383-1393.

Baughman, R. P., D. A. Keeton, et al. (1997). "Use of bronchoalveolar lavage semiquantitative cultures in cystic fibrosis." *Am J Respir Crit Care Med* 156(1): 286-291.

Boogaard, R., et al., Yield from Flexible Bronchoscopy in Pediatric Cystic Fibrosis Patients. *J Bronchol,* 2008. 15(4): p. 240-246

Brennan, S., C. Gangell, et al. (2008). "Disease surveillance using bronchoalveolar lavage." *Paediatr Respir Rev* 9(3): 151-159.

Cabello, H., A. Torres, et al. (1997). "Bacterial colonization of distal airways in healthy subjects and chronic lung disease: a bronchoscopic study." *Eur Respir J* 10(5): 1137-1144.

Cetin, I., U. Ozcelik, et al. (2004). "BALF nitrite as an indicator of inflammation in children with cystic fibrosis." *Respiration* 71(6): 625-629.

Chang, A. B., N. C. Boyce, et al. (2002). "Bronchoscopic findings in children with non-cystic fibrosis chronic suppurative lung disease." *Thorax* 57(11): 935-938.

Chhajed, P. N., C. Aboyoun, et al. (2005). "Sedative drug requirements during bronchoscopy are higher in cystic fibrosis after lung transplantation." *Transplantation* 80(8): 1081-1085.

Cobanoglu, N., U. Ozcelik, et al. (2010). "Anti-neutrophil cytoplasmic antibodies (ANCA) in serum and bronchoalveolar lavage fluids of cystic fibrosis patients and patients with idiopathic bronchiectasis." *Turk J Pediatr* 52(4): 343-347.

Cohen, M. and S. A. Sahn (1999). "Bronchiectasis in systemic diseases." *Chest* 116(4): 1063-1074.

Dahm, L. S., C. W. Ewing, et al. (1977). "Comparison of three techniques of lung lavage in patients with cystic fibrosis." *Chest* 72(5): 593-596.

Davis, S. D., L. A. Fordham, et al. (2007). "Computed tomography reflects lower airway inflammation and tracks changes in early cystic fibrosis." *Am J Respir Crit Care Med* 175(9): 943-950.

de Blic, J., F. Midulla, et al. (2000). "Bronchoalveolar lavage in children. ERS Task Force on bronchoalveolar lavage in children. European Respiratory Society." *Eur Respir J* 15(1): 217-231.

Della Rocca, G., Anaesthesia in patients with cystic fibrosis. *Curr Opin Anaesthesiol,* 2002. 15(1): p. 95-101.

Dikensoy, O., C. Usalan, et al. (2002). "Foreign body aspiration: clinical utility of flexible bronchoscopy." *Postgrad Med J* 78(921): 399-403.

Einarsson, J. T., J. G. Einarsson, et al. (2009). "Middle lobe syndrome: a nationwide study on clinicopathological features and surgical treatment." *Clin Respir J* 3(2): 77-81.

Fernald, G. W. (1978). "Bronchiectasis in childhood: a 10-year survey of cases treated at North Carolina Memorial Hospital." *N C Med J* 39(6): 368-372.

Flume, P. A., P. J. Mogayzel, Jr., et al. (2010). "Cystic fibrosis pulmonary guidelines: pulmonary complications: hemoptysis and pneumothorax." *Am J Respir Crit Care Med* 182(3): 298-306.

Gilchrist, F. J., S. Salamat, et al. (2011). "Bronchoalveolar lavage in children with cystic fibrosis: how many lobes should be sampled?" *Arch Dis Child* 96(3): 215-217.

Herlitz, G. N., D. I. Sternberg, et al. (2006). "Treatment of bronchomalacia in cystic fibrosis by silicone stent." *Ann Thorac Surg* 82(6): 2268-2270.

Hilliard, T. N., S. Sukhani, et al. (2007). "Bronchoscopy following diagnosis with cystic fibrosis." *Arch Dis Child* 92(10): 898-899.

Huffmyer, J. L., K. E. Littlewood, et al. (2009). "Perioperative management of the adult with cystic fibrosis." *Anesth Analg* 109(6): 1949-1961.

Ismail, Y. (2004). "Pulmonary tuberculosis--a review of clinical features and diagnosis in 232 cases." *Med J Malaysia* 59(1): 56-64.

Joseph, P. M., B. P. O'Sullivan, et al. (2001). "Aerosol and lobar administration of a recombinant adenovirus to individuals with cystic fibrosis. I. Methods, safety, and clinical implications." *Hum Gene Ther* 12(11): 1369-1382.

Karlet, M. C. (2000). "An update on cystic fibrosis and implications for anesthesia." *AANA J* 68(2): 141-148.

Knutsen, A. P. and R. G. Slavin (2011). "Allergic bronchopulmonary aspergillosis in asthma and cystic fibrosis." *Clin Dev Immunol* 2011: 843763.

Laufer, P., J. N. Fink, et al. (1984). "Allergic bronchopulmonary aspergillosis in cystic fibrosis." *J Allergy Clin Immunol* 73(1 Pt 1): 44-48.

Li, A. M., S. Sonnappa, et al. (2005). "Non-CF bronchiectasis: does knowing the aetiology lead to changes in management?" *Eur Respir J* 26(1): 8-14.

Linnane, B., P. Robinson, et al. (2008). "Role of high-resolution computed tomography in the detection of early cystic fibrosis lung disease." *Paediatr Respir Rev* 9(3): 168-174; quiz 174-165.

Linnane, B. M., G. L. Hall, et al. (2008). "Lung function in infants with cystic fibrosis diagnosed by newborn screening." *Am J Respir Crit Care Med* 178(12): 1238-1244.

MacGregor, G., R. D. Gray, et al. (2008). "Biomarkers for cystic fibrosis lung disease: application of SELDI-TOF mass spectrometry to BAL fluid." *J Cyst Fibros* 7(5): 352-358.

McLaughlin, A. M., E. McGrath, et al. (2008). "Treatment of lobar atelectasis with bronchoscopically administered recombinant human deoxyribonuclease in cystic fibrosis?" *Clin Respir J* 2(2): 123-126.

Molina-Teran, A., T. N. Hilliard, et al. (2006). "Safety of endobronchial biopsy in children with cystic fibrosis." *Pediatr Pulmonol* 41(11): 1021-1024.

Muhlebach, M. S., M. B. Miller, et al. (2006). "Are lower airway or throat cultures predictive of sinus bacteriology in cystic fibrosis?" *Pediatr Pulmonol* 41(5): 445-451.

Murray, J.F., Nadal, J.A. (2010) *Murray & Nadal's Textbook of Respiratory Medicine* (5th Edition) Saunders, Elsevier, ISBN: 978-1-4160-47100-0, Philadelphia, USA

Noah, T. L., P. C. Murphy, et al. (2003). "Bronchoalveolar lavage fluid surfactant protein-A and surfactant protein-D are inversely related to inflammation in early cystic fibrosis." *Am J Respir Crit Care Med* 168(6): 685-691.

O'Donnell, A. E. (2008). "Bronchiectasis." *Chest* 134(4): 815-823.

Pang, J. A., A. Cheng, et al. (1989). "The bacteriology of bronchiectasis in Hong Kong investigated by protected catheter brush and bronchoalveolar lavage." *Am Rev Respir Dis* 139(1): 14-17.

Pasteur, M. C., D. Bilton, et al. (2010). "British Thoracic Society guideline for non-CF bronchiectasis." *Thorax* 65 Suppl 1: i1-58.

Perricone, M. A., J. E. Morris, et al. (2001). "Aerosol and lobar administration of a recombinant adenovirus to individuals with cystic fibrosis. II. Transfection efficiency in airway epithelium." *Hum Gene Ther* 12(11): 1383-1394.

Price, J. F. (1986). "The need to avoid general anaesthesia in cystic fibrosis." *J R Soc Med* 79 Suppl 12: 10-12.

Priftis, K. N., D. Mermiri, et al. (2005). "The role of timely intervention in middle lobe syndrome in children." *Chest* 128(4): 2504-2510.

Quast, T. M., A. R. Self, et al. (2008). "Diagnostic evaluation of bronchiectasis." *Dis Mon* 54(8): 527-539.

Regamey, N., T. N. Hilliard, et al. (2007). "Quality, size, and composition of pediatric endobronchial biopsies in cystic fibrosis." *Chest* 131(6): 1710-1717.

Rosenfeld, M., R. L. Gibson, et al. (2001). "Early pulmonary infection, inflammation, and clinical outcomes in infants with cystic fibrosis." *Pediatr Pulmonol* 32(5): 356-366.

Rowe, S. M., S. Miller, et al. (2005). "Cystic fibrosis." *N Engl J Med* 352(19): 1992-2001.

Sheikh, S., K. Madiraju, et al. (1997). "Bronchiectasis in pediatric AIDS." *Chest* 112(5): 1202-1207.

Slattery, D. M., D. A. Waltz, et al. (2001). "Bronchoscopically administered recombinant human DNase for lobar atelectasis in cystic fibrosis." *Pediatr Pulmonol* 31(5): 383-388.

Stafler, P., J. C. Davies, et al. (2011). "Bronchoscopy in Cystic Fibrosis Infants Diagnosed by Newborn Screening." *Pediatr Pulmonol.*

Stern, R. C., T. F. Boat, et al. (1978). "Treatment and prognosis of lobar and segmental atelectasis in cystic fibrosis." *Am Rev Respir Dis* 118(5): 821-826.

Tan, Y. K., A. S. Lee, et al. (1999). "Rapid mycobacterial tuberculosis detection in bronchoalveolar lavage samples by polymerase chain reaction in patients with upper lobe infiltrates and bronchiectasis." *Ann Acad Med Singapore* 28(2): 205-208.

Tanaka, E., R. Amitani, et al. (1997). "Yield of computed tomography and bronchoscopy for the diagnosis of Mycobacterium avium complex pulmonary disease." *Am J Respir Crit Care Med* 155(6): 2041-2046.

Wagner, R. B. and M. R. Johnston (1983). "Middle lobe syndrome." *Ann Thorac Surg* 35(6): 679-686.

Wainwright, C. E., K. Grimwood, et al. (2008). "Safety of bronchoalveolar lavage in young children with cystic fibrosis." *Pediatr Pulmonol* 43(10): 965-972.

Wainwright, C.E.,S. Vidmar, et al. (2011). " Effect of Bronchoalveolar Lavage-directed therapy on Pseudomonas aeruginosa infection and structural lung injury in children with Cystic Fibrosis: A randomized trial ." *JAMA* 306(2):163-171.

Walsh, T.S. and C.H. Young, Anaesthesia and cystic fibrosis. *Anaesthesia,* 1995. 50(7): p. 614-22.

Watanabe, Y., S. Murakami, et al. (1997). "Treatment of bronchial stricture due to endobronchial tuberculosis." *World J Surg* 21(5): 480-487.

Watanuki, Y., S. Odagiri, et al. (1999). "Usefulness of bronchoscopy for the diagnosis of atypical pulmonary mycobacteriosis." *Kansenshogaku Zasshi* 73(8): 728-733.

Webb, W.R. (2009) *High Resolution CT of the lung* (4th Edition) Lippincott Williams & Wilkins, ISBN-13: 978-0-7817-6909-4, Philadelphia, USA

Weeks, A.M. and M.R. Buckland, Anaesthesia for adults with cystic fibrosis. *Anaesth Intensive Care,* 1995. 23(3): p. 332-8.

Weycker, D., J. Edelsberg, et al. (2005). "Prevalence and Economic Burden of Bronchiectasis." *Clinical Pulmonary Medicine* 12(4): 205-209.

Whitaker, P., K. Brownlee, et al. (2011). "Sequential Bronchoscopy in the Management of Lobar Atelectasis Secondary to Allergic Bronchopulmonary Aspergillosis." *Journal of Bronchology & Interventional Pulmonology* 18(1): 57-60

Whittaker, L. A. and C. Teneback (2009). "Atypical mycobacterial and fungal infections in cystic fibrosis." *Semin Respir Crit Care Med* 30(5): 539-546.

Wood, R. E., S. R. Lacey, et al. (1992). "Endoscopic management of large, postresection bronchopleural fistulae with methacrylate adhesive (Super Glue)." *J Pediatr Surg* 27(2): 201-202.

Section 4

Evolving Therapeutic Uses of Bronchoscopy

7

Endotracheal Intubation with Flexible Fiberoptic Bronchoscope (FFB) in Cases of Difficult Airway

Francisco Navarro, Raúl Cicero and Andrea Colli
Departament of Thoracic Endoscopy, Pneumology and Thoracic Surgery Service
General Hospital of México OD, Faculty of Medicine,
National Autonomous University of Mexico
México

1. Introduction

Endotracheal intubation is a procedure whereby a tube is inserted into the trachea to warrant and maintain adequate ventilation with good respiratory gas exchange in patients who undergo anesthesia for surgery or require invasive mechanical ventilation.Since 1967 the flexible fiberoptic bronchoscope was considered as an advanced device to intubate patients with difficult airway having surgery,"fiberoptic assisted tracheal intubation".[1]

In most cases,tracheal intubation is done by oral laryngoscopy performed with a rigid laryngoscope,[2] but there are cases in which the intubation attempt fails due to the presence of difficult airway. This problem occurs in 1/22,000 cases of general anesthesia and is the most frequent serious airway complication.[3] Among 37,482 intubation attempts by direct laryngoscopy for general anaesthesia, 161 (0.43%) cases could not be intubated because of being overly difficult as mentioned by Burke.[4] Other authors report 6/13,380 cases but in obstetric patients it has been reported to be 1/300 cases.[5]

The definition of difficult airway according to the American Society of Anesthesiologists Task Force on Management of the Difficult Airway is "a clinical situation in which a conventionally trained anesthesiologist experiences difficulty with face mask ventilation of the upper airway, difficulty with tracheal intubation or both."[6] Under these conditions, intubation must be attempted with another technique or must be postponed because a life-threatening situation may arise if the anesthesiologist is unable to intubate and cannot ventilate. Use of FFB is then indicated for tracheal intubation as an emergency measure.

2. General considerations

Evaluation of the patient's airway

A difficult intubation can be predicted and avoided with a proper and careful preoperative evaluation of the airway by a skilled anesthesiologist. The clinical record and history of previous episodes of failed intubation during anesthesia for surgical interventions are important.[7] A first question must be answered: Are the larynx and vocal cords visible? If

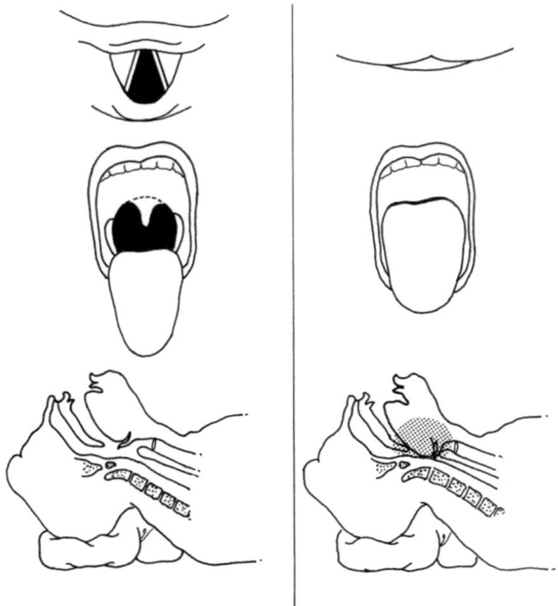

Fig. 1. Normal airway and difficult airway,Cormack-Lehane and Mallampati.The visualization or not of retropharynx and vocal cords is important to predict difficult airway.(Ref 14) Failure of intubation with rigid laryngoscope due to impossible visualization of the larynx is indication for FFB endotracheal intubation.

not, the possibility of difficult tracheal intubation may be identified during the pre-anesthetic evaluation.[8] However, a difficult tracheal intubation is sometimes unpredictable whether occurring in the operating room, the intensive care unit (ICU) or in the emergency department.[9] This is certainly true in cases of an oropharyngeal condition that does not allow epiglottis and vocal cord visualization. These cases were previously classified as difficult airway according to the original Mallampati[10] classification or the modified classification.[11] In cases with limited mouth opening or restricted mobility of the head and neck, evaluation of anatomic conditions is also mandatory. A more accurate evaluation may be done by computerized facial analysis in challenging intubations.[12] If a difficult airway is present, use of FFB may be anticipated.

3. Airway assessment

Anatomic conditions and mobility of the head and neck are important[13] as well as imaging with X-ray. Airway exploration must be made in all cases according to ASA recommendations, with particular attention to mouth opening, Mallampati classification, Cormak-Lehane, thyromental distance or other methods.[14] Patency of the nose is important, but under emergency situations it may be impossible to perform this assessment.

4. Common indications for endotracheal intubation with FFB

FFB intubation is indicated and appropriately scheduled in cases diagnosed as difficult airway or as an emergency procedure. Patients in whom previous evaluation of the airway suggests a difficult intubation are the primary candidates for scheduling FFB intubation. Some examples are morbid obesity,trismus, facial trauma, pharynx and larynx injury, limited flexion and extension of the neck, craniofacial disorders, jaw malformations, temporomandibular joint ankylosis, macroglossia, larynx tumors, laryngo-tracheobronchitis, glottic edema and epiglottitis along with other unexpected conditions. An emergency intubation carried out in the ICU or in the emergency department lacks proper previous evaluation of the airway.

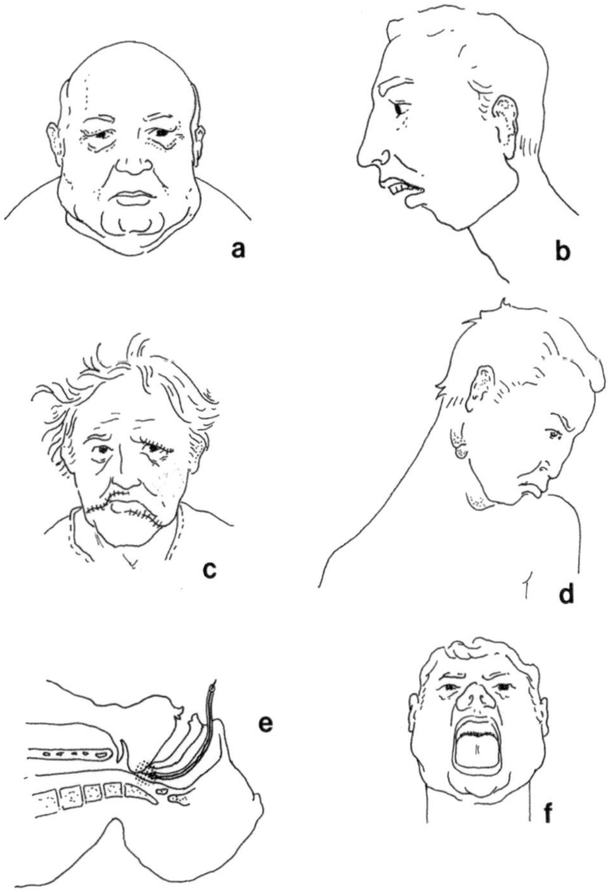

Fig. 2. Some examples of candidates for FFB endotracheal intubation. a) morbid obesity with short neck, b) prominent incisors teeth and micrognatia, c)facial trauma, d)cervical ankylosis, e)macroglossia, f) Mallampati IV (Ref 13)

FFB intubation is better performed with the assistance of a video magnification screen in the operating room.[15] In the ICU it is not always possible and must be done by direct vision in the FFB with a second observer device for the assistant Proper monitoring of electrocardiogram , oximetry, arterial pressure and capnography is always required.

In every case of intubation with FFB, the bronchoscopist must work in complete coordination and communication with anesthesiologists and intensive care physicians.

5. Awake intubation and anticipated intubation with the FFB

Awake intubation with FFB requires informed consent about the procedure and the risks along with complete cooperation of the individual during the procedure. Confidence between the operator and the patient is also essential.

In predicting difficult intubation,scheduled cases may be better subjected to the procedure in the supine position as a safer and more comfortable measure, with the use of supplemental oxygen.[16] Local anesthesia is easily applied with 2% lidocaine spray. In difficult cases, previous instillation of 3 to 5 mL of 2% lidocaine solution through the nose may be useful. Phenylephrine as vasoconstrictor is advisable to apply in the nose. A sedative such as midazolam or diazepam may be employed. If the mouth opening is limited or restricted, transnasal approach would be the appropriate choice. Gentle manipulation from the operator is required in patients with spontaneous breathing. Before initiating the procedure, the FFB is previously inserted into the selected endotracheal tube as recommended by Stubb and McDougal,[17] then is introduced through the mouth or nose .Instillation of lidocaine solution in the working channel is useful to avoid cough and nausea. Once the FFB is in the trachea the tube is slided over the endoscope. The FFB is removed and the tube is left in the trachea. Manipulation and transport of the patient must be done with extreme care to prevent an unexpected extubation. The approach with a nasopharyngeal trumpet to the glottis followed by the insertion of the FFB and the tube in the trachea may also be used.[18] Basic endoscopic equipment must always be available (Table 1).

1. Every operating room or intensive care unit must have the facilities for intubation under bronchoscopic visualization: FFB of different lengths and diameters should be available. FFB Olympus P60 and 1T60 with 6.0 mm outer diameter or MP60 4.4 mm are suitable in the majority of cases. Ultraslim 3C40 of 3,6 mm and N20 with 2.2 mm are used in cases with major grade of glottic stenoses. All endoscopic instruments must be tested to verify their good conditions.
2. Portable light source of halogen or xenon.
3. Tracheal tubes of different diameters must be available (4.0 mm to 10 mm) (Rush-Magill). Also, armored PVC spiral tubes must be considered.
4. Lidocaine solution 2%-4%. Lubricating the FFB with with lidocaine 2% gel warrants the sliding of the endoscope inside the tube.
5. Neuromuscular relaxants and sedatives.
6. Suction devices: A Yankauer cannula connected to a suction power source.
7. Tracheostomy cannulae, may be percutaneous, with proper equipment for its insertion in cases of impossible intubation.
8. Cardiac arrest equipment is always important

Table 1. Portable airway trolley: Basic equipment

6. Intubation with the patient under general anesthesia

Intubation under general anesthesia always requires 100% oxygen supply with an adaptor or jet injection device. It must be done carefully and quickly. Careful head and neck immobilization is necessary, preferably through oral access if there are no contraindications.

7. Emergency intubation after failure to intubate by direct laryngoscopy

This event occurs in the operating room. The patient must be oxygenated as quickly as possible. Monitoring by oximetry and capnography must be maintained. The head must be immobilized with a pillow placed under the neck. The bronchoscopist immediately introduces the FFB by mouth or nose, previously inserted in the selected tracheal tube and well lubricated. The FFB must be introduced until the glottis can be seen and the instrument inserted and the tracheal lumen visualized. The tube is slide gently and introduced into the trachea until reaching the distal tip of the FFB. Together these are pushed into the tracheal lumen, reaching the middle third of the trachea. The tube should be fixed firmly at the face of the patient before the FFB can be withdrawn(Table 2).

1.	Selecting FFB and endotracheal tube
2.	Insertion of the FFB into the lumen of the tracheal tube (lubrication is essential).
3.	Introduction of the FFB through the nose or oral cavity with a mouthguard.
4.	Advance of the FFB until the glottis is visible.
5.	Introduction of the FFB into the trachea.
6.	Slide the tube until reaching the distal tip of the FFB.
7.	Introduction of the FFB and the tube until reaching the middle third of the trachea.
8.	Extraction of the FFB, retaining the tube within the trachea.
9.	Fixation of the tube to the face, avoiding unplanned extubation.
10.	Finally, tracheal tube is immediately connected to the oxygen source.

Note: All steps must be done gently and quickly to recover efficient ventilation of the patient.

Table 2. Technique for tracheal intubation with FFB

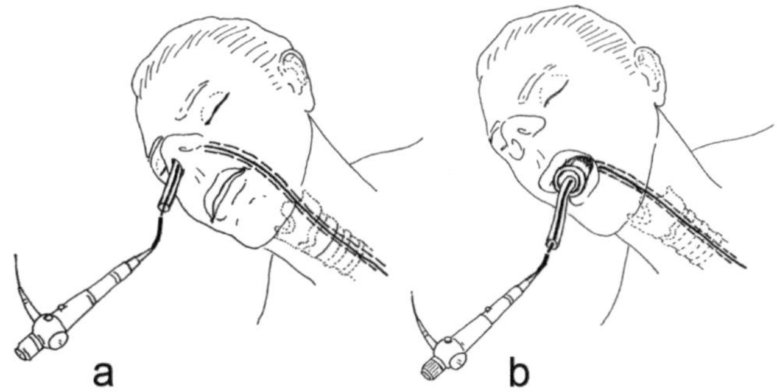

Fig. 3. Introduction of the FFB and the tracheal tube through the nose a)or mouth b) for FFB endotracheal intubation. The FFB is inserted in the tube.

8. Intubation in the ICU and emergency department

Failure to intubate occurred in 0.07% to 3.4% of all intubation attempts in the ICU.[19] Critically ill patients are unstable, cannot cooperate, and have no prior airway assessment. Some difficulties arise because the patient is surrounded by monitoring and mechanical respiration devices. The bronchoscopist may be in a cumbersome bedside situation at the time of the maneuver with the FFB. Use of neuromuscular blocking agents, induction drugs as etomidate, lidocaine and scopolamine are recommended.[20] An assistant must hold the endotracheal tube to prevent unplanned extubation. Despite these difficulties, the FFB can be easily introduced in the majority of cases. The FFB must be removed immediately after a successful tracheal intubation to prevent oxygen desaturation and increase of partial pressure of carbon dioxide ($PaCO_2$) because the presence of the endoscope within the endotracheal tube may obstruct proper ventilation.[21,22,23]

9. Oral or transnasal bronchoscopy?

Oral access has the advantage of introducing tubes with wider diameters. Transnasal approach requires the use of more thin tubes. These procedures are well tolerated and comfortable for the patient.

10. Patient recovery

Tracheal tubes cannot be removed until the patient is completely recovered with an effective cough reflex. If the patient must remain intubated, a bronchoscopic examination for testing the patency of the tube is indicated.

11. Complications

Use of FFB in tracheal intubation is generally safe. Epistaxis is a relatively common problem in transnasal insertion. Injury of the retropharyngeal wall, epiglottis or vocal cords may occur. Rarely, the working channel may be obstructed by thick secretions or clots. Laryngospasm, bronchospasm, nausea, vomiting, tachycardia and bradycardia due to vagal reflex may also be present.

Endoscopes can be damaged with improper manipulation.

12. Contraindications

If it is not possible to introduce the FFB in laryngeal and tracheal stenosis it is contraindicated to attempt FFB intubation. If a narrow tracheal channel persists, thin catheters may be introduced with the aid of an ultrathin FFB.

13. Removing the tracheal tube

Before removing a tracheal tube, a bronchoscopic examination may be required in order to identify complications related to intubation. It is advisable to remove the tube with the FFB inside to allow visualization of the complete tracheal lumen. Reintubation is a risk that must be taken into consideration in extremely difficult cases. Chest X-ray is advisable after extubation.

14. Advantages of using the FFB

FOB intubation is a nontraumatic procedure. Injury is a rare complication during careful introduction of the FFB and tracheal tube. Manipulation by a trained bronchoscopist generally is rapid and safe.

15. Conclusions

All patients classified as having a difficult airway must be considered as potential candidates for endotracheal intubation with FFB as well as patients with failed intubation in anesthesia, intensive care unit and the emergency department. Bronchoscopy must be performed by an experienced and skilled endoscopist. There is a high rate of success using this technique.

16. References

[1] Jabob AK, Kopp SL,Bacon DR, Smith HM. History of Anesthesia. In "Clinical Anesthesia" 6th ed. Barash PG, Cullen BK, Stoelting RK, Cahalan MK, Stock MG Editors. Philadelphia. Lippincott.William & Wilkins. Wolter Kluwer Business.2009:pp.3-26

[2] Brendan T, Finucane T, Santora AH. Principles of airway management. 3rd ed. New York, Springer Verlag; 2003. pp. 214-254

[3] Cook TM, Woodall N, Frerk C. Major complications of airway management in the UK. Results of the Fourth National Audit Project of the Royal College of Anaesthetists and the Difficult Airway Society. Part 1: Anaesthesia. Br J Anaesth 2011;106:617-631.

[4] Burke C, Walsh MT, Harrison BA, Curry TB, Rose BH. Airway management after failure to intubate by direct laryngoscopy: outcomes in a large teaching hospital. Can J Anesth 2006;52:634-640.

[5] Cormack RS, Lehane J. Difficult tracheal intubation in obstetrics. Anaesthesia 1984;39:1105-1111.

[6] American Society of Anesthesiologists. Practice guidelines for management of the difficult airway. An updated report by the American Society of Anesthesiologist Task Force on Management of the Difficult Airway. Anesthesiology (Special article) 2003;98:1269-1277.

[7] Samsoon GLT, Young JRB. Difficult tracheal intubation: a retrospective study. Anesth Analg 1987; 42:487-490.

[8] Wilson MF, Spiegelhalter D, Robertson JA, Lesser P. Predicting difficult intubation. Br J Anaesth 1988;61:211-216.

[9] Bair AE, Caravelli R, Tyler K. Feasibility of the preoperative Mallampati airway assessment in emergency department patients. J Emerg Med 2011;38:677-680.

[10] Mallampati SR, Gatt SP, Guggino LD, Desair S, Waraska B, Freiberger D. A clinical sign to predict difficult tracheal intubation. A prospective study. Can Anaesth Soc J 1985;32:429-434.

[11] Lee A, Fan LTY, Gin T, Karmakar MK, Kee WDN. A systematic review (meta-analysis) of the accuracy of the Mallamapati tests to predict the difficult airway. Anesth Analg 2006;102:1867-1878.

[12] Connor C, Segal S. Accurate classification of difficult intubation by computerized facial analysis. Anesth Analg 2011;112:84-93.

[13] Elizondo E, Navarro F, Pérez-Romo A, Ortega C, Muñoz H, Cicero R. Endotracheal intubation with flexible fiberoptic bronchoscopy in patients with abnormal anatomic conditions of the head and neck. Ear Nose Throat J 2007;86:682-684.

[14] Orozco-Díaz E, Álvares-Ríos JJ, Arceo-Díaz JL. Ornelas-Aguirre JM. Predictive factors of difficult airway with known assessment scales. Cir Cir 2010;78:393-399.
[15] Serocki G, Bein B, Scholz J, Dörges V. Management of the predicted difficult airway: a comparison of conventional blade laryngoscopy with video-assisted blade laryngosopy and the GlideScope. Eur J Anaesthesiol 2010;27:24-30.
[16] van Zwan JP, Kapteijns EFG, Lahey S, Smit HJM. Flexible bronchoscopy in supine or sitting position. A randomized prospective analysis of safety and patient comfort. J Bronchol Intervent Pulmonol 2010;17:29-32.
[17] Stubb SE, McDougall. Preparation of the patient for bronchoscopy. In Bronchoscpy. Ed. UBS Prakash. New York. Raven Press; 1995. p. 109.
[18] Heir JS, Kupferman ME. A simple approach to facilitating fiberoptic intubation in the difficult airway. Laryngoscope 2011;121:310-312.
[19] Fragoso Guerreiro da Cunhna E, Rosal Gonçalves JM. Role of fiber optic bronchoscopy in intensive care unit: current practice. J Bronchol Intervent Pulmonol 2011;18:68-69.
[20] Reynolds SF, Heffner J. Airway management of the critically ill patient. Chest 2005;127:1397-1412.
[21] Cook TM, Woodall N, Benjer J. Major complications of airway management in the UK. Results of the Fourth National Audit Project of the Royal College of Anaesthetist and the Difficult Airway Society. Part 2: Intensive care and emergency departments. Br J Anaesth 2011;106:632-642.
[22] Tai DYH. Bronchoscopy in the intensive care unit. Ann Acad Med 1998;27:552-558.
[23] Phua GC, Wahif MM. ICU procedures in the critically ill. Respirology 2009;14:1092-1097.

8

Bronchoscopic Balloon Dilation (BBD) for Benign Tracheobronchial Stenosis

Masayuki Tanahashi, Hiroshi Niwa, Haruhiro Yukiue,
Eriko Suzuki, Hiroshi Haneda, Naoko Yoshii and Hisanori Kani
Division of Thoracic Surgery, Respiratory Disease Center,
Seirei Mikatahara General Hospital
Japan

1. Introduction

Bronchoscopic balloon dilation (BBD) is a useful method of treating tracheobronchial stenosis. Tracheobronchial stenosis in adults can arise from benign or malignant disease. Benign stenosis causes include sarcoidosis, tuberculosis, Wegener's granulomatosis, trauma, berylliosis, and foreign body reaction. Furthermore, it can arise after prolonged endotracheal intubation, after sleeve resection or after lung transplantation. Despite adequate systemic therapy, airway stenosis may progress due to tuberculosis or sarcoidosis. In infants, prior use of endobronchial and tracheostomy tubes or congenital stenosis from complete cartilaginous rings are the primary reasons for such stenosis (McDonald & Stocks, 1965; Parkin ea al., 1976). Subglottic or tracheal sites are thus common and may continue to present serious and often fatal respiratory problems in infants. In adults, the etiologies are variable and the stricture can happen in any part of the airway. Tracheobronchial stenosis may produce symptoms such as dyspnea, cough, wheeze, stridor, or recurrent lower respiratory tract infections, and these symptoms cause the airway stricture to mimic asthma. There are various treatments including surgical resection, laser resection, and bougie dilation during rigid bronchoscopy. For lesions causing impending respiratory failure, surgical resection or stent placement is the most prudent treatment. In less urgent conditions, BBD has been considered a simple, rapid, and safe method to restore airway caliber. BBD has been used alone or in combination with other modalities such as laser resection, cryotherapy, and electrocautery. In 1984, Cohen et al. (Cohen et al., 1984) reported a successful balloon dilation through a tracheostomy tube under propylidone injection for a stricture after segmental resection of congenital stenosis in an infant. In 1987, Fowler et al. (Fowler et al., 1987) described bronchoscopic balloon dilation using a rigid bronchoscope for anastomotic stenosis in an adult who had had a sleeve resection for an endobronchial squamous cell carcinoma of the right main-stem bronchus 2 years earlier. The following year Carlin et al. (Carlin et al., 1988) reported two cases of bronchial stenosis successfully treated with a combination of bronchoscopic balloon dilation and Nd-YAG laser photoresection with a rigid bronchoscope. In 1991, balloon dilation using flexible bronchoscopy was described for the first time by Nakamura et al. (Nakamura et al., 1991). They treated two patients with tuberculous bronchial stenosis through a flexible bronchoscope under local anesthesia. Since then, several reports of BBD have been published (Ball et al., 1991; Keller &

Frost, 1992; Carre et al., 1994; Fouty et al., 1994; Ferretti et al., 1995; Sheski & Mathur, 1998). The major advantages of BBD are lower morbidity and mortality than surgery, stent placement, or bougienage. BBD has thus become an accepted treatment for benign tracheobronchial stenosis.

2. Indications and contraindications

Balloon dilation has an indication in almost all benign tracheobronchial strictures. The bronchial stenosis caused by tuberculosis finally heals with fibrous scarring through a submucosal infiltration by tubercles and lymphocytes, followed by ulceration and growth of granulation tissue (Bugher et al., 1937; Wilson, 1945; Auerbach, 1949; Judd, 1947). Stenosis from other medical causes such as Wegener's granulomatosis, sarcoidosis (Fouty et al., 1994; Olsson et al., 1979), berylliosis, post-tracheostomy, and complicated tracheobronchial anastomosis may also ultimately result in fibrous scars. Such fibrotic stenosis is a good indication for BBD. Visual characteristics such as pale or nonedematous mucosa may suggest a lesion with little inflammation and a greater likelihood of successful opening (Ferretti et al., 1995; Brown et al., 1987). In particular, inoperable long segmental stenosis is well treated by BBD. On the other hand, if the bronchial cartilage is destroyed, the success rate of BBD is low (Carre et al., 1994). An airway stricture with tracheobronchomalacia usually requires combination therapy with another therapeutic modality such as stent placement to maintain airway patency. Iwamoto et al. (Iwamoto et al., 2004) reported that endobronchial ultrasonography (EBUS) imaging was useful in making a diagnosis of cartilaginous tracheobronchomalacia and in aiding the decision as to whether or not a stent was needed. In lung transplantation, this endobronchial stenosis may be a result of airway rejection or due to ischemic changes at the site of the bronchial implantation. When there must be an ongoing process such as airway rejection or ischemia, even if repeated BBD is performed, endobronchial stenosis is often recurrent. In malignancy, balloon dilation is performed in combination with other modalities such as laser resection, stent placement, cryotherapy, and electrocautery (Hautmann et al., 2001). Assessment of the patient's coagulation status before the procedure is important because bleeding is a frequent complication of BBD. The decision to continue or withhold anticoagulant or antiplatelet drugs should reflect a balance of the consequences of periprocedural hemorrhage versus the risk of periprocedural vascular complications. Aspirin, NSAIDs, ibuprofen, clopidigrel, and warfarin should be discontinued at least 7-10 days, 3 days, 24 hours, 7-10 days, and 3-5 days before BBD, respectively (Douketis et al., 2008; Kearon et al., 1997; Larson et al., 2005). Nonacetylated NSAIDs can be continued in the periprocedual period. If the patient cannot stop taking any anticoagulant or antiplatelet medication, BBD should be performed prudently.

3. Technique

BBD is generally performed under topical anesthesia and conscious sedation, but BBD for tracheal stenosis will be performed better under general anesthesia with laryngeal mask ventilation or tracheal intubation, because long-term respiratory arrest is needed during inflation and this would cause great anxiety to the patient. Patients are maintained with 100% oxygen during the procedure and are hyperventilated immediately before balloon inflation.

After local or general anesthesia, bronchoscopy is first performed with a diagnostic bronchoscope (BF-260; Olympus, Tokyo) or a therapeutic bronchoscope (BF-1T60; Olympus, Tokyo) to assess and localize the airway stenosis before balloon dilation. Bronchoscopy provides information about not only the localization and extent of the stenosis but also the condition of the mucosa and influence of extra-bronchial lesions. Radiopaque markers are placed on the surface of the skin to identify the proximal and distal limits of the stenosis. A flexible, 0.035-inch guidewire (Jagwire™ Plus; Boston Scientific/Medi-tech, Natick, MA) is then inserted through the working channel of the bronchoscope and is passed through the stenosis (Fig. 1a). This is performed under fluoroscopy to ensure that the guidewire does not extend to the pleura. With the guidewire held in place, the bronchoscope is withdrawn. The placement of the guidewire should be confirmed with fluoroscopy after the bronchoscope has been removed. Next, a balloon catheter (CRE™ Fixed Wire & Wire Guided Balloon Dilators, Hurricane™ RX Biliary Balloon Dilation Catheter, Max Force™ TTS; Boston Scientific/Medi-tech, Natick, MA) is selected, based on balloon length and diameter in relation to the stenosis dimensions. These balloon catheters are made of polyamide and have radiopaque markers at the proximal and distal ends of the balloon. They are available in variety of size ranges. The balloon is constructed of such material that the nominal diameter of the balloon is proportional to the inflation pressure (3-12 atm). The balloon is inflated based on that particular balloon catheter's characteristics. The diameter of the balloon is chosen to be the same diameter as that of the lumen measured at the proximal region of the normal airway. The length of the balloon is at least 0.5cm greater than that of stenotic segment, since the entire stenosis will be dilated when the balloon is inflated. If the inflated balloon length is insufficient, the balloon can slip out of the stenosis. If the balloon length is too great, there is a potential for airway damage. This diameter and length of the balloon are measured by both bronchoscope and chest CT scans. The required width can be estimated from a comparison of the bronchoscope diameter to that of the stenosis. The required length of balloon is estimated by passing the bronchoscope through the stenosis and by measuring the distance between the proximal and distal limits of the obstruction. Three-dimensional CT is a useful noninvasive evaluation for BBD (Rooney et al., 2005). It allows for preoperative determination of balloon size and length, even if the bronchoscope cannot be passed through the obstruction. It can allow an accurate determination of the degree and length of stenosis, an evaluation of the airway distal to the stenosis and show the presence of multiple stenoses as well as the relationships with mediastinal structures. Furthermore, it is a useful noninvasive technique for postoperative follow-up. It can not only evaluate the effect of BBD, but also detect complications related to BBD such as a deep laceration, pneumomediastinum or mediastinal bleeding (Y. H. Kim et al., 2006). When the stenosis is too narrow for a balloon catheter, a smaller balloon catheter is used first to create a passage for the larger balloon catheter and a wider and longer balloon may be used by exchanging the balloon catheter for another over the guidewire. Under fluoroscopic guidance, an appropriately sized balloon catheter is then advanced over the guidewire and positioned such that the balloon markers are properly located with respect to the stenosis (Fig. 1b). The bronchoscope is again inserted to visualize the stenosis and the balloon catheter (Fig. 1c). The balloon is then inflated with a dilute nonionic contrast medium (Iopamidol; Bracco, Milan), and the results are observed via both fluoroscopy and bronchoscopy (Fig. 1d). The inflation time is between approximately 30 seconds and 2 minutes, depending on the clinical tolerance and consequences on cutaneous oxygen saturation. Occasionally the initial inflation times must be very short, but they can be increased as dilation proceeds. Nonionic

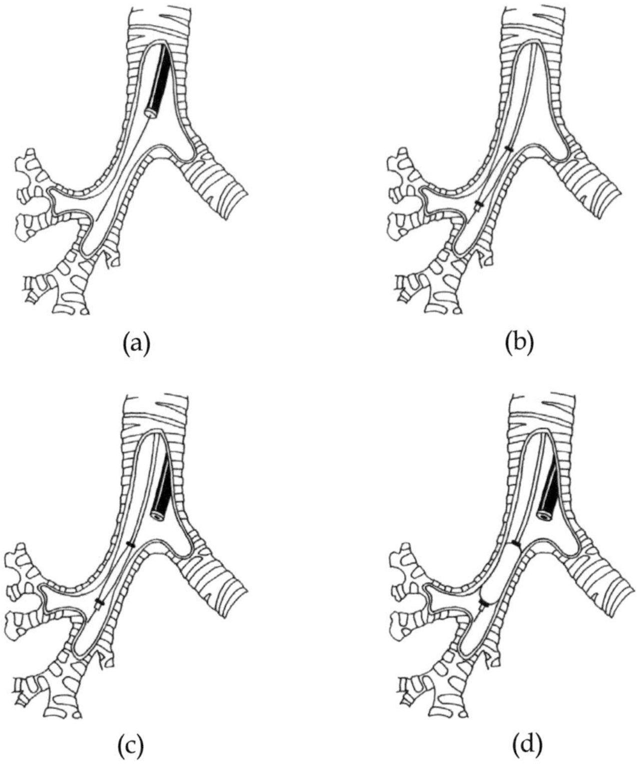

Fig. 1. a) A guidewire is passed beyond the stenosis, using bronchoscopy and fluoroscopy to ensure that the guidewire does not extend to the pleura and then the bronchoscope is withdrawn, leaving the guidewire in place. b) The balloon catheter is advanced over a guidewire and positioned under fluoroscopy. c) Proper positioning of the proximal end of the balloon is confirmed with visualization through the bronchoscope. d) Bronchoscopy allows direct monitoring of balloon inflation and deflation with fluoroscopy.

contrast media are safe for the bronchus because bronchography using nonionic contrast media instead of propylidone is performed safely (Morcos et al., 1989, 1990; Riebel & Wartner, 1990).

If the diameter of the deflated catheter is less than that of the working channel, a bronchoscope is not needed to remove before the balloon catheter is inserted. A balloon catheter is passed over the guidewire through the working channel and positioned within the narrowed segment of the airway under bronchoscopic visualization (Fig. 2a, Fig. 2b).

During inflation, a balloon inflation device with pressure-gauge monitor (Alliance™ Inflation Device; Boston Scientific/Medi-tech, Natick, MA) is used to inflate the balloon and to monitor the inflation pressure. Success is defined as loss of the typical waist made in the wall of the balloon by the stenosis as observed by fluoroscopy and a stable increase in tracheobronchial diameter of the stenotic segment by bronchoscopy. If necessary, the balloon catheter then can be repositioned or replaced by a larger sized balloon catheter, and the procedure repeated until the desired effect is obtained. Adjunctive treatments such as laser vaporization or stent placement may precede or follow balloon dilation. Patient who

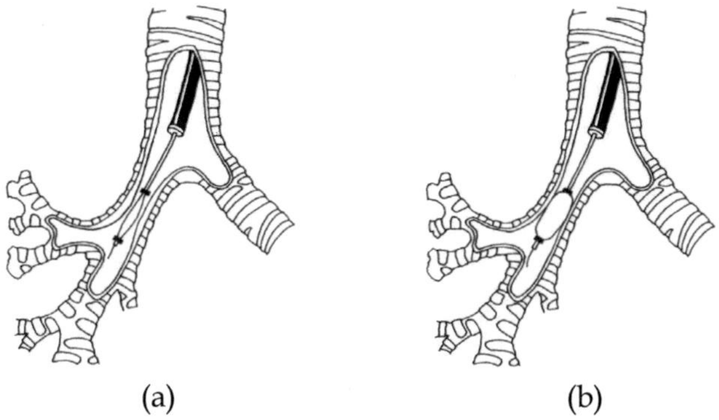

Fig. 2. a) If the diameter of the deflated catheter is less than that of the working channel, the bronchoscope need not be removed before the balloon catheter is inserted. A balloon catheter is passed over the guidewire through the working channel and positioned within the narrowed segment of the airway under bronchoscopic visualization. b) The balloon is inflated and deflated, and the results are observed via both bronchoscopy and fluoroscopy.

underwent BBD usually discharges the next day of the procedure. If a complication such as laceration occurs, the patient needs to be hospitalized for several days to monitor his conditions. Follow-up bronchoscopy is performed about 2-4 weeks after dilation. If the desired airway diameter is not attained or recurrent stenosis is observed, the balloon dilation is repeated until the desired effect is obtained.

4. Complications

During BBD, chest pain, bronchospasm and atelectasis have been reported (Brown et al., 1987; Elkerbout et al., 1993; Hebra et al., 1991). Excessive balloon inflation may lacerate or rupture the airway, causing bleeding, pneumothorax, pneumomediastinum, or mediastinitis. As far as we know, there are few reports describing lacerations of the tracheobronchial tree after balloon dilation. One case of rupture requiring surgical management has been reported (Knott et al., 2004). However, other lacerations except for this one healed spontaneously and there were no clinical problems (Y. H. Kim et al., 2006; J. H. Kim et al., 2007; K. H. Lee et al., 2002). No patients have died during or from problems related to BBD.

5. Results

Several reports of BBD in adults are available. Technical success is defined by successful passing of a balloon catheter through a stenosis. Short-term clinical success is defined as the loss of the typical waist made in the wall of the balloon by the stenosis by fluoroscopy, an increase in tracheobronchial diameter of the stenotic segment immediately after bronchoscopy, and improvement of the patient's clinical symptoms. Long-term success is based on the patient remaining asymptomatic. Recurrence is defined as the return of symptoms. Some patients have undergone radiographic evaluation with chest roentgenography or CT scan, pulmonary function testing, or bronchoscopy as part of follow-up care. The short-term results of balloon dilation to treat benign tracheobronchial stenosis have been favorable. Clinical success rates of 63% to 100% have been reported

(Carre et al., 1994; Ferretti et al., 1995; Sheski & Mathur, 1998; J. H. Kim et al., 2007; K. W. Lee et al., 1999; Mayse et al., 2004). However, the long-term efficacy of balloon dilation in a large group of patients has rarely been reported. According to the reports, recurrence rates range from 30% to 80% (Carre et al., 1994; Ferretti et al., 1995; Iwamoto et al., 2004; J. H. Kim et al., 2007; K. H. Lee et al., 2002; K. W. Lee et al., 1999).

Kim et al. (J. H. Kim et al., 2007) reported that a group of patients with tracheobronchial lacerations (n=64) showed better cumulative airway patency than a group without tracheobronchial lacerations (n=60) (medium patency duration, 24 vs. 4 months, respectively). They concluded that better clinical outcomes might occur following superficial or deep lacerations after BBD in patients with a benign tracheobronchial stricture. Lee et al. (K. H. Lee et al., 2002) reported that initial symptomatic improvement after BBD was achieved in 83% (49/59) of patients, however, during a mean of 32 months follow-up the recurrence rate of BBD was high (80%, 39/49). They also reported that the secondary patency rate with repeat balloon dilation at 32 months was 43%, a relatively acceptable long-term result. Lee et al. (K. W. Lee et al., 1999) reported that improvements in dyspnea after BBD for tuberculous bronchial stenosis occurred immediately in 73% (11/15), 73% after 1 month, 73% after 6 months, 64% after 1 year, 64% after 3 years, and 42% after 6 years. They concluded that the long-term results of BBD were acceptable.

We performed BBD in eleven sessions for benign tracheobronchial stenoses in 8 patients between December 1987 and March 2009. The patients were four males and four females, and ranged in age from 30 to 60 years. The indications were tuberculous stenosis (n=6), post-tracheostomy stricture (n=1) and post-bronchoplasty anastmous stenosis (n=1). The sites of stenosis were the trachea (n=4), left main bronchus (n=3), right main bronchus (n=2), left upper bronchus (n=1), and left lower bronchus (n=1). Stenoses ranged in diameter from pinhole (more than 90%) to 70%, and in length from 0.5 to 6 cm. They were followed up for 3-48 months (mean follow-up 26.7 months) with radiographic evaluation by chest roentgenography or CT scan, pulmonary function testing, or bronchoscopy after BBD. BBD was performed under local anesthesia in 3 patients and general anesthesia in 5 patients. For tracheal stenosis, 8-18 mm diameter balloons (55-80 mm long) were used. For bronchial stenosis, 4-12 mm diameter balloons (20-55 mm long) were used. The results in seven of eight treated patients were successful in maintaining airway patency. The only one unsuccessful patient was one of post-tracheostomy stenosis resulting in secondary tracheomalacia, and this patient needed T-tube stent placement to support the weakened cartilage and prevent dynamic airway collapse. As regards complications, there were four patients with longitudinal tracheal or bronchial lacerations, but all lacerations healed spontaneously after conservative treatment. Thus, a laceration should be regarded as an expected result of sufficient balloon dilation, not as a major complication. There were no recurrences during 3-48 months follow up period in our study. Tables 1 and 2 summarize our experience. Figures 3 to 12 show the patients with tracheobronchial stenosis who underwent BBD.

Respiratory functional improvement can be obtained after BBD, as well as improved tracheobronchial diameter. Lee et al. (K. H. Lee et al., 2002) reported significant improvements in the mean forced vital capacity (FVC), forced expiratory volume in 1 second (FEV1), and forced expiratory flow 25%-75% after technically and clinically successful balloon dilation in 49 patients. Lee et al. (K. W. Lee et al., 1999) reported that improvement of dyspnea occurred immediately in 11 of 15 patients (73%) after balloon

Patient	Age	Sex	C.C.	Etiology	Area	Length	Severity
1	42	F	DOE	Tb	Tr	4cm	70%
2	60	F	DOE	Tb	Tr	3cm	70%
3	30	M	#	Tracheostomy	Tr	6cm	70%
4	33	F	Cough, Sputum	Tb	Lt-MB	2cm	Pinhole
5	19	M	DOE	Tb	Lt-MB	2cm	Pinhole
					Lt-UB	0. 5cm	Pinhole
6	38	M	DOE	Bronchoplasty	Rt-MB	1cm	Pinhole
7	48	F	DOE	Tb	Tr	6cm	80%
					Rt-MB	2cm	pinhole
8	30	M	Cough, Stridor	Tb	Lt-MB	5cm	70%
					Lt-LB	1cm	Pinhole

C.C=Chief complaint, DOE=Dyspnea on excertion, #=Difficulty in removing tracheostomy tube, Tb=Tuberculosis, Tr=Trachea, Lt-MB left main bronchus, Lt-UB=left upper bronchus, Rt-MB=right main bronchus, Lt-LB=left lower bronchus

Table 1. Patients underwent bronchoscopic balloon dilation

Patient	Anes.	Balloon Catheter (d×l, mm)	Pressure (atm)	Complications	Patency
1	G	18×55	3	None	3 mos good
2	G	12~15×55	3	Laceration	4 mos good
3	G	18 × 80	2~4	Laceration	Fair
4	L	10 × 40	4	None	3 yrs good
5	L	10×40, 12×55	3~4	None	3 yrs good
	L	10×20	3~4	None	3 yrs good
6	L	10×20	6	None	3 yrs good
7	G	8~18×80	3~8	Laceration	4 yrs good
	G	8~12×55	3~8	Laceration	4 yrs good
8	G	6~10×55	3~10	Laceration	2 yrs good
	G	4~6×20	7~12	None	2 yrs good

Anes.=anesthesia, G=general anesthesia, L=local anesthesia, d=diameter, l=length, atm=atmosphere, BBDs=balloon dilations, mos=months, yrs=years

Table 2. Details and results of bronchoscopic balloon dilation

dilation and an increase of FEV1 or FVC of more than 15% after BBD was obtained in five of 13 patients after 1 or 2 days and that eight of the 13 patients (62%) showed improvement of FEV1 or FVC after 1 year. Hautmann et al. (Hautmann et al., 2001) reported that lung function analysis demonstrated a small but significant increase in FEV1, peak expiratory flow rate (PEFR), FEV1/FVC, and PaO2 within 72 hours after BBD in 42 patients with malignant tracheobronchial disease. In our study, the improvements in symptoms such as dyspnea, cough, and stridor following dilation were dramatic in most patients. Patients' respiratory status was evaluated before and after BBD by means of pulmonary function test and Hugh-Jones classification (Table 3). All patients showed improvements of FEV1, peak expiratory flow (PEF) and Hugh-Jones classification (Fig. 13). Thus, BBD is useful not only for increasing the tracheobronchial diameter of the stenotic segment but also for improving respiratory function and symptoms.

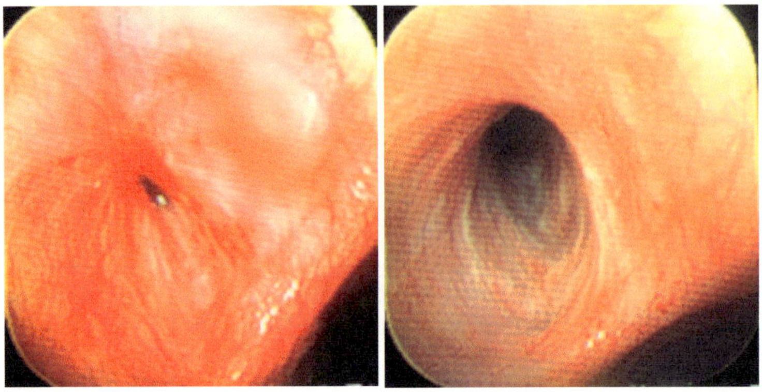

(a) (b)

Fig. 3. Tuberculous bronchial stenosis of a 19-year-old man (patient 5). a) Pre-balloon dilation bronchoscopic view shows severe stenosis at the left main bronchus. The orifice is almost obstructed. b) Bronchoscopy three years after balloon dilation shows an almost normal airway. His symptoms immediately improved and he has done well.

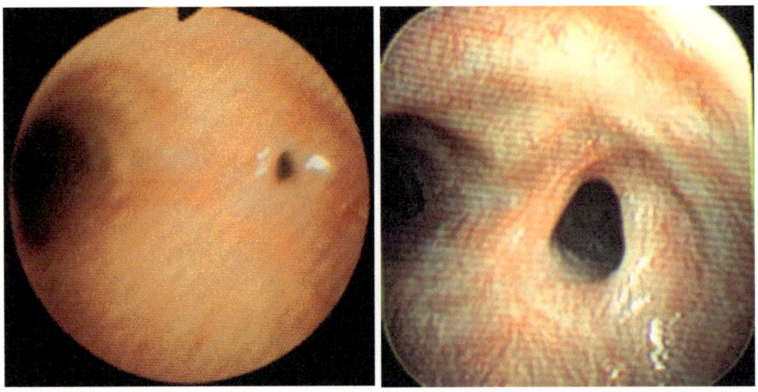

(a) (b)

Fig. 4. Post-bronchoplastic stenosis of a 38-year-old man (patient 6). a) Pre-balloon dilation bronchoscopic view shows pinhole size opening of the right main bronchus. b) At follow up bronchoscopy 3 years after BBD an almost normal lumen of the right main bronchus is maintained. He is doing well without evident respiratory symptoms.

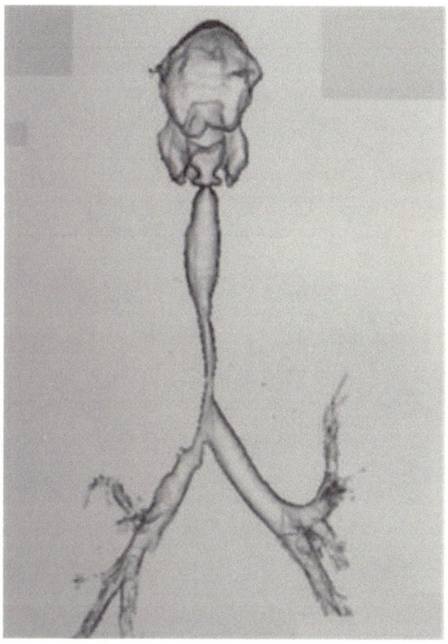

Fig. 5. Tuberculous tracheal and right main bronchial stenosis of a 48-year-old female (patient 7). She had progressive severe dyspnea at rest with continuous coughing and stridor. Three-dimensional reconstruction CT shows 60mm segment of 8mm diameter severe narrowing from upper trachea to right main bronchus.

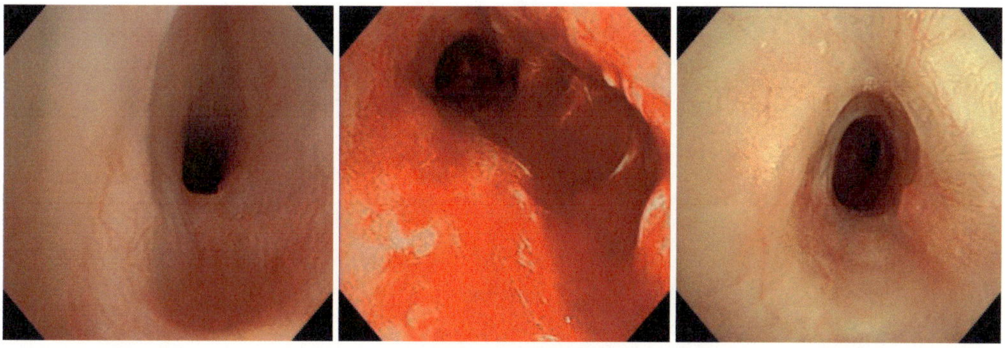

(a) (b) (c)

Fig. 6. a) Pre-balloon dilation bronchoscopic view of patient 7 shows severe long segmental stenosis at the trachea. b) Immediately after balloon dilation, a deep laceration is observed from the trachea to the right main bronchus at the membrane portion, but the patient is stable and asymptomatic. c) Two months later, the laceration is spontaneously healed and the airway is markedly wider than before dilation. Following the balloon dilation the patient is less dyspnetic at rest and can perform housework without becoming short of breath.

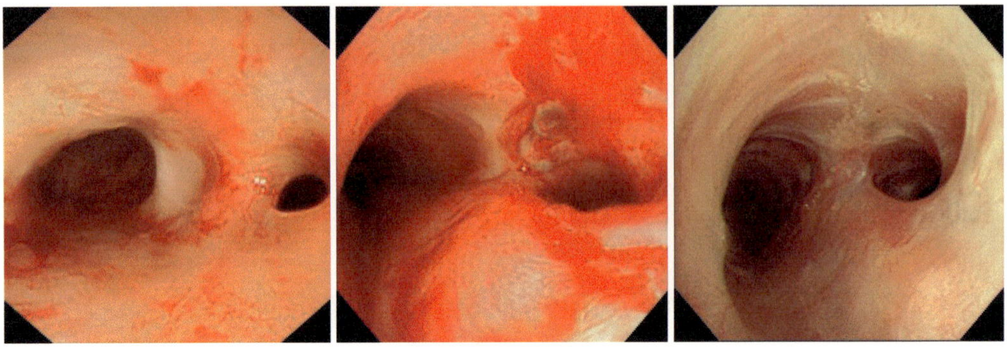

(a) (b) (c)

Fig. 7. a) Pre-balloon dilation bronchoscopic view of patient 7 shows severe stenosis of the right main bronchus. b) Immediately after balloon dilation, a deep laceration is observed at the right main bronchus. c) Bronchoscopic findings two months after dilation demonstrate that the laceration is spontaneously healed and the airway is significantly improved.

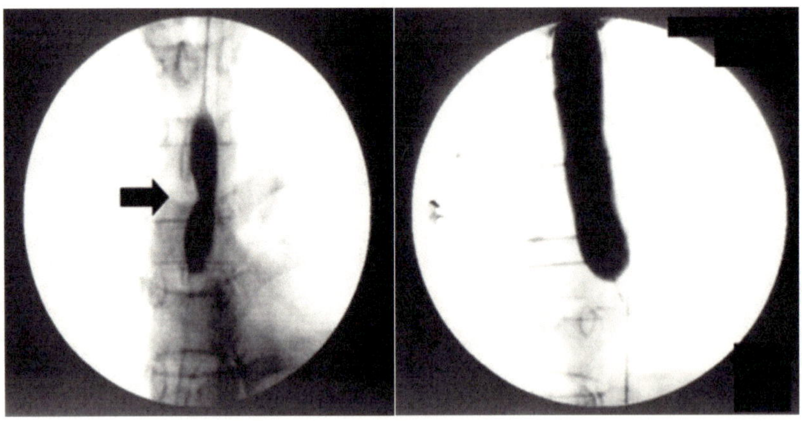

(a) (b)

Fig. 8. a) Fluoroscopic image of patient 7 obtained at the beginning of balloon inflation clearly demonstrates a waist (arrow) on the wall of the balloon at the level of the severe part of the stenosis. b) Fluoroscopic image obtained at the end of the dilation no longer shows a waist.

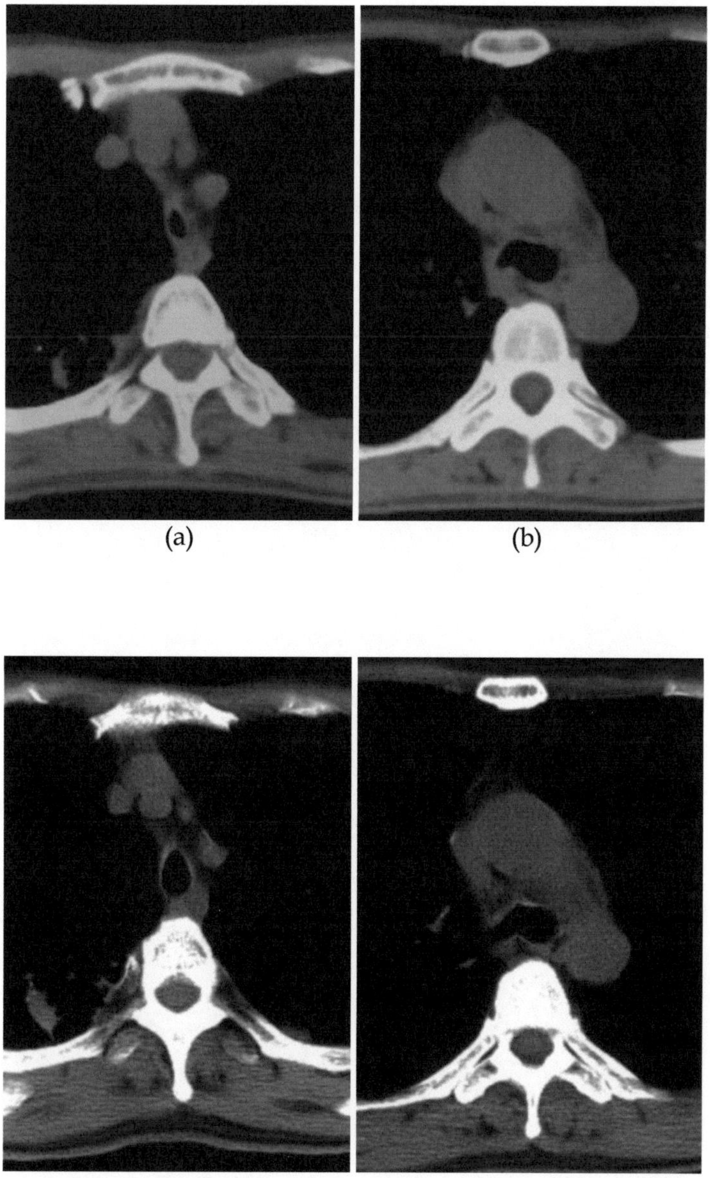

(a) (b)

(c) (d)

Fig. 9. Chest CT of patient 7 shows severe stenosis of the trachea (a) and the right main bronchus (b) before BBD. However, BBD brings a significant increase in the diameter of the trachea (c) and the right main bronchus (d).

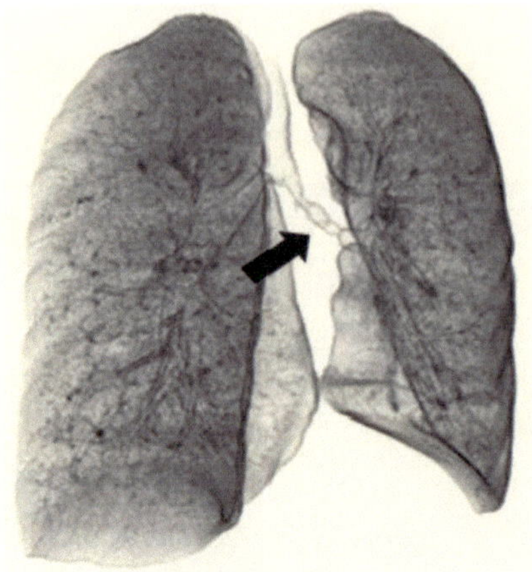

Fig. 10. Tuberculous stenosis of the left main bronchus and left lower bronchus of a 30-year-old male (patient 8). He developed continuous stridor and cough. Three-dimensional reconstruction CT shows irregular luminal narrowing from the left main bronchus to the left lower bronchus (arrow).

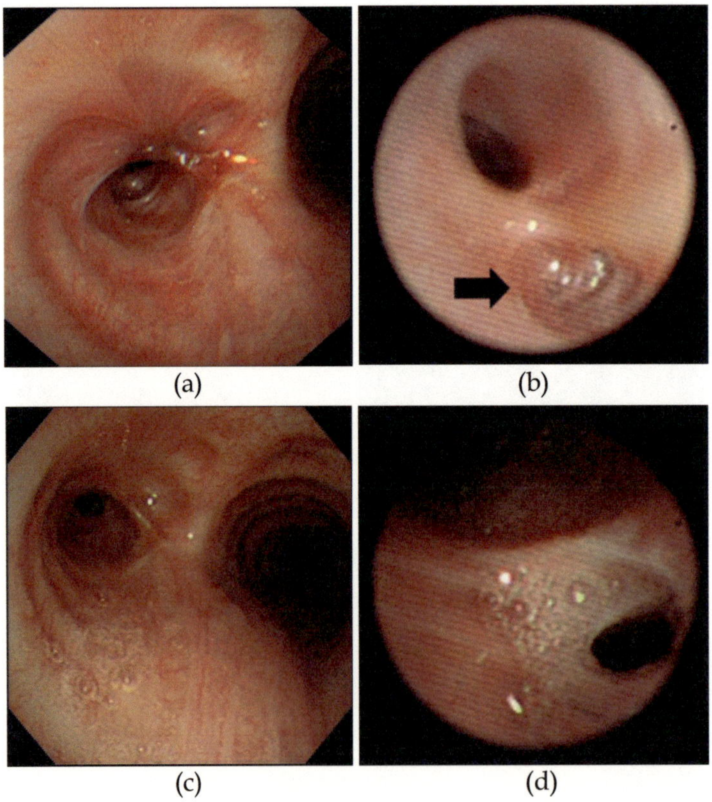

Fig. 11. a-b) Pre-balloon dilation bronchoscopic view of patient 8 shows severe stenosis at the left main bronchus (a) and the left lower bronchus (arrow in (b)). c-d) Bronchoscopic view shows improvement of the stenosis at the left main bronchus (c) and the left lower bronchus (d) after balloon dilation.

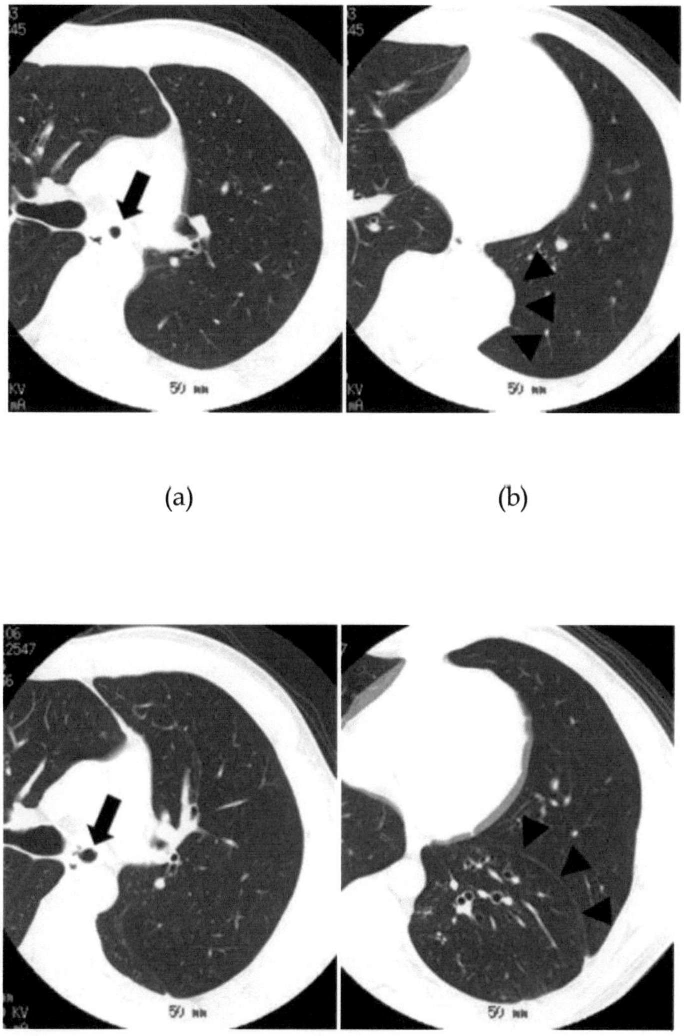

(a) (b)

(c) (d)

Fig. 12. a) Chest CT of patient 8 shows the stenosis of the left main bronchus (arrow). b) Chest CT shows the atelectasis of the left lower lobe caused by tuberculous bronchial stenosis (arrow heads). c) After balloon dilation. Chest CT shows increase of the diameter of the left main bronchus (arrow). d) After balloon dilation, the atelectasis is obliterated and the left lower lobe is expanded (arrow heads). He has been without symptoms and chest film evidence of atelectasis for 2 years.

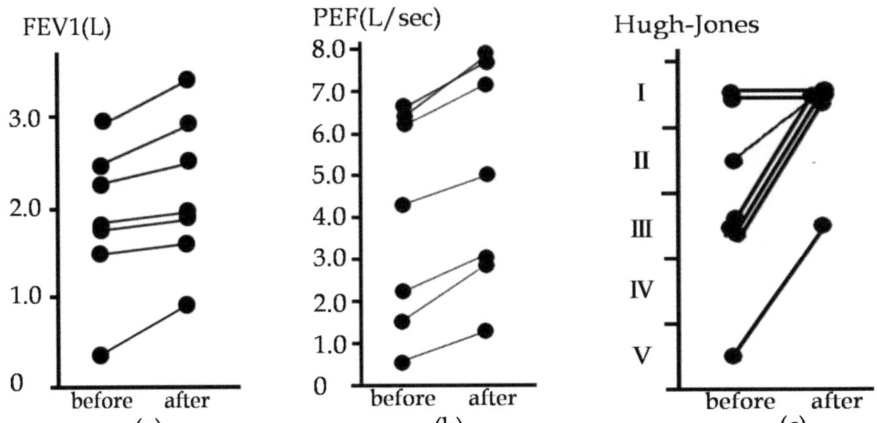

Fig. 13. All patients who underwent pulmonary function testing showed improvement of forced expiratory volume in 1 second (FEV1), peak expiratory flow (PEF) and Hugh-Jones classification.

I	The patient's breathing is as good as that of others of the same sex, age, and build while at work, on walking, or on climbing hills or stairs
II	The patient is able to walk with healthy persons of the same sex, age, and build on the level but is unable to keep up on hills or stairs
III	The patient is unable to keep up with healthy persons on the level but is able to walk a mile or more at a slower speed
IV	The patient is unable to walk more than about 100 yards on the level without a rest
V	The patient is breathless on talking or undressing or is unable to leave the house because of breathlessness

Table 3. Hugh-Jones classification

6. Conclusion

Bronchoscopic balloon dilation is a very useful therapy for benign tracheobronchial stenosis. The advantages of this procedure in comparison with other procedures are that it is minimally invasive, safe, and rapid. It can be performed under either local or general anesthesia. Balloon dilation can be performed safely and effectively because the balloon placement and inflation-deflation can be monitored via both fluoroscopy and bronchoscopy. A guidewire permits easy exchange of the balloon catheter. A relatively common complication is transmural laceration, but lacerations should be regarded as an expected result of sufficient balloon dilation and not as a major complication. No deaths have been attributed directly to balloon dilation alone. Only fibrous stenosis responds to balloon dilation alone; bronchial stenosis with coexisting tracheobronchomalacia usually requires combination therapy with another therapeutic modality such as stent placement to maintain bronchial patency. The procedure often needs to be repeated to achieve a satisfactory result.

7. References

Auerbach, O. (1949). Tuberculosis of the trachea and major bronchi. *Am Rev Tuberc*, Vol.60, pp. 604-620.

Ball, JB.; Delaney, JC.; Evans, CC.; Donnelly, RJ. & Hind, CRK. (1991). Endoscopic bougie and balloon dilatation of multiple bronchial stenoses: 10 year follow up. *Thorax*, Vol.46, pp. 933-935.

Brown, SB.; Hedlund, GL.; Glasier, CM.; Williams, KD.; Greenwood, LH. & Gilliland, JD. (1987). Tracheobronchial stenosis in infants: Successful balloon dilation therapy. *Radiology*, Vol.164, pp. 475-478.

Bugher, JC.; Littig, J. & Culp, J. (1937). Tuberculous tracheobronchitis: its pathogenesis. *Am J Med Sci*, Vol.193, pp. 515-525.

Carlin, BW.; Harrell, JH. & Moser, KM. (1988). The treatment of endobronchial stenosis using balloon catheter dilatation. *Chest*, Vol.93, No.6, pp. 1148-1151.

Carre, P.; Rousseau, H.; Lombart, L.; Didier, A.; Dahan, M.; Fournial, G.; Leophonte, P. & the Toulouse Lung Transplantaion Group. (1994). Balloon dilatation and self-expanding metal Wallstent insertion for management of bronchostenosis following lung transplantation. *Chest*, Vol.105, No.2, pp. 343-348.

Cohen, MD.; Weber, TR. & Rao, CC. (1984). Balloon dilatation of tracheal and bronchial stenosis. *AJR*, Vol.142, pp. 477-478.

Douketis, JD.; Berger, PB.; Dunn, AS.; Jaffer, AK.; Spyropoulos, AC.; Becker, RC. & Ansell, J. (2008). The perioperative management of antithrombotic therapy: American college of chest physicians evidence-based clinical practice guidelines (8th edition). *Chest*, Vol.133, No.6, pp. 299S-339S.

Elkerbout, SC.; van Lingen, RA.; Gerritsen, J. & Roorda, RJ. (1993). Endoscopic balloon dilatation of acquired airway stenosis in newborn infants: a promising treatment. *Arch Dis Child*, Vol.68, pp. 37-40.

Ferretti, G.; Jouvan, FB.; Thony, F.; Pison, C. & Coulomb, M. (1995). Benign noninflammatory bronchial stenosis: treatment with balloon dilation. *Radiology*, Vol.196, pp. 831-834.

Fouty, BW.; Pomeranz, M.; Thigpen, TP. & Martin, RJ. (1994). Dilatation of bronchial stenoses due to sarcoidosis using a flexible fiberoptic bronchoscope. *Chest*, Vol.106, No.3, pp. 677-680.

Fowler, CL.; Aaland, MO. & Harris, FL. (1987). Dilatation of bronchial stenosis with Gruentzig balloon. *J Thorac Cardiovasc Surg*, vol.93, pp. 308-315.

Hautmann, H.; Gamarra, F.; Pfeifer, KJ. & Huber, RM. (2001). Fiberoptic bronchoscopic balloon dilatation in malignant tracheobronchial disease: indications and results. *Chest*, Vol.120, No.1, pp. 43-49.

Hebra, A.; Powell, DD.; Smith, CD. & Othersen, HB. (1991). Balloon tracheoplasty in children: results of a 15-year experience. *J Pediatr Surg*, Vol.26, No.8, pp. 957-961.

Iwamoto, Y.; Miyazawa, T.; Kurimoto, N.; Miyazu, Y.; Ishida, A.; Matsuo, K. & Watanabe, Y. (2004). Interventional bronchoscopy in the management of airway stenosis due to tracheobronchial tuberculosis. *Chest*, Vol.126, No.4, pp. 1344-1352.

Judd, AR. (1947). Tuberculous tracheobronchitis: a study of 500 consecutive cases. *J Thorac Surg*, Vol.16, pp. 512-523.

Kearon, C. & Hirsh, J. (1997). Management of anticoagulation before and after elective surgery. *N Engl J Med*, Vol.336, No.21, pp. 1506-1511.

Keller, C. & Frost, A. (1992). Fiberoptic bronchoplasty: Description of a simple adjunct technique for the management of bronchial stenosis following lung transplantation. *Chest*, Vol.102, No.4, pp. 995-998.

Kim, JH.; Shin, JH.; Song, HY.; Shim, TS.; Ko, GY.; Yoon, HK. & Sung, KB. (2007). Tracheobronchial laceration after balloon dilation for benign strictures: incidence and clinical significance. *Chest*, Vol.131, No.4, pp. 1114-1117.

Kim, YH.; Sung, DJ.; Cho, SB.; Chung, KB.; Cha, SH.; Park, HS. & Um, JW. (2006). Deep tracheal laceration after balloon dilation for benign tracheobronchial stenosis: case reports of two patients. *Br J Radiol*, Vol.79, pp. 529-535.

Knott, PD.; Lorenz, RR.; Eliachar, I. & Murthy, SC. (2004). Reconstruction of a tracheobronchial tree disruption with bovine pericardium. *Int Cardiovasc Thorac Surg*, Vol.3, pp. 554-556.

Larson, BJ.; Zumberg, MS. & Kitchens CS. (2005). A feasibility study of continuing dose-reduced warfarin for invasive procedures in patients with high thromboembolic risk. *Chest*, Vol.127, No.3, pp. 922-927.

Lee, KH.; Ko, GY. Song, HY. Shim, TS. & Kim, WS. (2002). Benign tracheobronchial stenoses: long-term clinical experience with balloon dilation. *J Vasc Interv Radiol*, Vol.13, pp. 909-914.

Lee, KW.; Im, JG.; Han, JK.; Kim, TK.; Park, JH. & Yeon, KM. (1999). Tuberculous stenosis of the left main bronchus: results of treatment with balloons and metallic stents. *J Vasc Interv Radiol*, Vol.10, No.3, pp. 352-358.

Mayse, ML.; Greenheck, J.; Friedman, M. & Kovitz, KL. (2004). Successful bronchoscopic balloon dilation of nonmalignant tracheobronchial obstruction without fluoroscopy. *Chest*, Vol.126, No.2, pp. 634-637.

McDonald, IH. & Stocks, JG. (1965). Prolonged nasotracheal intubation. *Br J Anaesth*, Vol.37, pp. 161-173.

Morcos, SK.; Baudouin, SV.; Anderson, PB.; Beedie, R. & Bury, RW. (1989). Iotrolan in selective bronchography via the fiberoptic bronchoscope. *Br J Radiol*, Vol.62, No.736, pp. 383-385.

Morcos, SK.; Anderson, PB.; Baudouin, SV.; Clout, C.; Fairlie, N.; Baudouin, C. & Warnock, N. (1990). Suitability of and tolerance to Iotrolan 300 in bronchograhy via the fiberoptic bronchoscope. *Thorax*, Vol.45, pp. 628-629.

Nakamura, K.; Terada, N.; Ohi, M.; Matsushita, T.; Kato, N. & Nakagawa, T. (1991). Tuberculous bronchial stenosis: treatment with balloon bronchoplasty. *AJR*, Vol.157, pp. 1187-1188.

Olsson, T.; Bjornstad-Pettersen, H. & Stjernberg, NL. (1979). Bronchostenosis due to sarcoidosis. *Chest*, Vol.75, No.6, pp. 663-666.

Parkin, JL.; Stevens, MH. & Jung, AL. (1976). Acquired and congenital subglottic stenosis in the infant. *Ann Otol Rhinol Laryngol*, Vol.85, pp. 573-581.

Riebel, T. & Wartner, R. (1990). Use of non-ionic contrast media for tracheobronchography in neonates and young infants. *Eur J Radiol*, Vol.11, pp. 120-124.

Rooney, CP.; Ferguson, JS.; Barnhart, W.; Cook-Granroth, J.; Ross, A.; Hoffman, EA. & McLennan, G. (2005). Use of 3-dimensional computed tomography reconstruction studies in the preoperative assessment of patients undergoing balloon dilatation for tracheobronchial stenosis. *Respiration*, Vol.72, pp. 579-586.

Sheski, FD. & Mathur, PN. (1998). Long-term results of fiberoptic bronchoscopic balloon dilation in the management of benign tracheobronchial stenosis. *Chest*, Vol.114, No.3. pp. 796-800.

Wilson, NJ. (1945). Bronchoscopic observations in tuberculous tracheobronchitis-clinical and pathological correlation. *Dis Chest*, Vol.11, pp.36-59.

9

Endoscopic Percutaneous Tracheotomy in Prolonged Intubation of Mechanical Ventilated Patients Admitted in Cardio-Thoracic Intensive Care Unit

Rosa Mastropierro, Michela Bettinzoli and Aldo Manzato
Division of Cardiothoracic Intensive Care Unit, Spedali Civili Brescia
Italy

1. Introduction

Recent advances in surgical and anesthesia technology and biotechnology have made the intensive management of patients who have undergone open heart procedures more demanding.

New interventions and treatment strategies are desirable to improve the outcomes of this specific group of patients. Tracheotomy was performed mainly to prevent laryngeal and upper airway damage due to prolonged tracheal intubation after cardiac or thoracic surgery or medical illness.

In this chapter we will review and discuss the percutaneous dilational tracheotomy (PDT) approach in cardiac surgery patients who need prolonged mechanical ventilation. Available data were located regarding the technique, timing, advantages and complications of the PDT. We also underlined the utility of bronchoscopy control during the procedure. We describe also our experience performing PDT with bronchoscopy control procedure on patients admitted to Cardiothoracic Intensive Care Unit (CTICU) patients. In our CTICU we have a long-term experience of tracheotomy with bronchoscopy control that yields better clinical practice and outcome.

2. New cardiac surgery patient profile

The features of cardiac surgery patients are changing, mainly regarding the increasing numbers of the elderly patients, re-operated patients, patients with advanced heart disease, and with many severe co-morbidities. The number of patients undergoing simultaneous coronary artery by-pass grafting (CABG) and valve replacement, ventricular aneurysmectomy, aortic surgery, or carotid endoarterectomy has also increased, as well as the number of patients undergoing transplant and/or implantation of ventricular assist device as a bridge to transplant by the Intensive Care Units (ICU).

This new profile of cardiac surgical patient has lead to an increasing demand for high-tech medical interventions, such as mechanical ventilation in ICU.

Many of these patients are able to resume spontaneous ventilation as soon as they recovered from the anesthesia. The decision to extubate a patient depend on the recovery of physiological homeostasis, through return to normothermia, adequate heart and lung function, intravascular volume replacement, electrolyte normalization and optimization of pain relief. The extubation can be perform 24 hours a day as soon as these criteria are met.

The clinical and economic advantages of early extubation (within 4-8 hours after the ICU admission) are widely documented and show very positive results (Rajakaruna et al., 2005). This procedure has mainly reduced the adverse effects of positive pressure ventilation, including barotraumas. It has also decrease the potential incidence of infections and has minimized patient discomfort. Many studies have also shown that it reduces the length of intensive care unit, and therefore hospital stay and related costs (Rajakaruna et al., 2005).

However, approximately 2.6% to 22.7% of patients still require prolonged mechanical ventilation (PMV). This large variability depends on the selected criteria and guidelines adopted to define PMV. For example, Rajakaruna et al (Rajakaruna et al., 2005) conducted an observational study of 7553 patients and concluded that the PMV condition should be defined by a time period of more than 96 hours; while Alfieri et al (Pappalardo et al., 2004), studying the long-term survival and quality of life of 4827 adult cardiac surgical patients, define the PMV duration as more than seven days. Our literature review does not indicate a consensus regarding the exact definition of PMV.

3. Risk factors and clinical and economic effects of the PMV

Prolonged mechanical ventilation after cardiac and thoracic operations has become increasingly common over the past years. To rationalize the ICU work, improve the outcomes of this patients and contain the health care cost in literature (Trouillet et al., 2011) we identified a list of risk factors of PMV. Many authors (Cislaghi et al., 2009; Murthy et al., 2007; Trouillet et al., 2011) found implication of *preoperative* variables such as old age, higher BMI, diabetes mellitus, high pulmonary arterial blood pressure, New York Heart Association (NYHA) class higher than 2, ejection fraction under 50%, preoperative intraaortic balloon pump, creatinine clearance lower than 50 mL/min, operative priority. *Intraoperative* variables include the type of surgery (multiple valve replacement, aortic procedures, heart transplantation and reoperation), cardiopulmonary bypass (CPB) duration, intraaortic balloon pump. *Postoperative* variables include SAPS II higher than 45, neurologic event, lung injury, renal failure, internal bleeding, major arrhythmia.

Moreover several studies (Cislaghi et al., 2009; Trouillet et al., 2011) suggest that PVM is associated with higher in-hospital morbidity, mortality, and costs.

4. Technique

4.1 Lab studies

Many tracheotomies are electively performed on patients with secure airways (eg, for prolonged intubation) therefore it is reasonable to control hematologic parameters including hemoglobin (Hb), platelet count (PC) prothrombin time (PT), partial prothrombin time (PTT), and INR since it became available in 1998. A adequate correction must be eventually assured to take PC to a value greater than 50, and INR to a value of less than 1.5.

As with any procedure, the decision to perform an emergency tracheotomy is not influenced by lab parameters.

4.2 Setting and patient preparation

The old method of performing tracheotomy in critically ill patients requires transport from the intensive care unit (ICU) to the operating theatre, were the surgical team performed the tracheotomy. The percutaneous technique, for the limited dissection, results in less tissue damage and lower bleeding, and can be performed at the bedside on the ICU avoiding the risks related to the patients transportation. Furthermore, this technique can be successfully managed by intensivists, without specialized surgical training.

The patient usually has already a translaringeal endotracheal (TE) tube in place before tracheotomy. Continuous vital signs, pulse-oximetry, and complete ventilatory parameters are monitored throughout the procedure, antibiotic prophyaxis is necessary with a single dose of second generation cefalosporin.

General anesthesia is performed, using propofol, fentanyl, and pancuronium. Ten minutes before the tracheotomy procedure the positive end-expiratory pressure was reduced stepwise to 5 mm Hg if required, and all patients received positive-pressure ventilation with 100% oxygen throughout the tracheotomy.

4.3 Cricothyroidotomy

This approach requires to place a tube through the cricothyroid membrane.

Cricothyroidotomy can be used to gain emergency access to the airway, but as it is associated with numerous complications, it is suggested to replace this tube within 48-72 hours with a standard tracheotomy.

4.4 Open surgical tracheotomy

Elective surgical tracheotomy (ST) is ideally performed in the operation room. However, bedside tracheotomy can be performed.

The technique has changed very little since its original description by Chevalier Jackson (Jackson, 1909). Briefly, a 4 cm to 5 cm vertical or horizontal skin incision is made 1 cm below the cricoid cartilage over the second to fourth tracheal rings and the pretracheal tissues are dissected; the endotracheal tube is slowly withdrawn to just above the tracheotomy incision, but not removed, in case difficulty in tracheotomy placement requires its urgent reinsertion. Finally the tube is inserted into the tracheotomy under direct vision.

As animal experiments suggest, the injury to the cricoid cartilage was a major risk factor for subsequent subglottic stenosis, De Leyn recommended placing the tracheostoma well below the cricoid cartilage (De Leyn et al., 2007).

4.5 Percutaneous dilational tracheotomy

The theoretical basis for the development of all percutaneous procedures is represented by the Seldinger's method that, since 1953, planned the needle replacement over a wire-guided for arterial catheterization.

The wire-guided percutaneous technique for percutaneous tracheostomy was developed and reported in the same year by the American surgeon Ciaglia, who combined the Seldinger wire nephrostomy tube multiple-dilator placement technique with a special, low-profile tracheostomy tube (Ciaglia et al, 1985).

Several different methods of performing percutaneous tracheostomy have been subsequently described.

4.5.1 The main different percutaneous techniques

Ciaglia first described PDT in 1985. The technique is based on progressive dilatation of a small initial tracheal aperture created by a needle, using a series of graduated dilators.

In 1990 Griggs described the Guidewire Dilating Forceps (GWDF) technique of percutaneous tracheotomy. It is based on enlarging a small tracheal aperture with a forceps, having a blunt tip and blunt edges.

In 1997 Fantoni and Ripamonti introduced the retrograd translaryngeal technique (TLT), another minimally invasive procedure achieved using a single device under direct vision with a rigid tracheoscope (RCT), subsequently replaced by a flexible fiberoptic bronchoscope (FFB).

In 1998, a modification of the Ciaglia technique was introduced (Ciaglia Blue Rhino Percutaneous Tracheotomy Introducer Kit; Cook Critical Care Inc., Bloomington, IN), whereby the series of dilators was replaced with a single, sharply tapered dilator, permitting complete dilatation in one step. It has been shown that the single dilator technique decreased operative time compared with the serial-dilator technique without increasing the complication rate.

However in 2002 Frova and Quintel described another procedure named PercuTwist, consisting in a single-step rotating dilatation tracheotomy applied with the use of a screw-like dilatators. The device is threaded into the tracheal stoma using a lifting motion.

In the present study we want describe in detail the Single Dilatator Ciaglia Blue Rhino Percutaneous Tracheotomy Technique with endoscopic guidance.

4.6 Ciaglia technique

The patient has usually endotracheal tube in place (regarding lab study, general anesthesia and antibiotic prophylaxis see above); the whole procedure is performed in direct vision with flexible bronchoscopy (BF-P240 or BF-40; Olympus; Tokyo, Japan) via translaryngeal tube.

Ciaglia technique is performed using the Ciaglia single dilator kit (Ciaglia Blue Rhino, Cook Critical Care, Bloomington, Illinois).

Vital signs are continuously monitored throughout the procedure, personnel are positioned with the operator to the patient's right, the bronchoscopist at the head of the bed, a circulating nurse is available to administer medications and otherwise assist in the procedure.

At the start the patient's neck is slightly reclined, inspected in detail, landmark points are indentified. The surgical area is cleansed and prepared with surgical drapes in the typical manner.

The broncoscopic placed in the endotracheal tube, having deflated endotracheal tube cuff with tapes loosened, together are withdrawn slowly to just below the vocal cords. Then the assistant held the tube with his hands continuously throughout the whole procedure and handles manual ventilation on a regimen of 1.0 FIO_2. The anatomical landmarks is identified by fiberoptic transillumination and digital manipulation of the trachea, approximately 2 fingerbreadths below the cricoid or 1 fingerbreadths above the sternal notch (Byhahn et al., 2000).

After identification of the translaryngeal puncture point, a 16-gauge Teflon introducer needle is inserted midline through the anterior wall of the trachea, between the first and second or second and third tracheal rings. The needle is withdrawn and replaced by the J-tipped guide-wire which is advanced through the Teflon sheath, toward the carina. The catheter sheath is removed and beveled plastic single dilator, held like a pen, and forced into the tracheal wall over the guide-wire, to create a tracheostoma. Once the tracheostoma has been dilated to the appropriated size, the loading dilator is removed to permit insertion of a specially tracheotomy tube into the trachea over the same guide-wire, using one of the dilators as a obturator. The cuff is inflated and ventilation resumes through the tracheotomy tube which is secured with a strap tied around the neck.

The bronchoscope, removed from the endotracheal tube, is placed through the tracheotomy tube to check its right position, to remove blood or bronchial secretions and, if necessary to collect the bronchoalveolar lavage (BAL), quantitative tracheal aspirate, or protected brush specimens (PSB).

The translaringeal tube is withdrawn when adequate ventilation is verified.

A dry dressing is applied to the neck and routine tracheotomy care is conducted, with cleaning and suctioning as required.

In 30% of the PDT, the tube passes through the thyroid isthmus, but bleeding is very rare, because the tracheotomy tube, being tightly fitting to the wall, acts as tamponade bleeding of vessels.

4.7 Comparison from different PDT techniques

The percutaneous techniques are based on the principle of tracheal puncture, stoma creation by dilation of the soft tissues of the neck and insertion of the tracheal tube, using the Seldinger technique. The differences are the shape and the managing of the dilator. Only the TLT is a reversed method in which, in contrast to the others procedures, the Seldinger wire is advanced cranially towards the larynx.

Few trials were published comparing these techniques, and very little information is available concerning the comparison of their early and late complications. Problems may be represented by the lack of precise definitions of outcome and early and late complications, or by the way in which these complications have been examined.

The studies that have been published so far on this topic are generally limited, and not adequately randomized. The follow-up of the tracheotomy patients can be difficult because of physical and mental problems. Therefore complications have not been investigated extensively (An˜ n et al., 2004; Ambesh et al., 2002).

The largest prospective randomized trial, comparing the most widely used percutaneous tracheotomy technique, was conducted by G.B. Fikkers (Fikkers et al., 2004, 2011). The author performed a meticulous observation of the procedures and follow-up. He involved in its study 120 patients, comparing the guide-wire dilating forceps (GWDF) and the single step dilatational tracheostomy (SSDT) technique, showing a trend toward less major perioperative complications with SSDT compared to GWDF technique. All procedures were conducted with bronchoscopic guidance, so that the optimal position of the cannula between the rings in the midline was always facilitated. However, more patients would be needed to detect smaller differences between the methods.

The rotating dilation (PercuTwist) and Griggs' forceps dilational tracheotomy methods were compared by Montcriol, in a recent prospective randomized study, involving 87 critical ill patients. The author found the PercuTwist significantly longer to perform than forceps dilational tracheotomy technique (five minutes vs three minutes), the complications were 20/87 (23%), and 18/20 were minor complications. He didn't found significant differences between the two groups of patients and concluded that the PercuTwist technique is safest, despite the longer duration of the procedure (Montcriol et al., 2011).

Since single dilator technique decrees operative time compared to the serial dilator technique, and without increasing the complication rates, the modified Ciaglia Blu Rhino technique is suggested as the technique of choice (level 2C, according to levels of evidence by American College of Chest Phisicians) (De Leyn, et al., 2007). Therefore, this is the only technique used in our centre, always under bronchoscopic guidance.

5. Timing of the tracheotomy

Overall, advances in clinical treatment and ICU practices are based on suitable mechanical ventilation. Many critical ill patients benefit from a prolonged ventilatory support program and subsequently from a meticulous weaning protocol from mechanical ventilation. In addition, the best clinical practice should always ensure patient comfort, safety, ability to communicate, clean oral and airway, as well as shorter days of mechanical ventilation, ICU and hospital stays. For these reasons tracheotomy is very beneficial, in fact with the now widespread use of the percutaneous technique with broncoscopic control, tracheotomy has become a very common practice in modern ICUs and in recent years, it has increased by nearly 200%. This raises the following three questions. The first is whether it is better to place early or late tracheotomy. The second is how to define "early" or "late tracheotomy". Finally, the third is the major methodological challenge, regarding how to define and predict the need for prolonged ventilation in different and specific groups of the patients.

For the first question, the best timing of tracheotomy has been a subject of debate and, still today, it has not found unanimous agreement. An analysis of a large database showed considerable variation in the timing and incidence of tracheotomy. In 1989 the consensus conference indicated that tracheotomy should be carried out after 3 weeks of endotracheal intubation (Plummer & Gracey 1989).

After, several studies have reported that tracheotomies which were performed earlier provided many benefits that include more rapid weaning from mechanical ventilation, shorter hospital length of stay (LOS), less complications from translaryngeal intubation, better patient's comfort and safety, facilitating progression of care in and outside the ICU (Rumbak et al., 2004).

Yaseen Arabi et al., in a cohort study and review, analyzed 136 trauma ICU patients who required tracheotomies, confirmed all these benefits of early tracheotomy and moreover he found, with a multivariate analysis, that late tracheotomy was an independent predictor of prolonged ICU stay (Arabi et al., 2004).

However others studies, including the large multicenter TracMan (Tracheostomy management in critical care, 2011) trial have found no differences between early and late timing of the procedure.

In a large prospective trial, Trouillet et al., randomized patients who required prolonged mechanical ventilation after heart surgery, assigning to early tracheotomy (5 days after surgery) or prolonged intubation followed by tracheotomy 15 days after randomization. In this study early tracheotomy provided no benefits in term of mechanical ventilation duration, LOS, mortality rate, or frequency of infectious complications, but it was associated with a lower rate of agitation or delirium, with less sedative, analgesic and neuroleptic consumption and better patient comfort, fewer unscheduled estubation and re-intubation, earlier oral nutrition and bed-to chair transfer (Trouillet et al., 2009).

A systematic review, including randomized and non-randomized studies, has not been able to support the effects of tracheotomy on duration of mechanical ventilation in all patients (Griffiths et al., 2005). The effects of early tracheotomy on mechanical ventilation, VAP, hospital outcome and LOS, remaining hotly debated. Therefore, there is still no consensus about "early" or "late tracheotomy" definition, many clinicians use their own specific time window.

In 2001 Guidelines, created jointly by the American Association for Respiratory Care, the American College of Chest Physicians, and the American College of Critical Care Medicine, make no specific recommendations about tracheotomy timing, but suggest that the procedure should be considered if the patient will require prolonged ventilator assistance (De Leyn et al., 2007).

In 2005 surveys involving a large number of ICU from France and the United Kingdom documented variability for both the timing and the indications for tracheostomy (Blot & Melot 2005).

Contemporary the group of Rumbak in a prospective, randomized study, comparing early with late tracheotomy, he defined "early tracheotomy", if performed within 48 hours and "late tracheotomy" if performed at 2 weeks. The authors showed a decrease of mortality by 50% in first group (Rumbak et al., 2004).

The same authors in a 2007 study confirmed that early tracheotomy reduces time in the ICU, on mechanical ventilation, and in the hospital, whereas benefits regarding incidence of pneumonia and mortality are variable according to the different patient population ().

An analysis of the US National Trauma Databank showed that the rate and timing of tracheotomy varied significantly across ICUs (Nathens et al., 2006).

Finally in answer to the third question, the lack of the population homogeneity is frequently evocated as a limit for these studies which aim to define the criteria in order to determine if a patient will require prolonged mechanical ventilation, and then identify the best timing to perform the tracheotomy. However, up to now, despite many efforts, no scoring system has been able to correctly identify patients for whom MV duration will be prolonged and, therefore, the early tracheotomy might be justified.

Especially after cardiac surgery, several studies have investigated factors associated with prolonged MV and many models have been developed in attempt to predict when the patients are designed to prolonged MV more than 48 hours.

Some authors in their studies refer alternatively to preoperative, intraoperative and immediately postoperative parameters, others showed that hemodynamic status on ICU admission and early postoperative events were more important than intraoperative variables, to predict ventilatory dependence, defined as MV greater than 72 hours after cardiac surgery (Cislaghi et al., 2009; Rajakaruna et al., 2005).

Trouillet, in is prospective observational study, considers, with a simple score, the clinical answer of the patient to the medical treatments during the first 3 days of the MV is more indicative of the prognosis than of any data gathered in a pre-operative or post-operative period. None of these models has been fully validated yet (Trouillet et al., 2011). However the message is to achieve a valid score to avoid a probably unnecessary invasive procedure, such as early tracheotomy in patients with a strong likelihood of rapid and successful MV weaning. Instead tracheotomy might be a right option in patients requiring longer MV and the highest safety may be achieved if it is performed with bronchoscopic guidance.

In our opinion, waiting further studies aimed to answer these important questions, for optimal management of critical ill patients, the decision regarding the best timing to perform tracheotomy depends on the physician, that should balance three problems: what is the patient expected recovery course, the risk of prolonged translaryngeal intubation and the risk of tracheotomy procedure.

6. The bronchoscopic guidance features

A problem with the PDT is the lack of visualization, therefore some studies suggested that the safety of the procedure may be enhanced by the use of ultrasound or bronchoscopic guidance (De Leyn et al., 2007; Kollig et al., 2000). However few randomized controlled trials have shown the utility of the bronchoscopic guidance during the percutaneous tracheotomy procedure.

In a clinical review, P. De Leyn et al, indicate in level 1C of the grading scheme classified recommendations, to perform any technique of PDT under bronchoscopic control. (De Leyn et al., 2007).

Over blind PDT, several goals are recognized by the video bronchoscopic guidance of puncture/dilatation process. Before initiating the procedure, the endoscopic survey can show any anatomic airway anomalies that may be encountered (Bobo et al., 1998).

During bronchoscopy proximal repositioning of the TE before introducing the guide-wire needle into the trachea can facilitate the procedure, and reduce the risk of the tube impalement; it shows the correct central area of the puncture and the appropriate tracheal rings with wound transillumination (Kost et al., 2005).

Initial needle placement in a midline, intercartilaginous position can be verified and corrected, as overpenetration of the lumen to the posterior tracheal wall. In a blind technique, tangential needle positioning is likely to go unrecognized, increasing risks of complications such as false passage, pneumothorax and pneumomediastinum (Kost et al., 2005).

Using endoscopic vision, technical difficulties can be recognized and corrected before life-threatening complications occur (Kost et al., 2005).

Finally it is an excellent tool for teaching PDT technique.

Nevertheless, some limitations of bronchoscopic guidance are recognized. They include impairment of mechanical ventilation and oxygenation, in fact manual ventilation is recommended, then the need for additional personnel, and added procedural time and expense.

During the procedure a potential increase in partial carbon dioxide tension and reduction in partial oxygen tension can raise intracranial pressure in susceptible patients (De Leyn et al., 2007). However, in many studies some authors confirms that percutaneous dilatational tracheotomy with endoscopy is a safe and acceptable alternative to open surgical tracheotomy.

7. Advantages of tracheotomy versus translaryngeal intubation

In recent years, the tracheotomy positioning has gained increased popularity as a resource to facilitate the patients weaning from the mechanical ventilation.

Several studies argue that early tracheotomy (within 7 days of mechanical ventilation) in ICU patients may help to reduce the duration of mechanical ventilation and length of stay in ICU (Carrer et al., 2009).

The tracheostomy allows to reduce the duration of mechanical ventilation, because of improves secretions removal with suctioning, decreases resistance to breathing and dead space, betters patient comfort with less needed of sedation or analgesia, preserves the glottic competence reducing incidence of ventilatory-associated pneumonia (VAP) and others lung infection (Durbin Jr, 2005).

Tracheostomy offers others advantages, it reduces the laryngeal injury as laryngeal stenosis and voice damage, reduces the oral injury, allows a better oral hygiene, improves the ability to communicate, preserves more the swallow with earlier oral feeding (Durbin Jr, 2005).

7.1 Potential advantages of PDT versus surgical tracheotomy

PDT is a cost-effective and safe alternative to surgical tracheostomy (ST) in critically ill patients in the ICU, and can be performed with very low morbidity by skilled and experienced practitioners (De Leyn, et al., 2007).

The main advantage of PDT is the possibility to perform it at the bedside in the ICU, avoiding a potentially dangerous transport of critically ill patients to the operating room. It prevents the inconvenience of long waiting lists for operating room scheduling and significantly decreases the delay between the decision to perform tracheostomy and the actual operation (De Leyn, et al., 2007).

In a retrospective analysis performed on clinical and financial outcomes, PDT resulted associated to less costs compared to surgical tracheostomy (Bacchetta et al., 2005).

This is predominantly a result of avoiding operating room charges (De Leyn et al., 2007).

In general, PDT appears to be a less traumatic and minimally invasive procedure than ST. In fact the incision in PDT is very small, the tracheotomy tube is fitted tightly against the stoma, and less dissection, tissue trauma and devitalisation occur; furthermore cartilage rings usually remain more or less intact during PDT, while most surgeons incise one or more tracheal cartilage rings during ST.

These advantages are probably responsible for the favorable outcomes, fewer overall postoperative complications described in short-term and long-term follow-up studies of patients undergoing PDT (Nieszkowska et al., 2005; Sue & Susanto 2003), including less postoperative and perioperative bleeding, fewer wound infection and subglottic stenosis and an aesthetically more favorable scar (Grillo, 2004).

7.2 Tracheotomy and lung infections

A potential, important benefit, without agreement in literature yet, attributed to tracheotomy, especially when it is provided at an early stage, is a lower ventilator-associated pneumonia (VAP) rate (Nseir et al., 2007; Rodriguez et al., 1990; Rumbak et al., 2004).

Micro-aspiration of oral secretions past the tube cuff can contribute to the development of pneumonia. In addition, dental plaques, the oropharyngeal cavity and the stomach are potential reservoirs for microorganisms in critically ill patients requiring mechanical ventilation through an endotracheal tube or a tracheotomy cannula (El-Solh, 2004; Frost & Wise, 2008). The most important underlying mechanism for the onset of VAP is the aspiration of oropharyngeal microorganisms into the distal bronchi, followed by bacterial proliferation and parenchymal invasion, leading to bronchopneumonia (El-Solh, 2004). The presence of an endotracheal tube and the aspiration of oropharyngeal contents, containing a large bacterial inoculum can overcome the host defenses that are already compromised by the critical illness and lead to the development of VAP (Frost & Wise, 2008; Kollef, 1999).

Some studies indicate an increased incidence in lower respiratory-tract infections following tracheotomy. However no adjustment was performed for the duration of the MV, which is probably the most important risk factor for VAP.

In a large, randomized controlled trial of patients who require prolonged mechanical ventilation after cardiac surgery, Trouillet et al. showed that early tracheotomy did not modify the frequency of VAP during the first 60 days after randomization between early percutaneous tracheotomy and prolonged intubation groups possibly followed by late tracheotomy (Trouillet et al., 2011).

Other authors found tracheotomy protective against VAP using matching for several confounding factors, including duration of MV.

Considering the patophysiology of VAP in intubated patients, Nseir demonstrated in a retrospective case-control study, that tracheotomy was independently associated with a decreased risk of VAP compared to patients with translaryngeal intubation. The potential reasons include: liberation of the vocal cords in tracheotomised patients, that results in normal closure and reduces the risk related to aspiration of contaminated secretions from the orofaryngeal cavity; in a reduction in bacterial biofilm formation along the inside of the tracheotomy cannula, associated with regular changing of the tube, once or twice a week; finally in a shorter duration of mechanical ventilation due to facilitation of MV weaning (Nseir et al., 2007). Furthermore, the oral care is better in tracheotomised patients than in intubated ones: in fact, the endotracheal tube may obscure the view of the oral cavity and predispose to xerostomia, which contributes to poor oral hygiene.

So, since some hospitals propose oral care programs for the VAP prevention, the tracheotomy must be considered (Schleder et al., 2002).

8. Complications of percutaneous dilational tracheotomy

Complications of tracheotomy can be divided into early and late incidences.

8.1 Early complications

Hemorrhage has been reported as the most common complication of PDT and occurs in 0 to 28.6% of cases. It is usually controlled by simply packing or suture ligation (Bobo et al., 1998). With open tracheotomy this rate dramatically increases in 3 to 36% of cases.

Another common complication is stoma infection: a tracheotomy is considered a clean-contaminated wound and for this reason antibiotic prophylaxis is necessary. Instead this infection is quite uncommon with PDT, occurring in up to 4% of cases (Bobo et al., 1998) while with the surgical tracheotomy the rates are higher generally occurring in 17 to 36% of cases.

Subcutaneous or mediastinal emphysema is another additional complication when subcutaneous emphysema can be caused by positive pressure ventilation or by cough against a tightly sutured or packed wound. The emphysema disappears spontaneously within a few days. Instead mediastinal emphysema is very uncommon and occurs in very few cases as pneumothorax which is caused by a false passage and is evidenced by chest radiograph (De Leyn et al., 2007).

A further complication is a tube displacement, caused either by inadequate securement of the tube around the neck or rapid cervical swelling. After the reinsertion of the tube, a false channel in the subcutaneous tissue anterior to the tracheal ostium may compress the trachea and cause an emergency. Then orotracheal intubation is needed when the tract cannot be restored immediately (De Leyn et al., 2007; Heffner et al., 1986). Finally, tube obstruction which can be caused by mucus or blood clots even displacement. If it is not possible to clean the tube, it must be replaced.

8.2 Late complications

One of the most common complications of tracheotomy is pulmonary infections mainly for pneumonia. A large proportion of ventilatory-associated pneumonia (VAP) develops within the first week after tracheotomy. The most common pathogens isolated are Pseudomonas aeruginosa and Gram-negative enteric bacteria that colonize the tracheobronchial tree in patients with long-term tracheotomy. The colonization of the airways depends on the severity of the disease, nutritional status of the patient and depression of mucociliary clereance caused by tracheotomy. In this cases it is advisable to consider a periprocedural antibiotic prophylaxis (De Leyn et al., 2007; Heffner et al., 1986; Rello et al., 2003).

Tracheal stenosis occurs in 1 to 2% of cases and can affect the tracheal stoma differently, the cuff or the tip of the tracheotomy tube. This complication result from ischemic damage to the tracheal mucosa when the high-pressure cuff are used and the tracheal wall tension exceeds mucosal capillary perfusion pressure for significant periods of time. Within 15 minutes of a continuous tracheal wall pressure above 50 mmHg, destruction of columnar epithelium happens. Inflammatory histologic changes result within 24 to 48 hours with superficial tracheitis and mucosal ulcerations appearing after several days. If persists inflammation, chondritis develops with deterioration of cartilaginous support within two to three weeks. The granulation and fibrosis that appear during recovery, produce the tracheal stenosis. Clinical manifestations of tracheal stenosis after tracheotomy include dyspnea on effort, cough and difficult to remove secretions. The symptoms appear when there is a 75% of reduction in tracheal lumen diameter. The treatment of tracheal stenosis consists in surgical trachea resection or tracheal dilatation.

On the other hand, tracheo-innominate artery fistula is quite uncommon (<0.7%) and can be determined by high direct pressure of the cannula against the innominate artery or by a too low placed tracheotomy tube that erode directly into the artery, because the innominate artery crosses the anterolateral surface of the trachea at the level of the upper sternum. The result is airway bleeding in which a possible sudden massive hemmorhage can cause a life-threatening condition. The overall survival rate of this complication is 25%. Therefore in order to prevent such incidences, thacheotomy should be performed at the second or third cartilaginous ring and should avoid prolonged or excessive hyperextension of the neck, using a re-adjustable tracheotomy tube (De Leyn et al., 2007; Heffner et al., 1986). Tracheo-esophageal fistula is another complication which occurs in less than 1% of cases. Early onset results from poor surgical techniques with the incision of the posterior tracheal wall. Late onset results from tracheal necrosis caused by excessive cuff pressure. The patient presents excessive secretions, food aspiration and leaking around the cuff with abdominal distension, the respiratory parameters can worsen in such cases. Tracheoscopy or esophagography can be used for the diagnosis. The treatment consists in a cervical incision when the patient is clinically stable (De Leyn et al., 2007; Heffner et al., 1986).

Swallowing difficulties are caused by decreased laryngeal elevation, esophageal compression and obstruction from the tracheotomy tube cuff concur resulting in swallowing difficulties (De Leyn et al., 2007).

Granuloma may result from a foreign body reaction to the tracheotomy tube (De Leyn et al., 2007).

Finally, persistent stoma can result from epithelialisation between the skin and the tracheal mucosa when the tube is in place for a prolonged period (De Leyn et al., 2007).

9. Materials and methods

9.1 Study location and patient population

This study was conducted in the CTICU of the Civil Hospital, Brescia, Italy, and a 2400-bed, university-affiliated teaching hospital. This CTICU has 6 beds available, including 1 for emergencies. Any patients undergoing heart and thoracic surgery, and occasionally other medical and surgical patients, are admitted to this CTICU.

Between 2006 and 2010, 184 patients required PMV (≥ 4 days), among these, 134 patients underwent percutaneous dilatational tracheotomy (PDT) with endoscopic guidance were retrospectively evaluated.

9.2 Study design and data collection

For all patients studied, the following data was retrospectively collected from ICU database: age, sex, origin (other ICU or hospital ward), SAPS II (Simplified Acute Physiology Score), reason for and diagnosis at ICU admission, mode of surgery (elective, urgent, emergent), duration of mechanical ventilation, re-intubation, timing of tracheotomy, complications of tracheotomy including pneumonia or other lung infections, ICU stay duration and outcome (patients transferred or died).

9.3 Technique

The patients enrolled in the study were those who required tracheotomy due to failure to be weaned from mechanical ventilation. The physicians in the department established the timing of tracheotomy. All tracheotomies were conducted at the patient bedside by experienced physicians in the ICU using the Ciaglia percutaneous technique (Ciaglia Blue Rhino, Cook Critical Care, Bloomington, Illinois) described before, in the technique section.

10. Results

10.1 Patients

Among the 3648 consecutive patients admitted in the CTICU from January 2006 to December 2010, a total of 184 were still intubated 4 or more days after CTICU admission. Therefore, a tracheotomy was performed on 134 patients of these patients.

Table 1 shows the preoperative and surgical characteristics, including the demographic, descriptive data of the patients and their department of origin.

Characteristics		Value* n = 134
Age, years		69.8 ± 9.2
Gender		
	Male	94 (70.1)
	Female	40 (29.9)
Department of origin		
	Cardiac surgery	82 (61.2)
	Thoracic surgery	15 (11.2)
	Coronary care unit	14 (10.4)
	Other medical or surgical wards	12 (8.9)

Characteristics		Value* n = 134
	Emergency rooms	9 (6.7)
	Other ICU wards	2 (1.5)
SAPS II		46.2 ± 20.3
Length of stay in CTICU		20.8 ± 13.5
Overall mortality		65 (48.5)

CTICU, Cardiothoracic Intensive Care Unit; PDT, percutaneous dilational tracheotomy
* Values are expressed as means ± SD or n (%).

Table 1. Characteristics of 134 study CTICU admitted patients requiring PDT.

Of the 134 patients, 94 (70.1%) were male, and the mean age ± SD was 69.8 ± 9.2 years (range: 32-85 years).

The mean ± SD SAPS II score on admission was 46.2 ± 20.3.

The mean ± SD length of stay in the ICU was 20.8 ± 13.5 days (Fig. 1).

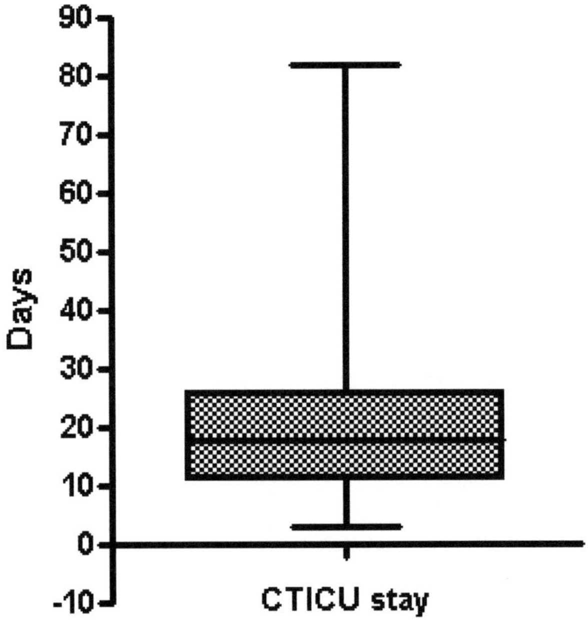

Fig. 1. ICU length of stay of patients received percutaneous dilational tracheotomy (PDT).

Of the 134 patients studied, 113 (84.3%) were surgical; of these, 39 (34.5%) underwent a valve replacement, 17 (15.0%) a coronary artery bypass graft (CABG), 22 (19.5%) a CABG with valve replacement, 16 (14.1%) an aortic surgery (ascending aortic surgery, aortic arch surgery, descending thoracic surgery), 12 (10.6%) a pulmonary resection for neoplasm, and 7 (6.2%) a surgery for miscellaneous conditions. Surgical intervention was performed in election in 92 (81.4%) cases, was urgent in 21 (18.6%) cases.

The twenty-one medical patients (15.7%) admitted to the ICU suffered from heart and/or respiratory failure.

10.2 Mechanical ventilation and tracheotomy

The mean ± SD duration of mechanical ventilation was 17.8 ± 12.2 days (Fig. 2).

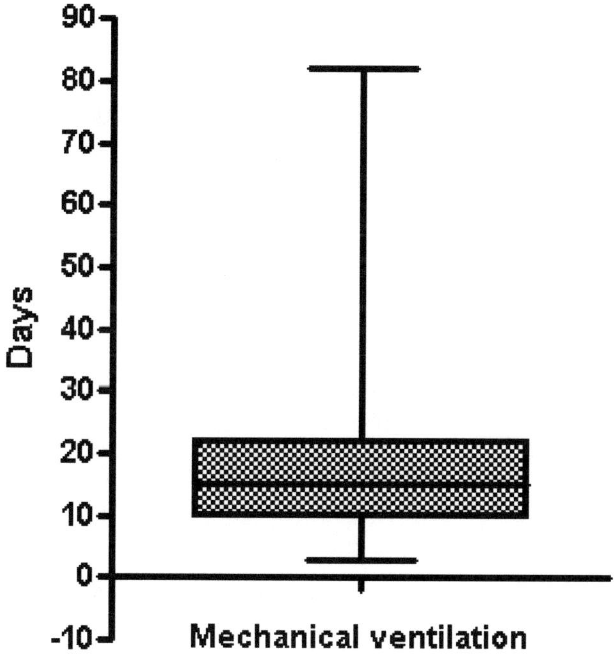

Fig. 2. Length of mechanical ventilation through endotracheal tube or tracheotomy.

Seventy patients (52.2%) were re-intubated.

The patients received a tracheotomy after a mean ± SD of 4.7 ± 2.5 days of endotracheal intubation (Table 2).

	Value*
During of ventilation, days	17.8 ± 12.2
Patients undergoing reintubation	70 (52.2)
Timing of tracheotomy, days	4.7 ± 2.5

* Values are expressed as means ± SD or n (%).

Table 2. Ventilation Data for 134 Patients Who Underwent Percutaneous Dilatational Tracheotomy

Any major side effect or technical problem that occurred during the procedure was recorded.

We assessed four minor complications: two episodes of tracheal rings fracture having no significant, and two minor stomal bleeding without transfusion requirements.

10.3 Pneumonia and other airway infections

Of the 134 patients, the cumulative incidence of VAP was 40.3% (n=54) and 19.4% of other airway infections (n=26).

10.4 Mortality and outcome

Overall, 65 patients (48.5%) died, while 69 patients (51.5%) who survived were transferred at day 2 or 3 after the tracheotomy to other departments, 42 (60.8%) requiring prolonged ventilation support, were weaned in a non-ICU department.

11. Conclusion

PDT is described as a safe technique, easier to perform with fewer overall postoperative complications, such as less pre and postoperative bleeding and fewer postoperative stomal infections than surgical tracheotomy (ST).

PDT is a procedure in rapidly evolving state regarding its technology and the number of the technique available. The safety of the procedure may be enhanced by the use of bronchoscopic guidance. The Tracheotomy Endoscope is just designed to prevent serious complications in dilational tracheotomies and facilitate their management, so that patients with tracheotomy, can be moved in SNF, even if ventilator support is necessary. It is also interesting that the method is very easy to learn.

The major indication of the PDT is prolonged mechanical ventilation (PMV), there are evidences supporting that PDT reduces work of breathing, facilitates the weaning and reduces length of MV.

Although there isn't agreement in literature about the PMV definition, many authors, so that in present study, judge "prolonged" the mechanical ventilation lasting for more than 96 hours, both continuously or after re-intubation.

Several authors showed that in medical ICU, PVM is a widely treatment that induces longer hospitalization and high costs. In CTICU, where it occurs in 2.6 to 22.7% according to various authors, is also associated with increased patient morbidity and mortality (range, 4.9-38%), its cost instead of 12% of the total.

Early weaning from MV, within 8-12 hours after open heart surgery, being associated with better cardiac function, and with a decrease in respiratory and infectious complications, should be the gold standard in the CTICU.

Continuously PMV begins necessary in selected, high-risk cardiac surgery patients, normally identified preoperatively, or recognized in the immediate postoperative.

Sometimes, in a not insignificant number of the patients without evident risk factors, activation of the inflammatory cascade due to the cardiopulmonary bypass (CPB), can be responsible for failing of the early extubation, making it necessary for re-intubation, and then for PMV.

As in most studies, our data showed a low rate of PMV in CTICU patients. Among 3648 admitted in our unit, over the past five years, 194 (5.3%) required PMV, of these 134 (69%) were underwent to PDT. Seventy PDT were performed to re-intubated patients.

We don't have data that could explain the reasons of PMV, why was not this the aim of the present study, therefore it will soon the object of the future work, to improve the management and the outcome of our patients.

It would be very important to find a score able to identify patients requiring PMV and consequently the best timing to perform tracheotomy. Many scores are developed, but due to their stiffness, poorly adapted to heterogeneous groups of admitted in ICU, none of these has been so far validated.

It is not shown in current literature yet, which is the right time when the tracheotomy must be performed, there is not even agreement regarding the exact definition of "early" and "late" tracheotomy.

Most well designed studies, focused on timing of tracheotomy, comparing tracheotomised with translaryngeal ventilator patients, showed a statistically significant reduction in mortality with "early" tracheotomy.

Rumbak et al., defined "early" (within 2 days from the MV) and "late" (days 14-16) tracheotomy, they compared the two methods and they showed a statistically significant reduction in mortality with early tracheotomy (31.7% vs 61.7% respectively) (Rumbak et al., 2004).

Driven by the need to not hinder the operating list and to optimize the resources, we performed tracheotomies after a mean ± SD of 4.7 ± 2.5 days from the beginning of the MV (Fig. 3), once a tracheostomy is in place, then we transferred patients to a skilled nursing facility (SNF), also with ventilator support.

Of all surviving, 69 (51.5%) were transferred to others departments at days 2 or 3 after tracheotomy, of these 42 (60.8%) requiring prolonged ventilation support, they were wean in non-ICU environment.

This appears rational and cost/effective, because if the tube is dislodged, no special equipment or skills are needed to replace it; after the stomal tract has matured, usually within 3–7 days, the tube can be easily reinserted without difficulty. The SNF are often able to wean from ventilator support.

Earlier transition of a patient from the ICU remains a major advantage of tracheostomy. To shorten ICU length of stay reduces health care costs.

The complication rates reported in most previously published large studies and meta-analyses ranging from 8.9 to 30%. They include severe complications in 1.5% of all cases and less dangerous complications that amounted to 6.5% (Bause et al., 1999). The most frequently complications related to the procedure concern malpositioning, tracheal stenosis, stomal infections, bleeding (rate of 3.2%) with transfusion requirements, respiratory failure (pneumothorax, pneumomediastinum) or need to change ventilator settings.

In this study, no serious side effects both during and after the procedure have occurred.

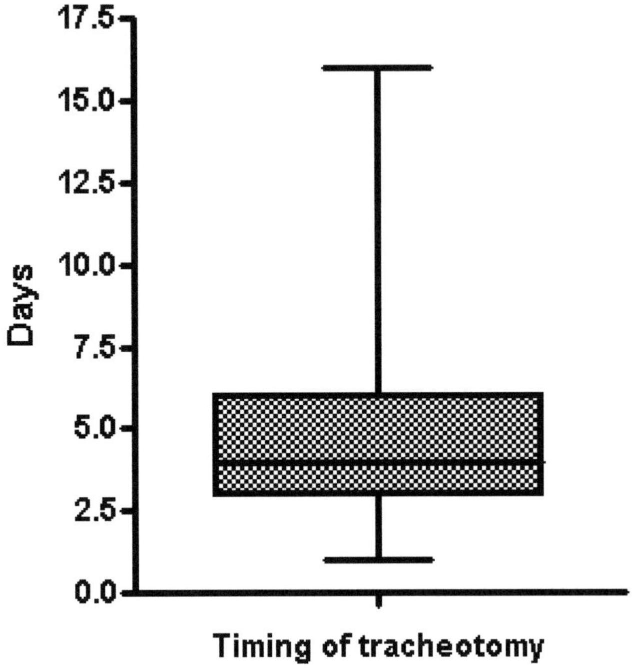

Fig. 3. Timing of tracheotomy after endotracheal intubation.

We assessed only four minor complications, regarding two episodes of tracheal rings fractures having no significant, and two minor stomal bleeding, without transfusion requirements.

One patient with enormous goitre was addressed directly to the ST, without consequence.

We attribute our low complication rates to careful evaluations of the right indications and the contraindications, and to the combination of the right timing of the procedure, and the fact that all procedures are performed in the CTICU by a team of experienced physicians, under bronchoscopic guidance.

In an our previous study (Mastropierro et al., 2009), we discovered bronchoscopy as an independent risk factor for VAP. Ever after, in our centre, the use of this technique is strictly controlled and decided by skilled and specialized health staff. Indications for this practice are well underlined in our protocols. PDT is a part of the indications, since, as demonstrated by literature and our experience, bronchoscopy has revealed to be useful for avoiding wrong insertions of tracheocannula and for finding possible endothracheal complications.

Among patients with tracheotomy, we detected an high mortality (48.5%), probably related to the high-risk profile of the patients referring to the heart and thoracic surgery, as preoperative comorbidities, complex surgery (19.5% was CABG combined with valve replacement), urgent surgery which was 18.6% of total. These factors increasing likelihood of prolonged MV, worsen the outcome. So the patients died with tracheotomy, but not for tracheotomy.

There is a paucity of clinical data describing the association of tracheotomy with patient outcomes, especially hospital mortality.

Marx et al. reported in their study a mortality rate of 0.39% (Marx et al., 1996).

Kollef in a prospective cohort study, describe outcomes of patients with respiratory failure in PMV, receiving a tracheostomy. They found the overall hospital mortality for patients receiving a tracheostomy (13.7%) was significantly less than the overall hospital mortality for patients with translaryngeal intubation (26.4%) (Kollef, 1999). Any reasons to explain this data are widely discussed.

Combining advances in technology and treatments with control healthcare costs, suggest that the effectiveness of patient care could be maintained or improved, and in meantime ICU expenses reduced.

The features of the cardiac surgery patients are changing, many of these suffering of multiple co morbidities. Concurrent with these changes, the needs for critical care service are increasing. Needham et al. estimated that the number of ICU patients who require MV will increase by 31% from 2000 to 2026 (Needham et al., 2005). PMV is commonly associated with substantially longer inpatient, ICU stay and higher cost.

In our experience PDT with broncoscopic guidance, that guarantees very low complications, must be considered as a best practice, aimed to reduce length of ICU and hospital stay, and to optimize healthcare resources.

Although we recognize some methodological limits in our study. First of all, it is an observational study and is not able to give strong messages. Missing data regard: the reasons of the failed early extubation in CTICU patients; the follow-up of the patients weaned from ventilator support in SNF, though there has always been a collaborative job between the CTICU and the SNF physicians. Current study also suggests to deepen the knowledge regarding both the incidence of VAP in patients with tracheotomy, performed with broncoscopic guidance and the real contribution of the early PDT to optimize healthcare recourses.

12. References

Al-Ansari, M.A. & Hijazi, M.H. (2005). Clinical review: Percutaneous dilatational tracheostomy. *Critical Care*, Vol.10, No.1, (2006), pp. 10-202

Ambesh, S.P.; Pandey, C.K.; Srivastava, S.; Agarwal, A. & Singh D.K. (2002). Percutaneous tracheostomy with single dilatation technique: a prospective, randomized comparison of Ciaglia Blue Rhino versus Griggs' guidewire dilating forceps. *Anesthesia & Analgesia*, Vol.95, No.6, (December 2002), pp. 1739-1745

An˜ n, J.M.; Escuela, M.P.; Go´mez, V.; Moreno A.; Lo´pez, J.; Dý´az, R.; Montejo, J.C.; Sirgo, G.; Herna´ndez, G. & Martý´nez, R. (2004). Percutaneous tracheostomy: Ciaglia Blue Rhino versus Griggs' guide wire dilating forceps. A prospective randomized trial. *Acta Anaesthesiologica Scandinavica*, Vol.48, No.4, (April 2004), pp. 451-456

Arabi, Y.; Haddad, S; Shirawi, N. & Al Shimemeri, A. (2004). Early tracheostomy in intensive care trauma patients improves resource utilization: a cohort study and literature review. *Critical Care*, Vol.8, No.5, (October 2004), pp. 347-R352

Arabi, Y.M.; Alhashemi, J.A.; Tamim, H.M.; Esteban, A; Haddad, S.H.; Dawood, A.; Shirawi, N. & Alshimemeri, A.A. (2009). The impact of time to tracheostomy on mechanical ventilation duration, length of stay, and mortality in intensive care unit patients. *Journal of Critical Care*, Vol.24, (2009), pp. 435–440

Armstrong, P.A.; McCarthy, M.C. & Peoples, J.B. (1998). Reduced use of resources by early tracheostomy in ventilator-dependent patients with blunt trauma. *Surgery*, Vol.124, No.4, (October 1998), pp. 763-767

Bacchetta, M.D.; Girardi, L.N; Southard, E.J; Mack, C.A.; Ko, W.; Tortolani, A.J.; Krieger, K.H.; Isom, O.W. & Lee, L.Y.(2005). Comparison of Open Versus Bedside Percutaneous Dilatational Tracheostomy in the Cardiothoracic Surgical Patient: Outcomes and Financial Analysis. *Annals of Thoracic Surgery*, Vol.79, No.6, (June 2005), pp.1879–1885

Barron, D.J.; Smith, D.C.; Tolan, M.J.; Livesey, S.A. & Tsang, V.T. (1996). Percutaneous dilational tracheostomy in post-cardiac surgery patients. *European Journal of Cardio-Thoracic Surgery*, Vol.10, (1996), pp.74-75

Bause, H.; Dost, P.; Kehrl, W.; Walz, M.K. & Schultz-Coulon, H.J. (1999). Puncture tracheotomy versus conventional tracheostomy. An interdisciplinary discussion. *HNO Journal* , Vol.47, No.1, (Jan 1999), pp.58-70.

Berkenbosch, J.W.; Graff, G.R.; Stark, J.M.; NER, Z. & TOBIAS, J.D. (2004). Use of a remifentanil–propofol mixture for pediatric flexible fiberoptic bronchoscopy sedation. *Pediatric Anesthesia*,Vol.14, (2004), pp. 941–946

Bobo, M.L & McKenna, S.J. (1998). The Current Status of Percutaneous Dilational Tracheostomy: An Alternative to Open Tracheostomy. *Journal of Oral and Maxillofacial Surgery*, Vol.56~58, (1998), pp. 681-685

Bouderka,M.A.; Fakhir, B.; Bouaggad, A.; Hmamouchi,B.; Hamoudi, D. & Harti, A. (2004). Early Tracheostomy versus Prolonged Endotracheal Intubation in Severe Head Injury. *The Journal of TRAUMA_ Injury, Infection, and Critical Care*, Vol.57, No.2, (August 2004), pp. 251-254

Byhahn, C.; Wilke, H.J.; Halbig, S.; Lischke, V. & Westphal, K. Percutaneous tracheostomy: ciaglia blue rhino versus the basic ciaglia technique of percutaneous dilational tracheostomy. *Anesth Analg*,Vol.91, No.4, (Oct 2000),pp.882-6

Carrer, S.; Basilico, S.; Rossi, S.; Bosu, A.; Bernorio, S. & Vaghi, G.M. (2009). Outcomes of percutaneous tracheostomy. *Minerva Anestesiologic*a, Vol.75, No.11, (November 2009), pp.607-15.

Ciaglia, P; Firsching, R & Syniec, C. (1985). Elective percutaneous dilatational tracheostomy. A new simple bedside procedure; preliminary report. *Chest*, Vol.87, No.6, (Jun 1985), pp. 715-9

Cislaghi, F.; Condemia, A.M. & Corona, A. (2008). Predictors of prolonged mechanical ventilation in a cohort of 5123 cardiac surgical patients. *European Journal of Anaesthesiology*, Vol.26, No.5, (2009), pp. 396-403

De Boisblanc, B.P.. Percutaneous dilational tracheostomy techniques. (2003). *Clinics In Chest Medicine*, Vol.24, (2003), pp. 399- 407

De Leyn, P.; Bedert, P.; Delcroix, M.; Depuydt, P. Lauwers, G.; Sokolov, Y.; Van Meerhaeghe, A. & Van Schil, P. (2007). Tracheotomy: clinical review and guidelines. *European Journal of Cardio-thoracic Surgery*, Vol.32, (June 2007), pp. 412–421

Delaney, A.; Bagshaw, S.M. & Nalos, M. (2006). Percutaneous dilatational tracheostomy versus surgical tracheostomy in critically ill patients: a systematic review and meta-analysis. *Critical Care*, Vol.10, No.2, (April 2006)

Di Pietro, A.; Coletta, R.P; Barbati, G. & Blasetti, A.G. (2006). Laryngeal mask vs. endotracheal tube in airway management during percutaneous tracheotomy using Blue Rhino technique, Our experience. *Acta Anaesthesiologica Italica*, Vol.57, (2006), pp. 51-63

Durbin, C. G. Jr. (2010). Tracheostomy: Why, When, and How?. *Respiratory Care*, Vol.8, No.55, (August 2010), pp.1056 -1068.

Durbin, C.G. Jr. (2005). Indications for and Timing of Tracheostomy. *Respiratory Care*, Vol.50, No.4, (April 2005), pp. 483- 487.

El-Solh, A.A.; Pietrantoni, C.; Bhat, A.; Okada, M.; Zambon, J.; Aquilina, A. & Berbary, E. (2004). Colonization of dental plaques: a reservoir of respiratory pathogens for hospital acquired pneumonia in institutionalized elders. *Chest*, Vol.126, No.5, (November 2004), pp.1575-1582.

Facciolongo, N.; Piro, R.; Menzella, F.; Castagnetti, C. & Zucchi, L. (2009). La broncoscopia in unità di terapia intensiva. *Rassegna di Patologia dell'Apparato Respiratorio*, Vol.24, (2009), pp. 212-219

Ferraro, F.; Capasso, A.; Troise, E.; Lanza, S.; Azan, G.; Rispoli, F. & Belluomo Anello, C. (2004). Modalità di ventilazione durante tracheostomia percutanea elettiva sotto guida endoscopica. Valutazione clinica di un nuovo metodo. *CHEST Edizione Italiana*, Vol.6, No.3, (Luglio-Settembre 2004), pp. 36-41

Fikkers, B.G.; Staatsen, M.; van den Hoogen, F.J.A. & van der Hoeven, J.G. (2011). Early and late outcome after single step dilatational tracheostomy versus the guide wire dilating forceps technique: a prospective randomized clinical trial. *Intensive Care Med*, Vo.37, No.7, (July 2011), pp.1103-1109

Fikkers, BG; Staatsen, M; Lardenoije, SG; van den Hoogen, FJ & van der Hoeven, JG. (2004). Comparison of two percutaneous tracheostomy techniques, guide wire dilating forceps and Ciaglia Blue Rhino: a sequential cohort study. *Crit Care*, Vol 8, No 5, (Oct 2004), pp. R299-305

François, B.; Clavel, M.; Desachy, A.; Puyraud, S.; Roustan, J. & Vignon, P. (2003). Complicanze della tracheostomia eseguita in Unità di Terapia Intensiva. Tracheostomia subtiroidea vs cricotiroidotomia chirurgica. *CHEST Edizione Italiana*, Vol.1, (Gennaio-Marzo 2003), pp. 75-81

Frost, P. & Wise, M.P. (2008). Tracheotomy and ventilator-associated pneumonia: the importance of oral care. *European Respiratory Journal*, Vo.31, No.1, (January 2008), pp.221-222

Griffiths, J; Barber, VS; Morgan, L & Young, JD. (2005). Systematic review and meta-analysis of studies of the timing of tracheostomy in adult patients undergoing artificial ventilation. *British Medical Journal*, Vol. 28, No 330, (May 2005), pp.1243

Grillo H.C. Tracheostomy: uses, varieties, complications. In: Grillo HC, editor. Surgery of the trachea and bronchi. Hamilton, London: BC Decker Inc.; 2004. p. 291—300. Chapter 10.

Heffner, J.E.; Miller, K.S. & Sahn, S.A. Tracheostomy in the intensive care unit. Part 2: Complications. (1986). *Chest*, Vol.90, No.3, (September 1986), pp. 430-436.

Jackson, C.M.D. Tracheotomy (1909). *Laryngoscope*, Vol.19, No.4 (April 1909), pp.285- 290.

Kollef, MH. (1999). Avoidance of tracheal intubation as a strategy to prevent ventilator-associated pneumonia. (1999). *Intensive Care Medicine*, Vol 25, No 6, (Jun 1999), pp. 553-5

Kollig, E.; Heydenreich, U.; Roetman, B.; Hopf, F. & Muhr, G. (2000). Ultrasound and bronchoscopic controlled percutaneous tracheostomy on trauma ICU. *Injury, International Journal of the Care of the Injured*, Vol.31, (2000), pp. 663–668

Kost, K. M. (2005). Endoscopic Percutaneous Dilatational Tracheotomy: A Prospective Evaluation of 500 Consecutive Cases. *Laryngoscope*, Vol. 115, (October 2005), pp.1–30

Lin, J.C.; Maley, R.H. & Landreneau, R.J. (2000). Extensive Posterior-Lateral Tracheal Laceration. Complicating Percutaneous Dilational Tracheostomy. *Annals of Thoracic Surgery*, Vo.70, (2000), pp.1194–11966

Marx, W.H.; Ciaglia P.& Graniero K.D. (1996). Some important details in the technique of percutaneous dilatational tracheostomy via the modified Seldinger technique. *Chest*, Vol.110, No.3, (Sept 1996), pp.762-766

Mastropierro, R.; Bettinzoli, M.; Bordonali, T.; Patroni, A.; Barni, C. & Manzato, A. (2009). Pneumonia in a cardiothoracic intensive care unit: incidence and risk factors. *J Cardiothorac Vasc Anesth*, Vol.23, No.6, (Dec 2009), pp.780-788

Montcriol, A.; Bordes, J.; Asencio, Y.; Prunet, B.; Lacroix, G. & Meaudre, E. (2011). Bedside percutaneous tracheostomy: a prospective randomised comparison of PercuTwist versus Griggs' forceps dilational tracheostomy. *Anaesthesia and Intensive Care*, Vol.39, No.2, (March 2011), pp. 209-216

Murthy, S.C.; Arroliga, A.C.; Walts, P.A.; Feng, J.; Yared, J.P.; Lytle, B.W. & Blackstone, E.H. (2007). Ventilatory dependency after cardiovascular surgery. *The Journal of Thoracic and Cardiovascular Surgery*, Vol.134, No.2, (August 2007), pp. 848-890

Needham, D.M.; Bronskill, S.E.; Calinawan, J.R.; Sibbald, W.J.; Pronovost, P.J. & Laupacis, A. (2005). Projected incidence of mechanical ventilation in Ontario to 2026: Preparing for the aging baby boomers. *Critical Care Medicine*, Vol.33, No.3, (March 2005), pp.574-579

Nieszkowska, A.; Combes, A.; Luyt, C.E.; Ksibi, H.; Trouillet, J.L.; Gibert, C. & Chastre, J.(2005). Impact of tracheotomy on sedative administration, sedation level, and comfort of mechanically ventilated intensive care unit patients. *Critical Care Medicine*, Vol.33, (2005), pp. 2527—2533.

Nseir, S.; Di Pompeo, C.; Jozefowicz, E.; Cavestri, B.; Brisson, H.; Nyunga, M.; Soubrier, S. & Durocher A. (2007). Relationship between tracheotomy and ventilator-associated pneumonia: a case–control study. *European Respiratory Journal*, Vol.30, No.2, (August 2007); pp.314–320

Pappalardo, F; Franco, A; Landonia, G; Cardano, P; Zangrillo, A & Alfieri, O. (2004). Long-term outcome and quality of life of patients requiring prolonged mechanical ventilation after cardiac surgery. *European Journal of Cardio-Thoracic Surgery*, Vol 25, No 4, (April 2004), pp. 548-552

Polderman, K.H.; Spijkstra, J.J.; de Bree, R.; Christiaans, H.M.T.; Gelissen, H.P.M.M.; Wester, J.P.J. & Girbes, A.R.J. (2003). Percutaneous Dilatational Tracheostomy in the ICU: Optimal Organization, Low Complication Rates, and Description of a New Complication. *Chest*, Vol.123, No.5, (May 2003), pp. 1595-1602

Rajakaruna, C.; Rogers, C.A.; Angelini, G.D & Ascione, R. (2005). Risk factors for and economic implications of prolonged ventilation after cardiac surgery. *Thoracic and Cardiovascular Surgeon*, Vol. 130, No.5, (November 2005), pp.1270-7

Rello, J.; Lorente, C.; Diaz, E.; Bodi, M.; Boque, C.; Sandiumenge, A. & Santamaria, J.M. (2003). Incidence, etiology, and outcome of nosocomial pneumonia in ICU patients requiring percutaneous tracheotomy for mechanical ventilation. *Chest*, Vol.124, No.6, (December 2003), pp.2239-2243

Rodriguez, J.L.; Steinberg, S.M.; Luchetti, F.A.; Gibbons, K.J.; Taheri, P.A. & Flint, L.M. (1990). Early tracheostomy for primary airway management in the surgical critical care setting. *Surgery*, Vol.108, No.4, (October 1990), pp.655-659.

Rumbak, M.J.; Newton, M.; Truncale, T.; Schwartz, S.W.; Adams J.W. & Hazard, P.B. (2004). A prospective, randomized, study comparing early percutaneous dilational tracheotomy to prolonged translaryngeal intubation (delayed tracheotomy) in critically ill medical patients. *Critical Care Medicine*, Vol.32, No.12, (December 2004), pp. 1689-1694.

Schleder, B.; Stott, K. & Lloyd, R.C. (2002). The effect of a comprehensive oral care protocol on patients at risk for ventilator associated pneumonia. *Journal of Advocate Health Care*, Vol.4, No.1, (Spring/Summer 2002), pp.27–30

Sharif-Kashani, B.; Shahabi, P.; Behzadnia, N.; Mohammad-Taheri, Z.; Mansouri, D.; Masjedi, M.R.; Zargari, L. & Salimi Negad L. (1998). Incidence of Fever and bacteriemia following flexible fiberoptic bronchoscopy: a prospective study. *Pneumologie*, Vol. 52, No.11, (November 1998), pp. 629-34.

Shirawi, N. & Arabi, Y. (2006). Bench-to-bedside review: Early tracheostomy in critically ill trauma patients. *Critical Care*, Vol.10, No.1, (2006), pp.201

Steinfort, D.P. & Irving, L.B. (2010). Patient Satisfaction During Endobronchial Ultrasound-Guided Transbronchial Needle Aspiration Performed Under Conscious Sedation. *Respiratory Care*, Vol.55, No.6, (June 2010), pp.702-706

Sue, R.D. & Susanto, I.. Long-term complications of artificial airways. (2003). *Clinics in Chest Medicine*, Vol.24, (2003), pp. 457—471.

Terragni, P.P.; Antonelli, M.; Fumagalli, R.; Faggiano, C.; Berardino, M.; Bobbio Pallavicini, F.; Miletto, A.; Mangione, S.; Sinardi, A.U.; Pastorelli, M.; Vivaldi, N.; Pasetto, A.; Della Rocca, G.; Urbino, R.; Filippini, C.; Pagano, E.; Evangelista, A.; Ciccone, G.; Mascia, L.; Ranieri, V.M. (2010). Early vs Late Tracheotomy for Prevention of Pneumonia in Mechanically Ventilated Adult ICU Patients. *JAMA*, Vol.303, No.15, (April 2010), pp.1483-1489

Trouillet, J.-L. MD; Luyt, C.-E. MD, PhD; Guiguet, M. PhD; Ouattara, A. MD, PhD; Vaissier, E. MD; Makri, R. MD; Nieszkowska, A. MD; Leprince, P. MD, PhD; Pavie, A. MD; Chastre, J. MD & Combes, A. MD, PhD. (2011). Early Percutaneous Tracheotomy Versus Prolonged Intubation of Mechanically Ventilated Patients After Cardiac Surgery. *Annals of Internal Medicine*, Vol.154, No.6, (March 2011), pp. 373-383

Trouillet, J.-L.; Combes, A.; Vaissier, E.; Luyt, C.-E.; Ouattara, A.; Pavie, A. & Chastre, J. (2009). Prolonged mechanical ventilation after cardiac surgery: outcome and predictors. *Journal of Thoracic and Cardiovascular Surgery*, Vol.138, No.4, (October 2009), pp: 948-53

Trouillet, J.-L.; Luyt, C.-E.; Guiguet, M.; Ouattara, A.; Vaissier, E.; Makri, R.; Nieszkowska, A.; Leprince, P.; Pavie, A.; Chastre, J. & Combes, A. (2011). Early Percutaneous

Tracheotomy Versus Prolonged Intubation of Mechanically Ventilated Patients After Cardiac Surgery. *Annals of Internal Medicine,* Vol.154, No.6, (March 2011), pp. 373-383.

Yung-Lun Ni, Y.-L.; Lo, Y.-L.; Lin, T.-Y; Fang, Y.-F. & Kuo, H.-P. (2010). Conscious Sedation Reduces Patient Discomfort and Improves Satisfaction in Flexible Bronchoscopy. *Chang Gung Med Journal,* Vol. 33, No. 4, (July-August 2010), pp. 443-452

Section 5

Pediatric Bronchoscopy

10

Pediatric Bronchoscopy

Selma Maria de Azevedo Sias,
Ana Cristina Barbosa Domingues and Rosana V. Mannarino
Pediatric Pulmonology and Bronchoscopy of Antonio Pedro University Hospital, Fluminense Federal University, Pediatric Pulmonology of Jesus Hospital - SMS/RJ and Pediatric Bronchoscopy of Cardoso Fontes Federal Hospital - MS/RJ, Neonatal ICU and Pediatric Pulmonology and Bronchoscopy of Gafrée Guinle University Hospital - UNIRIO
Brazil

1. Introduction

Particular aspects of upper airways anatomy in the child

The small size of the child's airway, differences in the anatomy of the larynx and the different pathologies according to age group, are characteristics that shows the endoscopic examination of the child quite unique and different from adults.

The infant larynx presents some different aspects compared to the adult. Its location is higher in the neck, the cricoid cartilage being located approximately at the fourth cervical vertebra. With the growth of the child the cricoid cartilage will gradually descend to the level of the seventh cervical vertebra, which is the location in adulthood. The size of the larynx in the newborn is about 1 / 3 of the adult. Their structures such as the vocal process of arytenoid, cuneiform cartilage, the arytenoids and the soft tissue that makes up the supraglottic larynx are also bigger. The epiglottis is proportionally more posterior and narrower and more tubular or omega-shaped (Figure 1).

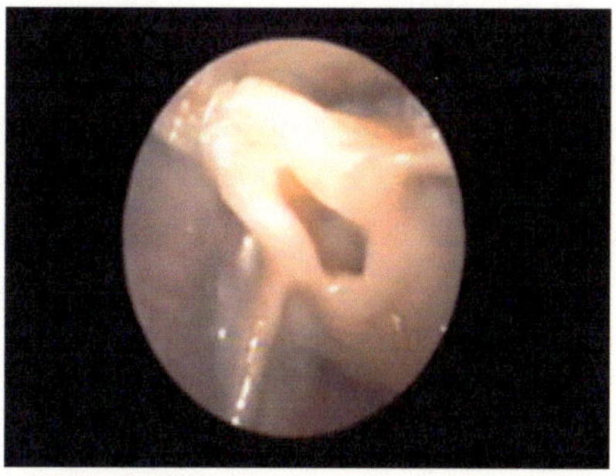

Fig. 1. Tubular or omega-shaped epiglottis of children.

The normal glottis of the infant, has a very small opening, about 7 mm in anteroposterior dimension and 4 mm in the posterior transverse dimension, so that 1 mm of edema may cause an obstruction of the airway in 35% of normal. Similarly, cartilage, muscle and submucosal tissues are softer and friable, providing a greater inflammatory reaction with edema and significant reduction of airway lumen. The cricoid region has been described as narrowest of the airways, but recent studies in anesthetized children have shown that the glottis is narrower than the cricoid in all age groups.

2. Anesthesia for pediatric bronchoscopy

Anesthesia for invasive procedures on the airways has always been a challenge. The success of pediatric bronchoscopy relies on careful planning and constant communication between the bronchoscopist and the anesthetist throughout the procedure. In most cases the pediatric patient does not tolerate bronchoscopy whilst alert. Flexible bronchoscopy is usually performed with the use of sedation or sometimes local anaesthetic in infants and neonates, while rigid bronchoscopy requires general anesthesia. Our aim is to analyze some aspects that directly affect the actions and decisions of the anesthesist involved in the assistance.

The pre-anesthetic evaluation for this procedure consists of the child's history, physical examination and laboratory tests. The anesthetist should explain to parents how the anaesthesia will be administered and must be sure the child has been fasting. Infants under 1 year are recommended to fast for 6 hours if fed on formula, 4 hours if breast-fed and 2 hours after the ingestion of clear fluids only. Children over 1 year must fast for 6h after the ingestion of food or milk and 2h if only clear fluids were ingested. Only healthy children with no risk of slow gastric emptying may be allowed to have clear fluids before the procedure.

The best anesthetic technique and the most appropriate anesthetics should be considered according to some factors such as the child's physical status; an assessment of airways to identify chemical and /or physical lesions; the presence of lower respiratory infection with concomitant bronchospasm, secretions and edema, hypoxia and acidosis (due to severely compromised respiratory function); any co-existent disease; the needs of the bronchoscopist (some procedures during the bronchoscopy such as bronchoalveolar lavage or removal of foreign body increase the time of the examination) and the skills of the anesthetist. The consideration of all these aspects is essential to ensure the safety of the child, with minimal risk of complications. The risk of adverse events related to general anesthesia is associated with the physical status of the patient, thus being prudent to apply the scale of classification of physical status, established by the American Society of Anesthesiologists (Table 1).

In many cases, the pre-anesthetic use of bronchodilators and or anti-cholinergic drugs can improve the oxygen saturation and alveolar ventilation besides preventing, or attenuating, vagal responses of bradicardia and bronchoconstriction during the airway manipulation as well as reducing secretions.

ASA I	Patient is entirely fit and healthy.
ASA II	A mild systemic disease is present, but does not limit activity.
ASA III	Patient has a severe systemic disease that limits activity, but is not incapacitating.
ASA IV	Patient has a chronic condition, which is a constant threat to life.
ASA V	Patient is likely to die within 24h, with or without treatment.
ASA VI	A declared brain-dead patient whose organs are being removed for donor purposes.

*ASA: American Society of Anesthesiologists

Table 1. ASA* classification of physical status

It is important to make sure the equipment for advanced life support is available and to be aware that these data on requires as much care as general anesthesia. The minimal mandatory monitoring equipment includes: pulse oximetry, stethoscope, capnograph, electrocardiogram (rhythm and rate more important than ST-T wave changes), non-invasive blood pressure (Doppler assistance useful for small children) and temperature. It is also crucial to closely monitor skin color, skin perfusion, respiratory rate and pattern, diaphragmatic and intercostal activity and any evidence of airway obstruction such as croup, retractions, tracheal tugging or stridor.

As a general rule, the smaller the children, the more incomplete their metabolism, specially concerning drugs. This group is more sensitive to depressant cardiovascular effects and to take longer to recover from anesthetics (exception must be made to the faster metabolism of remifentanil on neonates). Neonates and small children have reduced intracellular stores of calcium and reduced muscular mass of the myocardium, being susceptible to cardiac depressant effects of anesthetics. Neonates, especially prematures, are prone to post-anesthesia apnea, the greater incidence occurring in those < 60 weeks post-conceptual age. They also have reduced demands of inhalational agents to produce adequate levels of anesthesia. In children above 2 years, the larger fraction of cardiac output to kidneys and liver in proportion to their weight is responsible for a faster elimination rate of drugs.

The available devices for bronchoscopy are the facemask, the nasopharyngeal prong, the laryngeal mask (LM) and the endotracheal tube. Both endotracheal tubes and laryngeal masks have proved to be safe, but, according to some studies, the LM (reusable) is more appropriate than other supraglottic devices, and in children above 2 years, it causes less morbidity.

After the bronchoscopy has finished and if the child is stable, the patient will be moved to a recovery room and kept in the left lateral position. The child should still be monitored until awake and in control of the airway.

The most common complication is laryngospasm, related to light plane of anesthesia, pain, manipulation of the airway or cough. Hipoxemia can be caused by prolonged bronchoscopy, secretions or blood in the airway, bronchospasm or decreased cardiac output. Anesthetic agents can cause hypotension, especially in younger children. Bronchospasm can occur during the procedure. Malignant hyperthermia is rare.

3. Indications and contraindications of bronchoscopy in children

Bronchoscopy is indicated in any chest or lung disease where the tracheobronchial tree may be involved directly or indirectly. You should always consider whether the benefits of information and / or therapy provided by the examination outweigh the risks because it is not free of complications. It can be performed using rigid or flexible devices. The best bronchoscopic techniques should be chosen according to each case individually.

Indications for flexible and rigid bronchoscopy are similar. However, in the evaluation of congenital malformations, the rigid bronchoscope provides better visualization, manipulation of anatomical structures, measurements of length and diameter of stenosis, preoperative evaluation, as well as photographic documentation. In cases of removal of foreign bodies, preference is also rigid bronchoscopy.

3.1 Rigid bronchoscopy

The rigid bronchoscopes are straight metal tubes with side ventilation holes at the distal end. They have lighting system projecting light on its distal end. Rigid bronchoscopy can be performed under direct vision, but it is limited due to the small caliber of the airways of the child. Proximal illumination for rigid bronchoscopy is provided by prismatic light deflectors. An optical system magnifies the view. It can be coupled to a micro-camera generating the image on the display screen. Video monitoring can be used. This allows the team to anticipate needs and problems and to feel more a part of the procedure. A videorecorder can be used for bronchoscopy documentation (Figure 2). Tables 2 and 3 provide the indications for rigid bronchoscopy.

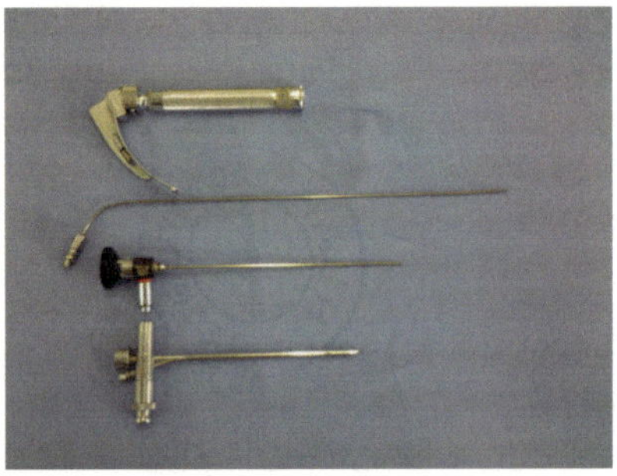

Fig. 2. Endoscopic instrumentation described from bottom to top: rigid bronchoscope (Storz) size 3.0 (20 cm), the optics of straightforward 0° telescope, metallic suction tube and laryngoscope.

Persistent unexplained cough or wheeze
Unexplained dyspnea or stridor
Suspected congenital anomalies
Hemoptysis
Recurrent infections of the airways or lungs
Persistent abnormalities on chest radiograph
Atelectatic lung, lobe or segment
Diagnostic bronchoalveolar lavage
Suspected tracheoesophageal fistula or broncoesofageal fistula
Mediastinal tumor
Chemical or thermal burns of the tracheobronchial tree
Suspected foreign body in tracheobronchial tree
Tracheobronchial stenosis
Lung abscess
Assessment of endotracheal tube placement
After airway reconstruction
Thoracic trauma

Table 2. Major indications for diagnostic bronchoscopy

Bronchial toilet, retained secretions, mucous plug, clots
Tracheobronchial mucosa necrotic
Removal of foreign bodies in tracheobronchial tree
Hemoptysis
Strictures and stenosis
Bronchogenic cysts (drainage)
Mediastinal lesions
Endotracheal tube placement and replacement
After airway reconstruction
Cystic Fibrosis
Asthma
Thoracic trauma

Table 3. Major indications for therapeutic bronchoscopy

In the last century, rigid bronchoscopy was performed by chest surgeons or otorhinolaringologist. But with the advent of the flexible bronchoscope in the 70's, rigid bronchoscopy has been used less, although it is still considered an indispensable tool, especially in the removal of foreign bodies in the airway.

Although bronchoscopy training should include both the device and the floppy drive, it has been observed in most services increased use of flexible bronchoscopy.

In Brazil, 45% of the members of the Department of Respiratory Endoscopy of the Brazilian Thoracic Society, who perform bronchoscopy feel able to perform rigid bronchoscopy. Less than 15% of them had some experience with therapeutic bronchoscopy.

In children, usually rigid bronchoscopy needs to be performed under general anesthesia and assisted ventilation. Even one of the most important advantages of rigid bronchoscopy is to allow control of the airway because the device is already inside the trachea, allowing adequate ventilation. However, manipulation with the rigid bronchoscope that is introduced orally, increases the risk of subglottic edema. This situation can be minimized by choosing the appropriate size of the bronchoscope according to age group (Table 4).

Patient age: mean (range)	size	outside diameter (mm)
Premature infant	2,5	3,7
Term newborn (birth - 3 mo)	3	4,8
6 mo (3 - 18 mo)	3,5	5,7
18 mo (1 - 3 y)	3,7	6,3
3 y (1 ½ - 5 y)	4	6,7
5 y (3 - 10 y)	5	7,8
10 y (> 10 y - adolescent)	6	8,2

Table 4. Size of the rigid bronchoscope according to age

Another advantage is the possibility of using various accessories instruments introduced through the bronchoscope such as suction tubes, forceps for biopsy, tumor resection and removal of foreign bodies (Figure 3, 4). There are four types of forcepscupped forceps (biopsy), alligator forceps, scissors and punch or cutting forceps (biopsy). Forceps for flexible bronchoscopes are more limited in size and strength than forceps for rigid bronchoscopes. They include biopsy forceps, baskets, claws and ballons.

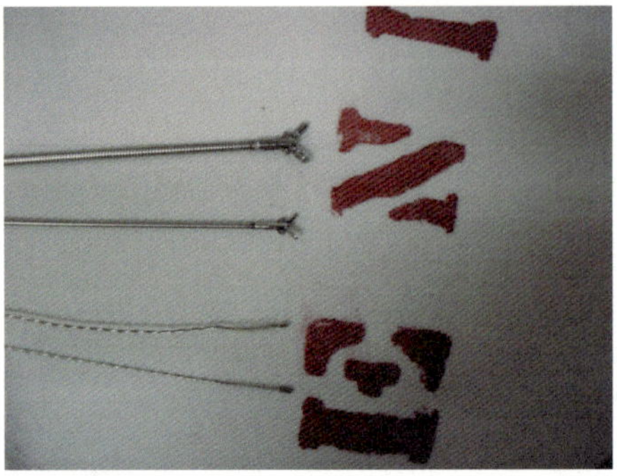

Fig. 3. Forceps and brush washed.

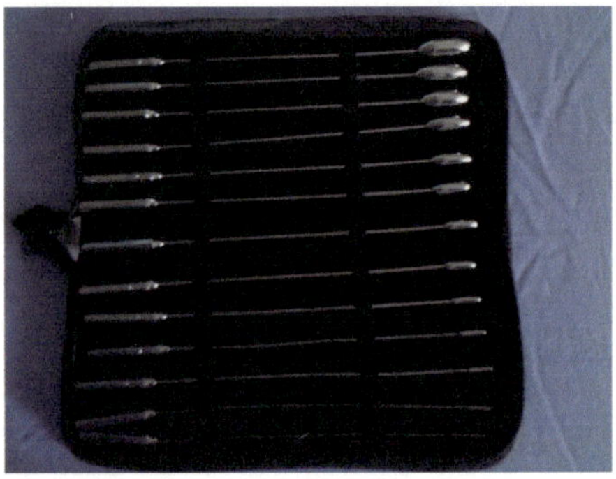

Fig. 4. Tracheal dilators can be used in children for dilation of subglottic stenosis.

Another limitation of rigid bronchoscopy is the difficulty in accessing the bronchi of smaller caliber, as well as the upper lobe bronchus. Table 5 shows the advantages and disadvantages of rigid bronchoscopy.

Advantages	Disadvantages
Excellent control of the airway	Need for general anesthesia
Inside diameter allowing use of instruments accessories	Difficulty in assessing the dynamics of normal vocal cords
Greater ability to suction secretions, blood or tissue biopsy	Increased risk of trauma to the airway
Performed in the operating room facilitating management of complications	Inability to reach into the the upper lobes and segmental bronchi
Lower cost	Difficulty in obtaining BAL
Better image quality	

Table 5. Advantages and disadvantages of rigid bronchoscopy

Rigid bronchoscopy is most suitable for therapeutic procedures in particular the extraction of foreign bodies in the airways, tracheobronchial structures for dilation, stent placement for airway, control of hemoptysis and CO2-laser therapy (Figure 5, 6).

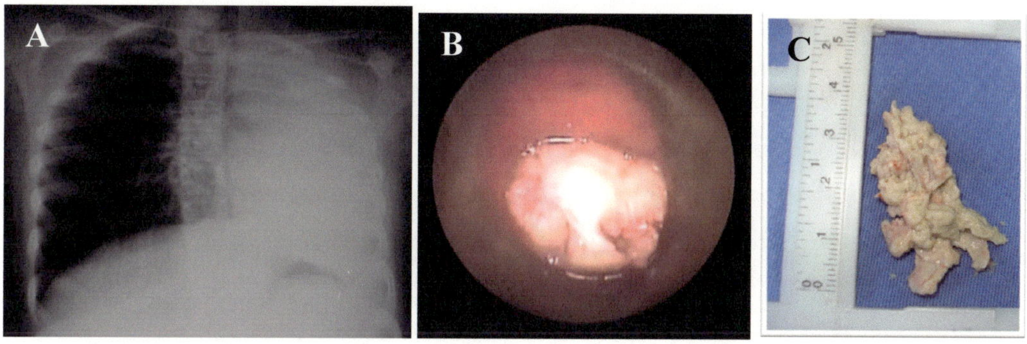

Fig. 5. Total left pulmonary atelectasis (A) due to bronchial casts filling the left bronchus (B) that was removed (C).

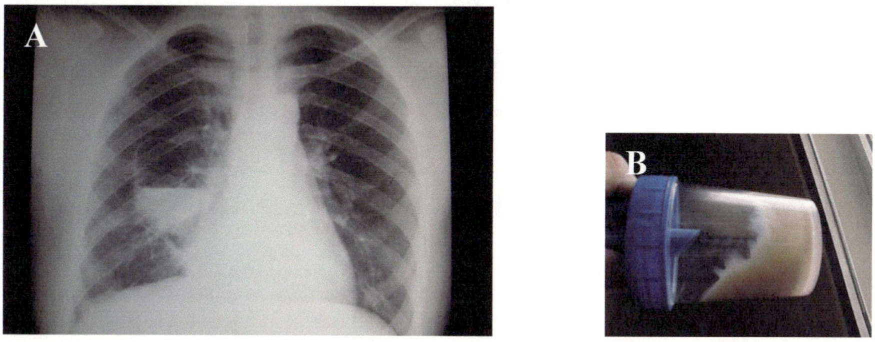

Fig. 6. Chest radiograph shows pumonary abscess (A) and pus aspirated by bronchoscopy (B).

3.2 Flexible bronchoscopy

Since 1981, the flexible bronchoscope (FB) has been used routinely in pediatric patients. Robert Wood was the forerunner in the use of this type of bronchoscope in children. FB are made of flexible fiber optic rods that transmit light and generate a magnified image through a lens system (Figure 7, 8).

Table 6 shows the types of flexible bronchoscopes used in children. In adults, the FB has an outer diameter of 6 mm and 2.2 mm working channel while the most commonly used in children has an outer diameter of 3.6 mm and working channel of 1.2 mm. Currently there is available a flexible bronchoscope with a 2.2 mm outside diameter can be used in preterm infants, but do not have a working channel. The small diameter working channel prevents the introduction of accessories instruments. FB is indicated in sample collection and in the exploitation of airway. However some treatment can be indicated in FB as alveolar proteinosis and lipoid pneumonia due to aspiration of mineral oil.

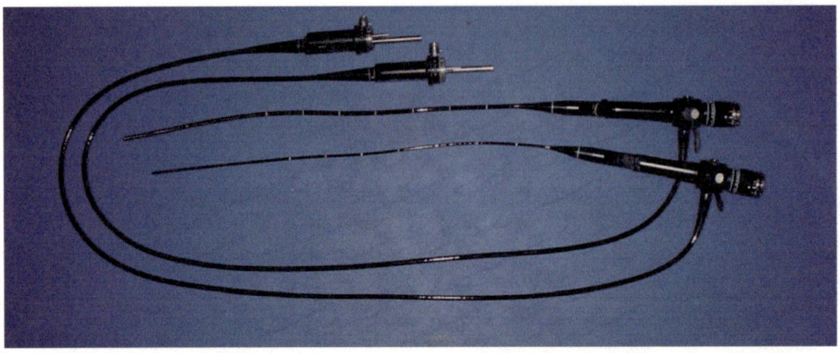

Fig. 7. Flexible bronchoscope 3,6 mm and 4,9 mm (OD).

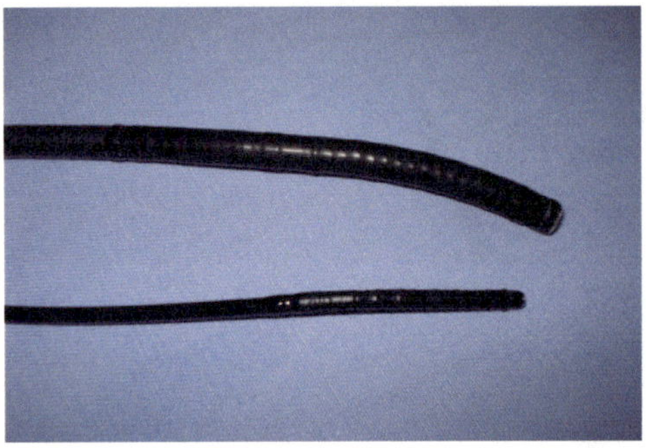

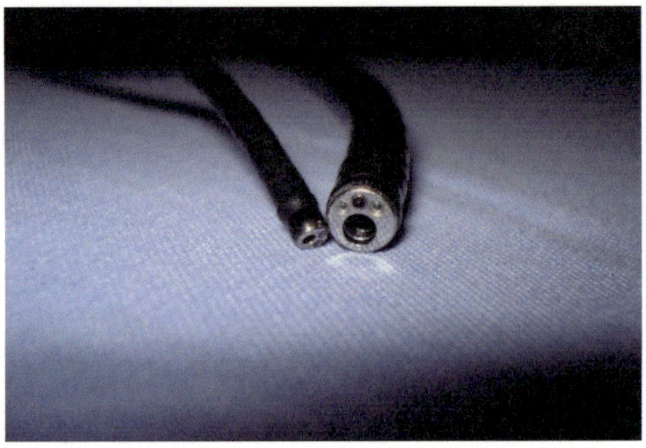

Fig. 8. Flexible bronchoscope showing the various dimensions (3,6 mm and 4,9 mm OD).

Outside diameter (OD)	4,9 mm	3,6 mm	2,8 mm	2,2mm
Working channel	2,2 mm	1,2 mm	1,2 mm	Nenhum
Viewing angle	100°	95°	90°	75°
Endotracheal tube	≥5,	≥4,5	≥4,5	≥3,5
Age of child	> 4 y	standard pediatric	< 4 y	newborn

Table 6. Flexible Bronchoscopes used in pediatrics

In most cases, the flexible bronchoscopy can be performed without general anesthesia using lidocaine and topical anesthesia with sedation. Then it can be performed outside the operating room. The FB can be inserted through the nostrils, laryngeal masks, endotracheal tubes, tracheostomy tube or through the rigid bronchoscope. It also has the advantage of allowing the examination of segmental and subsegmental bronchi, optimizing the exploitation of the distal airway.

It is suitable for exploration of the airways, for intra-operative assessment and also post-operative assessment, for obtain biological samples such as bronchoalveolar lavage, transbronchial biopsy and bronchial brushing, for diagnosis of pneumonia in immunocompromised patients, interstitial pneumonia, hemosiderosis, sarcoidosis, alveolar proteinosis, Langerhans, endoluminal obstructive disease and aspiration syndromes (Figure 9).

The therapeutic application is more limited compared with rigid bronchoscopy, but can be used in endobronchial secretions aspiration, instillation of drugs, guide in difficult

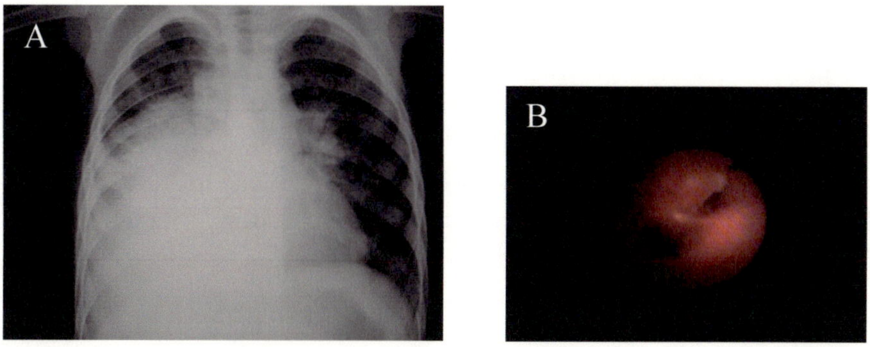

Fig. 9. Chronic pneumonia in the right lung (A). Bronchoscopy image shows enlargement of the main carina and narrowing of the right main bronchus due to extrinsic compression (B). BAAR and culture of BAL isolated *M.tuberculosis.*

intubations, monitoring and patient follow-up, to help as tracheotomy, and the extraction of same cases of foreign bodies (table 7).

Nowadays came a new generation of bronchoscopes that have a chip on its distal end. These are the videobroncoscopes, with higher resolution and image storage in digital format. Pediatric models are available in size with outside diameter of 3.6 y 4.9 mm. The disadvantage is the high cost of equipment.

New techniques are being developed, such as endobronchial ultrasound since 1999 and most recently ultrasonic bronchoscope with transbronchial needle, but without experience in the child population.

Stridor
Persistent atelectasis
Recurrent or / and persistent infiltrations
Pulmonary lesions of unknown etiology
Chronic cough
Hemoptysis
Removal of some foreign body
Evaluate the position, patency, or other changes related to ETT or tracheostomy
Assess the damage of inhalation or aspiration
Samples
Bronchoscopic lung biopsy
Remove secretions or mucus plaques
BAL therapy

Table 7. Indications for flexible bronchoscopy in pediatrics

3.3 Contraindications

In general there is no absolute contraindication to bronchoscopy. Wood RE related that the only absolute contraindication to bronchoscopy is the lack of a rational indication. However it is contraindicated in cases of unstable cardiovascular status or life-threatening cardiac arrhytmia, extremely severe hypoxemia and an inadequately trained bronchoscopist and bronchoscopy team.

Rigid bronchoscopy is relatively contraindicated in micrognathia, microstomia, cervical spine instability and mandibulomaxillary trauma or disease.

Flexible bronchoscopy is relatively contraindicated in some foreign body aspiration, hemorrhagic diathesis, severe hipoxemia and respiratory distress. Trombocytopenia is not a contraindication to pediatric bronchoscopy.

4. Bronchocoalveolar lavage in children

Since the 80's with the advent of a flexible bronchoscope, bronchoscopy is being increasingly used as a diagnostic tool in several lung diseases in children.

The bronchoalveolar lavage (BAL) is a resource used in bronchoscopy that has helped to increase the sensitivity and specificity of the bronchoscopy. Several studies have been published using the BAL for the diagnosis of various lung diseases, especially persistent or recurrent pneumonia, interstitial infiltrates, severe pneumonia in patients in intensive care units and pulmonary infiltrates in immunocompromised patients. Examination of BAL fluid can identify the etiologic agent in these types of pneumonia. BAL is considered a safe procedure and fast, with low percentage of complications, even in infants, and in many cases makes open lung biopsy unnecessary.

In children the BAL is commonly used for diagnosis of opportunistic infections in immunocompromised patients. BAL has a sensitivity and specificity comparable to those of open lung biopsy. However, unlike this, has much lower morbidity and mortality, although it is also an invasive procedure.

Another indication is in the cases of recurrent or persistent pulmonary infiltrates of unknown etiology. BAL is an diagnosis tool for children under age 6 who have difficulty, because of the age, to collect sputum for microbiological studies. Molecular biology allows identification of pathogens from small samples. In addition, analysis of cellular and non cellular components of BAL fluid can define the diagnosis of non-infectious causes of pulmonary infiltrates. Thus, the diagnosis of diseases such as alveolar proteinosis, hemosiderosis, lipid aspiration pneumonia, interstitial pneumonia, can be done by BAL.

The study of BAL has also contributed to understanding the pathogenesis of interstitial lung diseases and it has now been used to evaluate the treatment and prognosis of these diseases. Analysis of BAL solutes, including proteins and inflammatory mediators can be studied.

The BAL can be indicated as therapy in cases of alveolar proteinosis, for removal of secretions in cystic fibrosis and, in severe cases of status asthmaticus. BAL can be both a diagnostic or therapeutic tool even in critically ill children.

4.1 Techniques of BAL and the laboratory processing

Flexible bronchoscopy with bronchoalveolar lavage should be done safely in intensive care unit, special procedures areas and operating rooms.

In children bronchoscopy is performed under intravenous sedation (0.05 - 0.3 mg/kg Midazolan) and topical lidocaine anesthesia of the upper airways (4% lidocaine gel to the nasal passage and 1% lidocaine through the bronchoscope to the glotic region) using a flexible bronchoscope (external diameter of 2.8 / 3.6mm for small children and a diameter of 4.6 / 4.9 mm for >9 yrs of age).

Each child should have an intravenous access and should be monitored with pulse oximetry, and heart rate and administered O2 by nasal catheter. Immediate access to supplemental oxygen, resuscitation equipment and antagonists for sedative agents (naloxone and flumazenil) should be readily available. A swivel Y connector should be used in endotracheal tube, in intubated children. Cough can be controlled if small amount of 1% lidocaine is administered through the channel of bronchoscopio when it reaches the trachea.

It is carried out careful inspection of the tracheobronchial tree and the FB is wedged into the involved segments previously indicated by CT scan or if the disease is diffuse, the most suitable segments are the right middle lobe or the lingula.

BAL is carried out using normal sterile pyrogen-free saline previously warmed to body temperature (37°C) with a syringe attached to the suction channel of the FB for controlled aspiration with a suction trap. Negative pressure of 120 mmHg is adequate for obtaining return of BAL. It is instilled 3 aliquots of 1 ml/kg body weight in each compromised segment or lobe previously indicated by CT scan. Each instillation must be followed by sufficient air to ensure that the channel's dead space is empty and it should be immediately recovered by manual suction through a syringe or using the mechanical aspiration. The first aliquot collected should be used for culture because it probably represents bronchial origin. The others are pooled and processed for cytological studies and analysis of BAL solutes (Table 8).

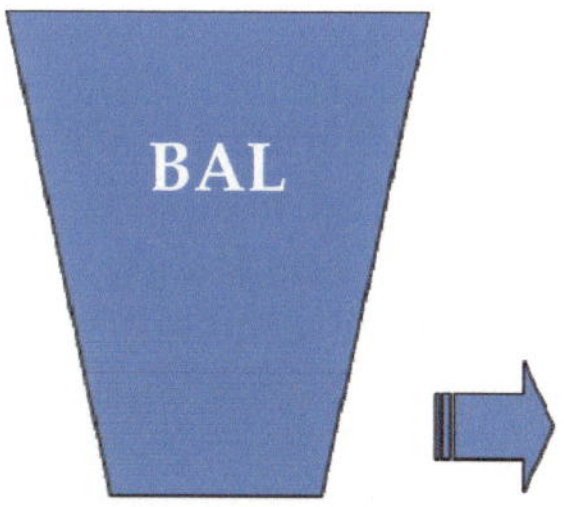

MICROBIOLOGY: Culture, molecular biology

CITOLOGY: total cell, cell count differential, Stains: Gram, H&E, Sudan, Silver methenamine, PAS, Pearls

SUPERNATANT (- 20 to - 70º):
Proteins, inflammatory mediators

Table 8. Laboratory processing of BAL

Some authors use functional residual capacity (FRC) to get the BAL. The total volume has been used at a rate of 5 to 15% of FRC, which is proportional to the total volume per FRC used in adults. BAL can be considered technically adequated if the recovery is more than 40% and contains few epithelial cells. BAL fluid must be transported under refrigeration and processed in a maximum of 1 hour.

The macroscopic aspect of the BAL should be evaluated because it may suggest some diseases. In lipoid pneumonia the BAL fluid has milky appearance, floating fat globules and numerous Sudan positive foam macrophages. (Figure 10). In hemorrhagic syndromes the BAL can be xanthochromic.

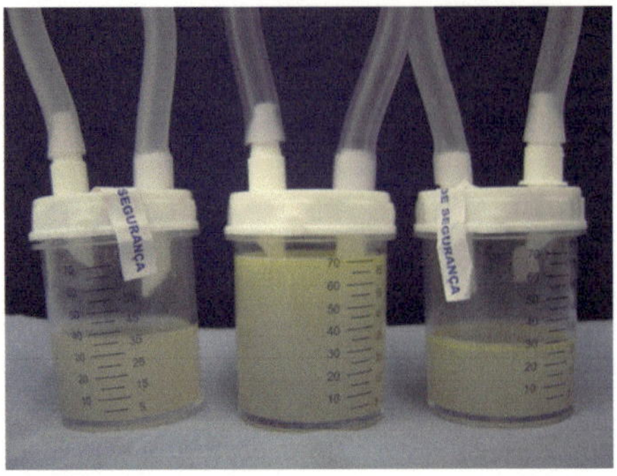

Fig. 10. Macroscopic aspect of BAL in children with Lipoid pneumonia: milky appearance with floating fat.

Routine laboratorial analysis for bacteria (routine aerobic, *Legionella, Nocardia, Mycobacteria* including *Mycobacterium tuberculosis,* Virus (CMV, RSV, Influenza, Parainfluenza, Enterovirus) and or cultivation of anaerobes, anaerobic transport media containing reducing agents may be used and the BAL fluid must not be exposed to air.

Cell counts are determined in Neubauer chamber and cell viability by trypan blue exclusion dye.Cytospins prepar after 5 min at 200g speed, are stained for bacterial (Gram), lipid-laden macrophages (Sudan or Oil red), lipoproteins in pulmonary alveolar proteinosis (PAS—periodic acid-Schiff), hemosiderin in idiopathic pulmonary hemosiderosis, Wegener's granulomatosis and Goodpasture's disease (Pearls), pulmonary histiocytosis X (monoclonal antibody OKT-6), fungi (Silver methenamine or Gomori-Grocott), *Mycobacterium tuberculosis* (Ziehl Neelsen) and Papanicolaou and May-Grunwald-Giemsa. Glutaraldehyde fixation for electron microscopy is performed if is necessary. (Figure 11, 12, 13).

The BAL cytology in healthy children is similar to that observed in healthy adults. In children the total cell counts tende to be higher in younger children (Table 9).

The interpretation of the differential cytology of BAL fluid can suggest the diagnosis of different types of lung diseases. Macrophages are the predominant cells followed by lymphocytes while the percentage of neutrophils appears to be higher in children under than 12 months. In general, in the absence of infection, the BAL of children have higher percentages of macrophages (upper to 90%) while those suffering from viral or bacterial infection have greater increases in the percentage of neutrophils. Unlike the adult the CD4/CD8 ratio in children has been found to be lower. The predominance of eosinophils in BAL suggests eosinophilic pneumonia or drug toxicity.

Although LBA prolongs the duration of bronchoscopy, because the bronchoscope stays longer in the airways, there is an increased risk of complications when compared with bronchoscopy simple. The main complications of the procedure are temporary, such as tachypnea without cardiac decompensation, and fever spikes 4 to 6 hours after the procedure. Other possible complications include hypoxemia that is most often minimized by concomitant administration of oxygen during the procedure and transient bronchospasm.

BAL has become a valuable procedure because, unlike lung biopsy is less invasive, well tolerated by patients, insurance and low percentage of complications, even in infants.

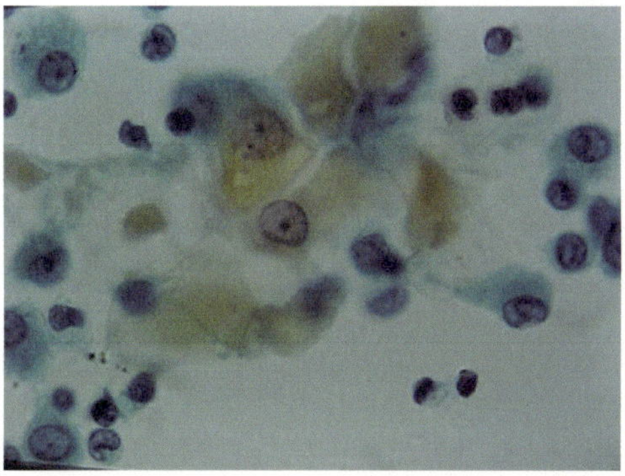

Fig. 11. BAL with large amounts of PAS-positive material in and out of cells (PAS 100 x).

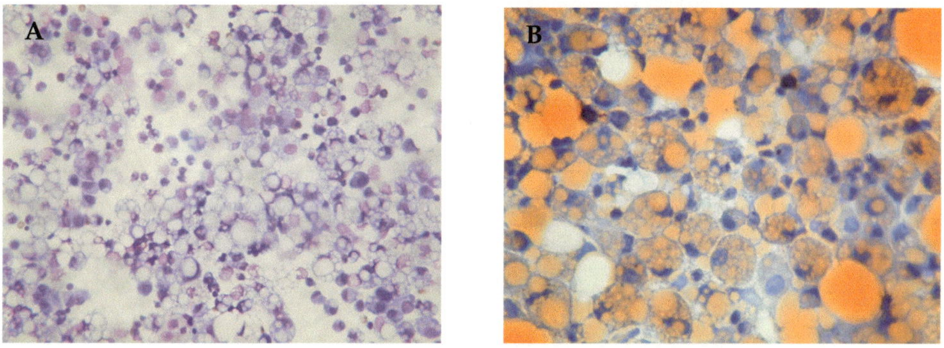

Fig. 12. BAL with large number of cells with predominance of foamy cytoplasm macrophages (A) (Giemsa 400X) and numerous macrophages with foamy cytoplasm stained orange (B) (Sudan 400X).

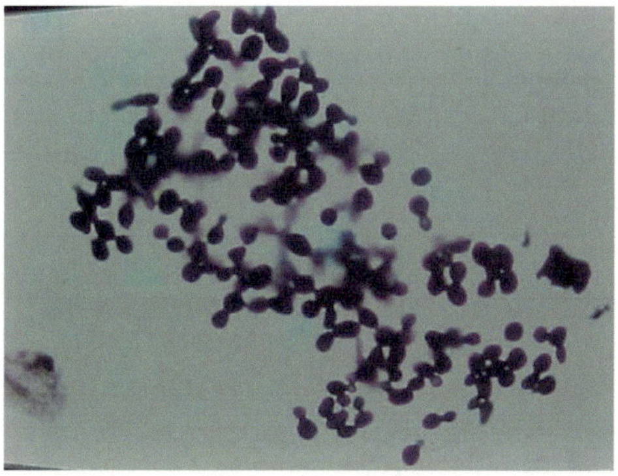

Fig. 13. BAL of immunocompromised child with chronic pneumonia shows a group of fungi (Gomori-Grocott 400x).

The presence of microorganisms in BAL fluid does not necessarily indicate they are the causative agents of pneumonia due to the possibility of contamination with the flora of the nasal or oropharynx. However, the growth of bacteria in the BAL should be enhanced through the use of protected a catheter or protected or by the quantitative bacteriological culture.

	Clement et AL 1987	Ratjen et al 1995	Riedler et al 1995	Midulla et al 1995	Tessier et al 1996
No. of children	11	48	18	16	11
Age range	1-15	3-5	1#-10	2#-3	4-16
Sedation	LA	GA	GA	LA	LA
No. of aliquots	6	3	3	2	6
Vol.saline	10% FRC	$3ml.Kg^{-1}$	$3ml^{-1}$	20ml	10% FRC
BAL fluid recovered %					
mean ± SD	NR	58±15	NR	43.1±12.2	69.7±9.6
median	NR	NR	62.5	42.5	68
range	NR	NR	42.5-71.5	20-65	52-87
X 10^4 $cells.mL^{-1}$					
mean±SD	25.5 ± 13.6	10.3 ± 11.1	ND	59.9 ± 32.9	35.1 ± 18.4
median	24	7.3	15.5	51	30.5
range	7.0±50	0.5±57.1	7.5±25.8*	0 20±130	9±68
Alveolar Macrophage %					
media±SD	89.7±5.2	81.2±12.7	NR	86±7.8	89.9±5.5
mediana	89	84	91	87	92.5
range	85-97	34.6-94	84.2-94*	71-98	77-98
Lymphocyte %					
media±SD	8.7±4.6	16.2±12.4	NR	8.7±5.8	8.9±5.6
median	10	12.5	7.5	7	8
range	1-17	2-61	4.7-12.8*	2-22	2-22
Neutrophil %					
media±SD	1.3±0.9	1.9±2.9	NR	5.5±4.8	1.2±1.2
median	1	0.9	1.7	3.5	1
range	0-3	0-17	0.6-3.5*	0-17	0-3
Eosinophil %					
media±SD	NR	0.4±0.6	NR	0.2±0.3	0
median	NR	0.2	0.2	0	0
range	NR	0-3.6	0-0.3*	0-1	0

Age range is given in years, except where indicated by #; *: First interquartile to third interquartile. LA: local anaesthesia; GA: general anaesthesia; FRC: functional residual capacity; ND: not done.

Table 9. Normal BAL cell count parameters in healthy children

5. Other special procedures in pediatric bronchoscopy

5.1 Bronchial biopsy

Bronchial biopsy is performed in the mucosa or in an endobronchial lesion allowing the assessment of the epithelium, the basal membrane and even the smooth muscle.

This procedure is safely used in research studies of respiratory disorders including asthma, recurrent wheezing, and cystic fibrosis, and has already revealed its usefulness for the diagnosis of either infectious or non-infectious granulomatous diseases (tuberculosis, sarcoidosis), endobronchial tumors, chronic fungal diseases, and for the management of difficult-to-control asthma. Although bronchial biopsy is appropriate for harvesting ciliated cells for the diagnosis of primary ciliary dyskinesia, nasal brushing remains the recommendable technique to be performed in this disorder due to its simplicity, with equal results.

Bronchial biopsies can be performed under direct vision although some endoscopists has been preferred to use flexible bronchoscope. Adult flexible bronchoscope (4.9 mm OD) is also used for biopsies because a 2.0mm instrumentation channel is needed for most biopsy forceps. Standard 1.8 mm diameter forceps are also used to obtain bronchial samples, although the 1,1 forceps has been successfully used, too. We have to keep in mind that the size of the samples obtained with the 1,1 forceps are obviously smaller, and the successful rate of the technique could decrease because of that. An adequate sample for analysis must show at least 1mm of basal membrane, sufficient subepithelial stroma for inflammation assessment, areas of smooth muscle and submucosal glands. In general the number of biopsies performed for a trustworthy analysis varies from a minimum of 1 up to 6.

In general the technique is well tolerated and no important bleeding or pneumothorax has been reported. Different from transbronchial biopsy, routine chest radiography is not necessary as we don't go through bronchial wall during the procedure. The risk of major bleeding increases in biopsies of very vascularized lesions. In these cases, 1-2 ml of adrenalin at 1 / 20.000 should be instilled previous to the procedure. General anesthesia or deep sedation is usually used to avoid patient movement during the procedure and to increase safety, specially in children.

5.2 Transbronchial biopsy

Transbronchial biopsy (TB) is a procedure performed to obtain lung fragments, using an appropriate flexible biopsy forceps, which is inserted through the bronchoscope. The aim of this procedure is to collect material from the lung parenchyma using a minimally invasive procedure. Although, TB is routinely used in adult patients with a good diagnostic yield in many situations since the 70s, its role in children took longer to be established. Issues related to the techniques used, the yield results and the safety of the procedure possibly contributed to this fact.

Currently, TB has a well-defined role for the monitoring of pediatric patients who underwent a lung or a heart-lung transplantation, when it is performed with well-established protocols during the first year after transplantation to assess the presence of rejection or infection.

Transbronchial biopsy in this setting was able to detect asymptomatic rejection in up to 24% of cases (Faro et al., 2004). It must also be performed when there is any abnormality of the heart`s transplant patient presented with cough, dyspnea or fever associated with radiological findings or in the presence of decline in lung function. Although the diagnostic yield of TB in patients with other medical conditions, with or without immunodeficiency, may reach 67%, ERS Task Force considers the role of TB in non-transplanted patients are still controversial. Some studies also demonstrate the use of TB for the diagnosis of other diseases such as lung disease in immunosuppressed patients, sarcoidosis, eosinophilic granuloma and lymphoma.

Transbronchial biopsy can be performed either through a flexible or rigid bronchoscope. For the flexible bronchoscope, it is generally used the adult model with an outer diameter of 4.9 mm and a 2.2 mm working-channel diameter, which is not often a problem for older children (figure 14). For the younger children, smaller diameter bronchoscopes may be used with working-channels as narrow as 1.2 mm, which also involves the usage of smaller forceps, which could lessen the chances of obtaining adequate samples for analysis, potentially decreasing the diagnostic yield· The rigid bronchoscope could also be used for these younger children, thus allowing the use of larger forceps with no significant differences in technique·

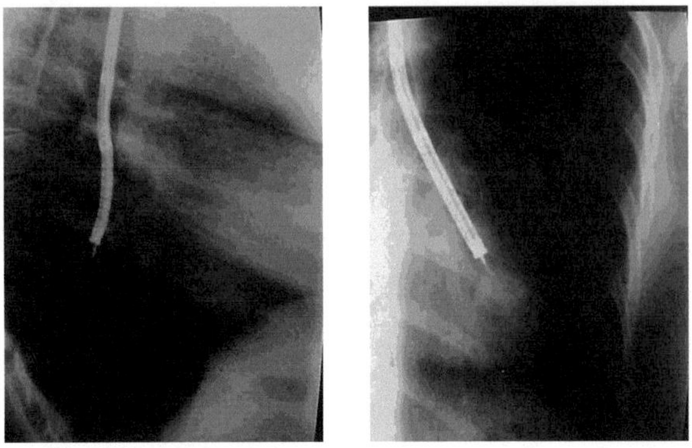

Fig. 14. Flexible bronchoscope with biopsy forceps on its distal end.

The technique for obtaining fragments from distal airways is the same as described by the ERS Task Force· In the absence of localized disease, at least two lobes should be approached. However, only one lung should be sampled to minimize the risk of bilateral pneumothorax. The minimum number of fragments to be harvested is still uncertain, ranging from 3 to 4, depending on the experience of each service· The use of fluoroscopy can be a great value for the procedure, since it allows a more accurate location of the biopsy forceps, and also the assessment off its operation during the procedure, despite the limitations of the two-dimensional image generated. ERS Task Force considers the use of fluoroscopy mandatory to perform TB.

Overall, TB is a safe procedure when performed by experienced professional. Less serious complications include transient hypoxemia, fever and dyspnea . Serious complications include bleeding and pneumothorax, and occur in around 5% of the patients submitted to TB, although series of patients reported the incidence of pneumothorax up to 12%. Recent publications reported the incidence of pneumothorax and bleeding around 2%· The complications rate appears to be higher than that observed in adult patients. The use of positive pressure ventilation can theoretically contribute to a higher incidence of pneumothorax. Therefore, TB should be performed during spontaneous ventilation whenever it's possible· TB seems to be a technique that deserves better use, still being underused in clinical pediatrics·

6. Foreing body aspiration

Accidents in childhood are important causes of morbidity and mortality worldwide , requiring prompt recognition and early treatment to minimize the risk of serious fatal consequences. Among the accidents, there is a foreign body aspiration (FBA) of the airway. United States of America statistics show that 5% of deaths from accidents with children under 4 years are due to FBA, which is also the main cause of accidental death at home in children under 6 years. In Brazil, the FBA is the third leading cause of accidents with death.

Currently, the foreign body aspiration remains an emergency, presents itself the same way as in earlier times, but with diminishing considerable morbidity and mortality.

The majority victims are infants and children, early in life, with the predominant age of 4 years. The male over female prevails in most published works, probably the most curious and impulsive nature of the boys. According to Reilly et al, children younger than 4 years are more susceptible to FBA injuries due to their lack of molar teeth, oral exploration, and poor swallowing coordination. Usually the coordination between chewing and swallowing is completed around 5 years old. The caregiver was present at the time of injury in 48.9%of cases (82.3% while the children were eating, and 33.8% while playing).

Foreign body aspiration in children is associated with a failure of the laryngeal closure reflex, poor control of swallowing and habit of putting objects in the mouth. The negligence of some parents with certain objects might can be aspirated, as small toys and some foods are predisposing factors.

Foreign bodies may be organic or inorganic material. The origin of organic vegetables are more common: peanuts, beans, corn, fruits and seeds. Beans and peanuts are the most frequently aspirated. However the type of foreign body aspiration varies according to regional food habits. Dried vegetables stimulates an inflammatory reaction within a few hours, making the extraction extremely hard. Foreign bodies can be found from animal sources like chicken bone, and teeth fragments. The non-organic may be metal or plastic. The most frequent non-organic FBA are plastic pen cap, earring, pin, plastic toy, nib, nail, hair clip, earring tuners, small plastic parts. In recent years, children have been increasingly exposed to the electronic technologies containing buttons and batteries (Figure 15).

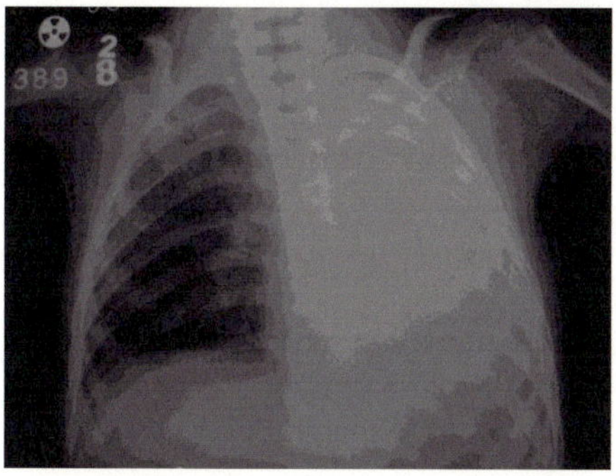

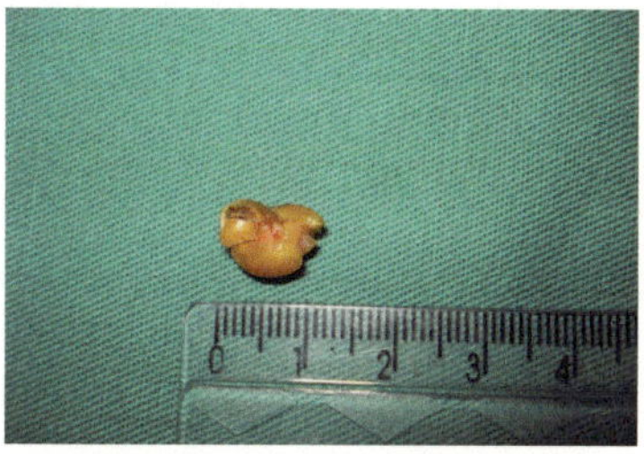

Fig. 15. Total atelectasis caused by corn removed from the left main bronchus.

Clinically, FBA manifests as a coughing, followed by choking, which may or may not be valued by parents. Most often, this is currently not seen by parents or guardians, a fact that delays the diagnosis, unless the aspiration is followed by complete obstruction of the airway.

Clinical findings depend on the type, size and location of foreign body and including persistent cough, located air intake, localized or diffuse, wheezing and breathing difficulties. Approximately 40% of the patients are asymptomatic and no changes in physical examination. The FBA can also be suspected in the first sudden onset of wheezing.

Foreign bodies may be located in the larynx, trachea and bronchi. The most commonly found is in the right main bronchus, due to anatomical position of this bronchus.

The symptoms will depend on the location:

Larynx: supraglottic (cough, dysphagia or difficulty to swallow food or saliva swallowing, inspiratory stridor); glottal (dysphonia, inspiratory stridor) (Figure 16) and subglottic (dyspnea or shortness of breath accompanied by chest indrawing, supraclavicular, suprasternal or universal).

Trachea: wheezing audible sound from the shock of the foreign body against the subglottis during expiration or coughing, cyanosis, retractions suprasternal, supraclavicular, intercostal, biphasic stridor, dysphagia, suffocation and sudden death.

Bronchi: clinical manifestations depend on the caliber that the foreign body occupies within the bronchial lumen. When there is atelectasis and a significant portion of the lung is involved can occur tachypnea, retractions, dullness to percussion and decreased breath sounds. Crackles may be present if there is infection.

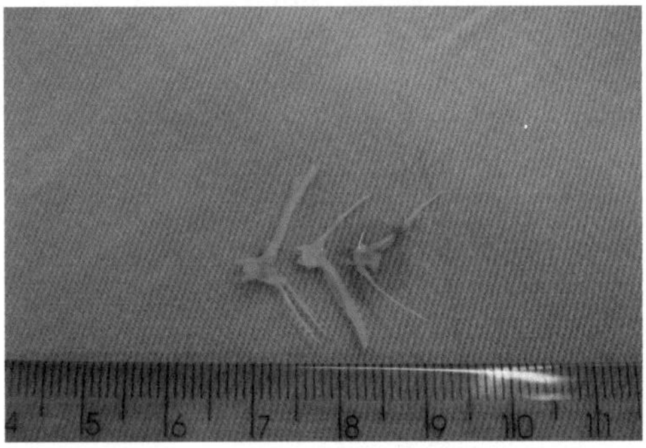

Fig. 16. Fish bone in 2-year-old boy presenting dysphonia and inspiratory dyspnea.

Although the radiographic study should be performed in almost all cases, it is reiterated that the decision for endoscopic investigation is always warranted before a history and physical examination suggestive of aspiration.

Radiological study using the technical inspiration and forced expiration, is altered in most cases. The main radiological abnormalities are lung hyperinflation and atelectasis. Normal chest radiograph, consolidations, and radiopaque foreign bodies are reported less frequently.

Chest X-ray should remain the initial imaging modality for patients with clinically suspected of FBA. Nevertheless, in cases with normal chest X-ray and clinical suspicion of FBA, multi-slice computed tomography possibly integrated with virtual bronchoscopy should be considered to avoid unnecessary bronchoscopy.

The early diagnosis of FBA is essential. Large number of patients are treated for weeks and months due to recurrent respiratory diseases before the suspicion of FBA. Late diagnosis or wrong results in respiratory complications such as recurrent pneumonia, lung abscess, and obstruction of the airway which can be fatal.

Bronchoscopy is the procedure of choice for foreign body removal. The authors prefer the rigid bronchoscope because it has less risk of complications.

Patients are submitted to rigid bronchoscopy under general inhalation anesthesia and assisted ventilation. The foreign body extraction is performed by special clamps for each type of foreign body, aided by optical rigid. In some cases fragments of foreign bodies are removed through small size bronchial lavage with saline solution and suction aspiration cannulas. Subsequently should be performed the review of tracheobronchial tree.

A radiological control should be done. Antibiotics and steroids are necessary in some patients due to inflammatory reaction triggered by plant and animal aspiration.

In cases of foreign body be larger than the opening of the glottis tracheostomy will be necessary. Thoracotomy is indicated when it is not possible to extract the foreign body by bronchoscopy after several attempts. The review of the tracheobronchial tree should be done in 2 to 4 weeks depending on the case.

Peri-operative complications, such as bronchospasm, bleeding, pneumotorax and desaturation can occur.

FBA are a life-threatening event in children that require early diagnosis and prompt successful management. Prevention is the most critical element in reducing morbidity and is considered the most effective treatment of FBA injuries. Changes in product design, campaigns of prevention of accidents in childhood, education of parents and carers are strategies that have been used to reduce morbidity and mortality caused by foreign body aspiration.

7. Stridor and congenital airway anomalies

Stridor is acute respiratory noise that results of a turbulent airflow due to blockage of airway. It is the most frequent indication for bronchoscopy.

The incidence of stridor ranging from 13.5% to 96% of endoscopies. It is higher in newborns and infants, with an average age of 4 months. In newborns and infants, the caliber of the airway is more narrow, and any obstruction can result in a blockage to the passage of air, resulting in a turbulent airflow. The preponderance of males over females is not clear. The most common is the inspiratory stridor, with origins in the larynx, upper trachea or hypopharynx.

The child with stridor should be examined carefully, starting with detailed history, followed by physical examination, radiological and endoscopic examination. Is very important to a good history, emphasizing a history of intubation, its duration and size of the endotracheal tube, history of trauma during intubation and the number of times that the child was intubated. Information such as age of onset of stridor, the duration of the stridor, the association with triggering agents, such as tears and pain, the association with the position (prone, supine, or sitting), the quality or nature of crying, the presence of other symptoms such as paroxysmal cough, cyanosis and aspiration are important and should be investigated.

If symptoms worsen in the supine position and improve in prone, may be caused by laryngomalacia, or tracheal compression by the innominate artery. In the prone position, the structures obstruct the airway and stridor increases. It is important to evaluate the morphology of the skull in relation to malformations, the presence of micrognathia or retrognathia, cyanosis, signs of infection in the oral cavity, the presence of excessive salivation or oral secretions, use of accessory respiratory muscles, throbbing of the nose, chest wall retraction and the child's level of consciousness.

Chest X-ray should be mandatory in all patients. Images of the neck and upper airway are useful for evaluating the air columns above and below the larynx and the lung parenchyma, allowing us to follow the evolution of local collapse and obstruction. High kilovoltage techniques are useful to observe the larynx, vocal cords and subglottic region. Fluoroscopy, barium swallow, computed tomography, and electromagnetic resonance may be useful in the diagnosis of structural and / or dynamic changes of the tracheobronchial tree, such as tracheomalacia, tracheal or bronchial compression by anomalous vessel, patients with swallowing disorders, laryngeal cleft, vascular ring, tracheoesophageal fistula and radiolucent esophageal foreign bodies. Although these tests can contribute to the differential diagnosis of stridor, bronchoscopy is establishing a definitive diagnosis.

The main causes of stridor are congenital and occur more frequently in the larynx, followed by the trachea and bronchi. Table 10 shows the causes of stridor by anatomical location.

Upper airway	Choanal atresia Tumors, cysts and masses Craniofacial anomalies
Larynx	Laryngomalacia Paralysis of vocal cords (congenital and adquired) Infections conditions (croup and epiglottitis) Subglottic stenosis (congenital and adquired) Hemangioma Saccular cysts e laryngoceles Webs, atresia Cleft larynx Laryngeal pappilomatosis Trauma Foreign body
Lower airway	Tracheomalacia, Bronchomalacia Tracheoesophageal fistula Vascular anomalies (aberrant innominate artery, double aortic arch, pulmonary artery sling) Tracheal web, cysts and stenosis Accessory bronchi and lobes Infections conditions Pulmonary sequestration Asthma, bronchiolitis, bronchitis Foreign body

Table 10. Most common causes of stridor in children

Laryngomalacia is the most common congenital anomaly of the larynx and the most important cause of stridor, predominantly in males in the ratio 1.6 / 1 (Figure 17). May be isolated or associated with other abnormalities of the airways such as tracheomalacia, bronchomalacia, vocal cord paralysis, subglottic stenosis, hypertrophy of adenoids.

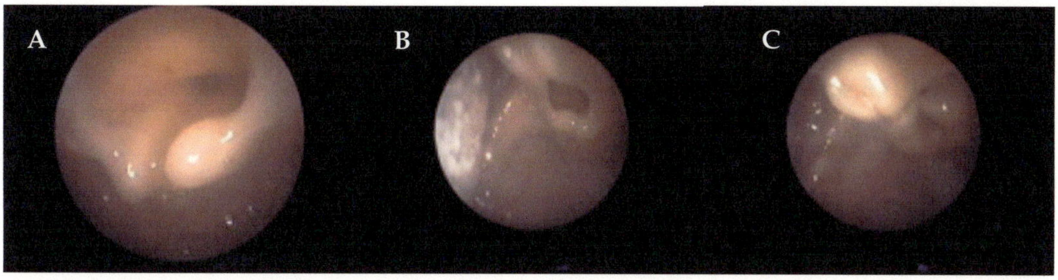

Fig. 17. Inspiratory collapse of cuneiform cartilages (A), anterior collapse of the cuneiform cartilages (B) and long tubular epiglottis (C).

The vocal cord paralysis is another frequent cause of stridor (Figure 18). Vocal cord paralysis secondary to congenital disorders of the central nervous system is common and often is associated with multiple anomalies, as Arnould-Chiari syndrome. The vocal cord paralysis can be acquired as a result of iatrogenic repair of cardiovascular disorders, most common cause of unilateral paralysis of vocal cords. Paralysis of vocal cords acquired from trauma and infections, is rare.

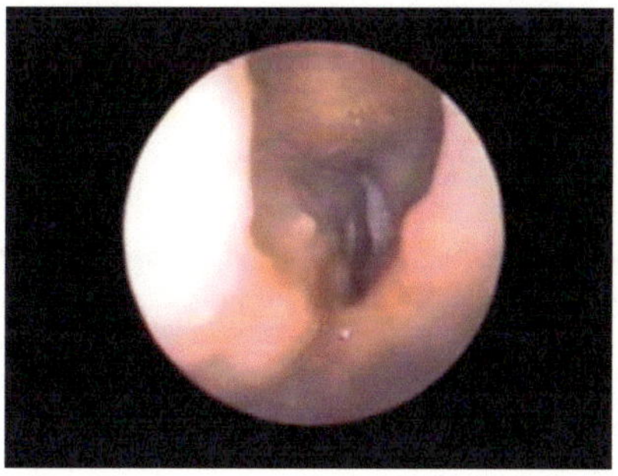

Fig. 18. Left vocal cord paralysis.

Acquired subglottic stenosis is also a frequent cause of stridor, usually secondary to intubation (Figure 19). The incidence of acquired subglottic stenosis is increasing due to improved care of premature.

Differential diagnosis of base of tongue mass includes lingual thyroid, thyroglossal duct cyst, lymphoid hyperplasia, hemangioma, teratoma, adenoma, salivary gland tumor, fibroma, dermoid cyst, and carcinoma.

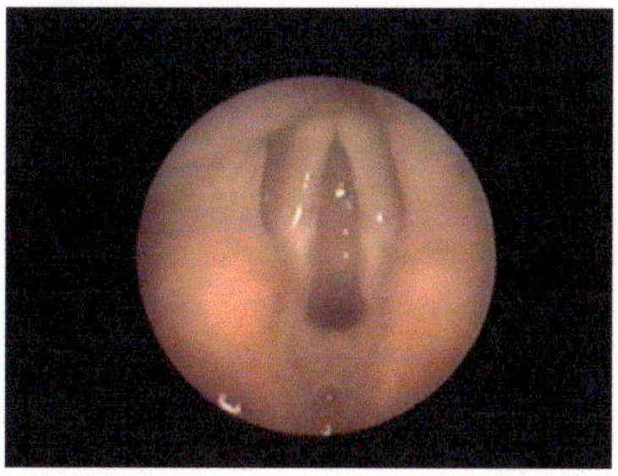

Fig. 19. Acquired subglottis stenosis.

The ectopic thyroid may be present in the tongue, although it is a rare injury, can occur in infants. The hygroma generally affects the hypopharynx and the supraglottic region, causing sometimes very important obstructions to breathing. Hemangiomas are the most common tumors of childhood , the incidence ranged from 1% to 3%. Papilloma is the most common laryngeal tumor.

The most patients affected by laryngeal trauma are those undergoing mechanical ventilation. The severity of the injury is related to the number and duration of endotracheal intubation.

The craniofacial anomalies may have severe impairment of the airways. The cause of airway obstruction in micrognathia is ptosis of the tongue. The children in prone position improved significantly. In more severe cases the tracheostomy is indicated.

In general the stridor caused by extrinsic compression of the trachea and bronchi is expiratory. The endoscopic examination can show pulsatile compression of the anterior wall of the trachea caused by double aortic arch, pulmonary sling and aberrant innominate artery. Symptoms such as dysphagia, recurrent vomiting, and chronic respiratory failure may be associated with stridor.

Respiratory infections also can cause stridor. They are most often of viral etiology. The most common are croup, epiglottitis and tracheitis. In general in cases of bacterial etiology there are high fever associated with toxemia. Endoscopy is indicated when the child does not respond to medical therapy, has prolonged or recurrent seizures and low age.

Congenital laryngeal membrane is unusual. The majority is glottic and is extending into the subglottis.

Atresia and stenosis are common congenital abnormalities in the nose, with an incidence of 1 in 7000 newborns, predominantly in males. Unilateral atresia is twice as common than bilateral and is associated with other craniofacial abnormalities facias.

Bronchial abnormalities most common are additional, stenosed and collapsed bronchus. Generally, bronchial abnormalities may be associated with other visceral anomalies, including inversus situs, intestinal malrotation and cardiac malformations.

Congenital tracheal stenosis is rare. The diagnosis is made by bronchoscopy that is the best procedure to define the extent of the stenosis.

8. Acknowledgment

We thank to Dr. Guilherme Millward for kind enough to give some photographic material.

9. References

Baker, PA. (2010). A prospective randomized trial comparing supraglottic airways for flexible bronchoscopy in children. *Paediatr Anaesth*, Vol.20, No.9, (September 2010), pp 831-838, ISSN 1460-9592

Barbato, A. (1997). Use of the paediatric bronchoscope, flexible and rigid, in 51 European centres. *Eur Respir J*, Vol.10, No.8, (August 1997), pp 1761-6, ISSN 0903-1936

Becker, HD. Bronchoscopy: the past, the present, and the future. *Clin Chest Med*, Vol.31, No.1, (March 2010), pp 1-18, ISSN 1557-8216

de Fenoyl, O. (1989). Transbronchial biopsy without fluoroscopy: a five year experience in outpatients. *Thorax*, Vol.44, No.11, (November 1989), pp 956-959, ISSN 0040-6376

Fan, LL. (1997). Diagnostic value of transbronchial, thoracoscopic, and open lung biopsy in immunocompetent children with chronic interstitial lung disease. *J Pediatr*, Vol.131, No.4, (October 1997), pp 565-569, ISSN 0022-3476

Fraga, AMA. (2008). Foreign body aspiration in children: clinical aspects, radiological aspects and bronchoscopic treatment. *J Bras Pneumol*,Vol.34, No.2, (February 2008), pp.74-82, ISSN 1806-3756

Greene, CL. (2008). Role of clinically indicated transbronchial lung biopsies in the management of pediatric post-lung transplant patients. *Ann Thorac Surg*, Vol.86, No.1, (July 2008), pp 198-203, ISSN 1552-6259

Holinger, LD & Green CG. (1997). Anatomy. In: *Pediatric Laryngology & Bronchoesophagology*, Lolinger LD, Lusk RP & Green CG, pp 19-33, Lippincott-Raven, INSB 0-397-51650-9, Philadelphia

Holinger, LD & Green CG. (1997). Instrumentation, epquipment and standardization. In: *Pediatric Laryngology & Bronchoesophagology*, Holinger LD, Lusk RP & Green CG, pp 65-80, Lippincott-Raven, INSB 0-397-51650-9, Philadelphia

Holinger, LD (1980) Etiology of stridor in the neonate, infant and child. *Ann Otol Rhinol Laryngol*, Vol.89, No.5 Pt.1, (September-October 1980), pp 397-400, ISSN 0003-4894

Holinger, LD (1997). Evolution of stridor and wheezing. In: *Pediatric Laryngology x Bronchoesophagology*. Hollinger, LD; Green, C; Lusk, R. pp 41-48, Lippincott-Raven , ISBN 0-397-51650-9, Philadelphia

Hui, H. (2008). Therapeutic experience from 1428 patients with pediatric tracheobronchial foreign body. *J Pediatr Surg*. Vol.43, No.4, (April 2008), pp 718-721, ISSN 0022-3468

Jaggar SI & Haxby E. (2002). Sedation, anaesthesia and monitoring for bronchoscopy. *Paediatr Respir Rev*, Vol.3, No. 4, (December 2002), pp 321-327, ISSN 1526-0542

Korlacki, W. (2011). Foreign body aspiration and therapeutic role of bronchoscopy. *Pediatr Surg Int*, Vol.27, No.8, (August 2011), pp 833-837, INSS 1437-9813

Malherbe, S. & Ansermino, JM. (2010). Total intravenous anesthesia and spontaneous ventilation for foreign body removal in children: how much drug? *Anesth Analg*, Vol.111, No.6, (December 2010), pp 1566, ISSN 1526-7598

Mancuso, RF. (1996). Stridor in Neonates. *Pediatr Clin North Am*, Vol.43, No.6, (December 1996), pp 1339-1356, ISSN 1557-8240

Meduri, GU. (1991). Bilateral bronchoalveolar lavage in the diagnosis of opportunistic pulmonary infections. Chest, Vol.100, No.5, (October 1991), pp 1272-1276, ISSN 1931-3543

Mendonça Picinin, IF (2011) Cell count and lymphocyte immunophenotyping of bronchoalveolar lavage fluid in healthy Brazilian children. *Eur Respir J*, Vol.38, No.3, (September 2011), pp 738-739, ISSN 1399-3003

Muntz, HR. (1992). Pediatric transbronchial lung biopsy. *Ann Otol Rhinol Laryngol*, Vol.101, No.2 Pt 1, (February 1992), pp 135-7, ISSN 0003-4894

Naguib, ML. (2005). Use of laryngeal mask airway in flexible bronchoscopy in infants and children. *Pediatr Pulmonol*, Vol.39, No.1, (January 2005), pp 56-63, ISSN 8755-6863

Newman, B. (1996). Left pulmonary artery sling: diagnosis and delineation of associated tracheobronchiasl anomalies with MR. *Pediatr Radiol,* Vol.26, No.9, (September 1996), pp 661-668, ISSN 1432-1998

Nicolai, T. The role of rigid and flexible bronchoscopy in children. *Paediatr Respir Rev,* Vol.12, No.3, (September 2011), pp 190-195. ISSN 1526-0550

Passàli, D. (2010). Foreign body inhalation in children: a update. *Acta Otorhinolaryngol Ital,* Vol.30, No., (February, 2010), pp.27-32. INSS 1827-675X

Prakash, UBS & Holinger LD. (1994). Pediatric Rigid Bronchoscopy. In: *Bronchoscopy,* Udaya BS Prakash, pp 329-343, Raven Press, INSB 0-7817-0095-7, New York

Regelmann, WE & Elliot, GR. (1993). Bronchoalveolar lavage. In: *Pediatric Respiratory Disease. Diagnosis and treatment.* Hilman BC. pp 116-122, WB Saunders Company, ISBN 0-7216-4683-2, Philadelphia

Riedler, J. (1995). Bronchoalveolar lavage cellularity in healthychildren. *Am J Respir Care Med,* Vol152, No.1, (July 1995), pp 163-168, ISSN 1535-4970

Saki, N. (2009). Foreign body aspirations in infancy: a 20-year experience. *Int J Med Sci,* Vol.6, N°6, (October, 2009), pp 322-328, INSS 1449-1907

Sias, SMA. (2009). Clinical and Radiological Improvement of Lipoid Pulmonary with Multiple Bronchoalveolar Lavage. *Ped Pulmonol,* Vol.44, No.4 , (April 2009), pp 309-15, ISSN 1099-0496

Tunkel, DE & Zalzal, GH. (1992) Stridor in infants and children: ambulatory evaluation and operative diagnosis. *Clin Pediatr (Phila),* Vol.31, No.1, (January.1992), pp 48-55, ISSN 0009-9228

Visner, GA. Role of transbronchial biopsies in pediatric lung diseases. *Chest,* 126 No.1, (July 2004), pp 273-780, ISSN 0012-3692

Wintrop, AL & Superina RA. (1990). The diagnosis of pneumonia in the immunocompromised child: use of bronchoalveolar lavage. *J Pediatr Surg,* Vol.25, No.8, (August 1990), pp 87-80, ISSN 1531-5037

Wood, RE & Prakash, UBS. (1994). Pediatric Flexible Bronchoscopy. In: *Bronchoscopy,* Udaya BS Prakash, pp 345-356, Raven Press, INSB 0-7817-0095-7, New York

Wood, RE & Prakash, UBS. (1994). Pediatric Flexible Bronchoscopy. In: *Bronchoscopy,* Prakash UBS, pp 345-356, Raven Press, INSB 0-7817-0095-7, New York

Wood, RE. (1990). Pitfalls in the use of the flexible bronchoscope in pediatric patients. *Chest,* Vol.97, No.1, (January 1990), pp 199-203, ISSN 0012-3692

11

Manual Jet Ventilation Using Manujet III for Bronchoscopic Airway Foreign Body Removal in Children

Shaoqing Li, Yuqi Liu and Fang Tan
The Eye, Ear, Nose and Throat Hospital, Fudan University, Shanghai
China

1. Introduction

Aspiration of a foreign body (FB) into the airway was often a life-threatening event in children. A particular challenge to anesthesiologists was that the airway must be shared with the surgeon during FB removal. It was difficult to maintain adequate ventilation, oxygenation and anesthetic depth without disturbing the operation. Also, the methods of anesthetic management and modes of ventilation during bronchoscopic FB removal varied greatly among institutions and anesthetists.

Since the introduction of the rigid bronchoscope, the rate of successful removal of FB has increased dramatically and the safety of the operation has improved. However, Intraoperative or postoperative hypoxemia was still found to be the most frequent adverse event, and it could lead to a life-threatening outcome if not promptly treated. The occurrence of hypoxemia occurrence may depend on a variety of factors including the property of the FB, the surgeon's experience, anesthetic method, and patient's condition. Our study identified five factors that strongly correlated with increased rate of intraoperative hypoxemia: age of patient, plant seeds as FB, pneumonia before procedure, long duration of FB removal surgery, and ventilation mode.

Of all the factors related to hypoxemia or other complications in our study, ventilation mode was strongly associated with intraoperative hypoxemia. An extensive medical literature search revealed that the optimal ventilation mode during rigid bronchoscopy for FB removal is still actively controversial. In general, spontaneous ventilation(SV) was more popular and was advocated before the mid 1990s, whereas more recently reports in favor of control ventilation(CV) have appeared. In a review by Farrell, the advantages and disadvantages of SV and CV were discussed; however, no personal preference was suggested. Jet ventilation in rigid bronchoscopy was first introduced by Sanders in 1967. Since then, it has been modified and widely used in suspended laryngoscopy. Its use in pediatric FB removal has not been widely advocated. In our study, we developed a MJV method using Manujet III in which a small catheter was placed transnasally into the trachea for oxygen delivery. This technique produced fewer episodes of intraoperative hypoxemia than any other ventilation mode. The value of MJV became more pronounced when the bronchoscope had to be inserted distal to the FB. In this instance, ventilation became limited to the lung distal to the FB. In this situation, MJV became advantageous over the other ventilation modes, because MJV provided continuous ventilation in the noninvolved lung with a catheter separated from the bronchoscope. Thus, compared to other modes of ventilation, MJV significantly reduces the risk of hypoxemia.

This chapter was to narrate The Application and Possible Complications of manual jet ventilation using Manujet device for bronchoscopic removal of airway FBs in children, and discuss in detail the application and possible complication.

2. Manujet III

The Manujet III (VBM Medizintechnik GmbH, Germany, Figure 1) is a portable and easily regulated device that can be used for manual jet ventilation with a low volume of mechanical dead space, is specially made for Jet Ventilation in circumstances of problem airways and can be used in areas that have a high pressure oxygen air outlet. If there is an acute obstruction of the upper airway, the Manujet, in connection with a Jet Ventilation catheter acc. Ravussin or the Endojet adaptor, allows the patient to be ventilated.

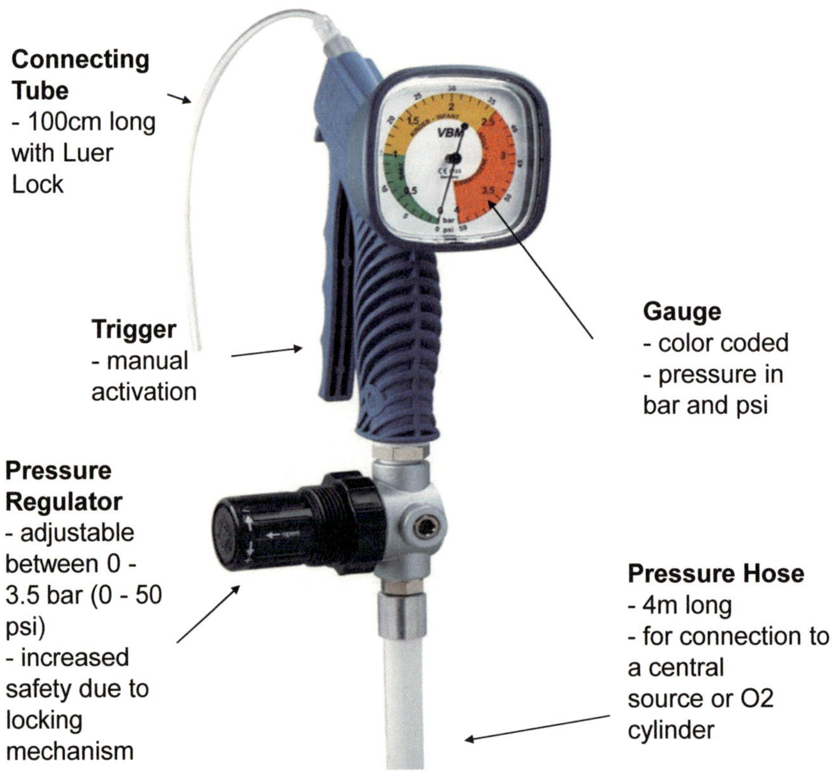

Fig. 1. The Manujet III device (from VBM medical, INC.)

the Manujet Includes:

- Case with 4 m pressure hose
- Luer lock connecting tube

- Bronchoscope adaptor
- Endojet adaptor with Endojet catheter
- One of each Jet Ventilation catheter acc. to Ravussin for infant, child and adult(13G, 14G, 16G)

Connecting Tube—100cm long with Luer Lock

Endojet Adapter—for connection to the Endotracheal Tube,15mm

Bronchoscope Adapter—for connection to the rigid bronchoscope, 15mm

Endojet Adaptor—The Endojet adaptor allows jet ventilation on the endotracheal tube, laryngeal mask or face mask. The catheter can be pushed forward through the endotracheal tube or laryngeal mask as far as required and can be fastened with the screw.

The features of Manujet III are: faster and simple, lightweight, portable and immediately ready for use.

3. Manual Jet Ventilation (MJV)

Since jet ventilation was first used in endolaryngeal procedures in 1971, there have been many improvements based on Sanders' ventilation technique. Based on the position of the catheter, jet ventilation can be categorized as follows: supraglottic jet ventilation, subglottic jet ventilation and percutaneous transtracheal jet ventilation. Based on the frequency, jet ventilation is also classified as low-frequency jet ventilation (LFJV that is administered at <60 times/minute) and high-frequency jet ventilation (HFJV that is administered at >60 times/minute). Because it can provide ventilation at low peak airway pressure, HFJV plays an important role in both airway surgeires and pulmonary protective ventilation, while LFJV is easily to be performed manually using a manual jet ventilator. This article reviews the application of manual jet ventilation (MJV) in airway surgeries.

Gas entrainment as a result of the "Venturi effect" is described in medical textbooks as the basis of jet ventilation. It is thought that the high-speed stream of gas directed into the airway by the jet nozzle causes a pressure gradient betwen the surrounding atmosphere and the gas stream, this pressure gradient drives the entrainment of the air in the surrounding atmosphere into the airway. However, Dr Ihra G believed that there was no "Venturi effect" in jet ventilation, because during jet application, positive pressures can be measured inside the jet stream and inside the injector. Other consideration involves that the pressurized jet stream causes an acceleration of the quiescent air, as a consequence the viscosity and friction between the moving and static layers of the air increases, thus drawing the surrounding air into the airway, resulting in the always larger actual tidal volume than the set shooting volume.

MJV has several advantages over HFJV. MJV can be more easily performed as the MJV device and oxygen source are the only equipment required. The pressure and frequency of ventilation can be easily and instantaneously adjusted according to actual situation during the procedure. Another advantage of the MJV is that the frequency and inspiration/expiration ratio are both similar to physiological conditions, so that carbon dioxide expiration is easier. While, in HFJV, the positive end expiratory pressure (PEEP) caused by this technique benefits oxygenation but makes carbon dioxide expiration more difficult. In some cases, the increase in respiratory frequency may result in a decrease in alveolar ventilation. Vourc'h, et al made a comparison of MJV (20 times/minute) with HFJV (300 times/minute) which were used in tracheobronchial stenosis patients who received laser surgery under general anesthesia. Within the first 10 minutes of the operation, there was no significant difference between the two ventilation techniques as determined by blood gas analysis. However, those patients who received HFJV suffered from mild hypercapnia. It was thought that MJV is suitable better choice for patients who had tracheobronchial stenosis.

3.1 The application of MJV using Manujet III in rigid bronchoscopy for FB removal

MJV has been rarely reported to be used in airway foreign body removal. In our hospital, MJV using Manujet III has been applied in tracheobronchial foreign body removal in more than 2000 cases with satisfactory results since 2004. Our latest report concluded that, in addition to the fact that MJV provided a good condition for bronchoscopic manipulation, the occurrence of hypoxia during the operation was decreased. This conclusion was drawn after a comparison of the three ventilation techniques in 360 cases had been made; the techniques studied included spontaneous respiration, mechanically controlled ventilation and MJV. The effectiveness of the above three techniques were compared in the study with additional information including compliance to bronchoscope placement, successful rate of foreign body removal, occurrence of hypoxia and etc. From another study done by our group involving 384 patients, we concluded that the ventilation method was one of the risk factors in causing intraoperative hypoxemia. Specifically, spontaneous respiration tended to increase the occurrence of hypoxemia, while MJV decreased the occurrence. To perform this ventilation technique, a catheter (1.5 mm in I.D.) was placed transnasally into the trachea under the guidance of a laryngoscope and connected to the Manu-jet device (Figure 2) after anesthesia induction. Jet ventilation was manually controlled throughout the operation with the driving pressure of 15 psi in children aged less than 12 months or 15–35 psi (usually less than 25 psi) in children aged more than 1 year at a frequency of 20–35 times/minute. One outstanding advantage of this ventilation method is that the ventilation route is separate from the route used for bronchoscopy. This method can provide a steady oxygen supply

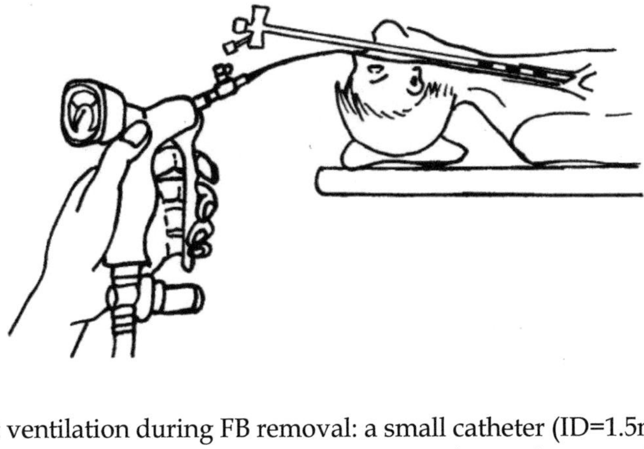

Fig. 2. Manual jet ventilation during FB removal: a small catheter (ID=1.5mm) was inserted transnasally into the trachea and connected to Manu-jet device during rigid bronchoscopy.

during the process of bronchoscope placement, which provides surgeons with ease in placing the bronchoscope. Constant and steady ventilation can also be achieved in the non-involved lung via a catheter separated from the bronchoscope when it is inserted into the distal side of bronchi of the involved lung. Even after the bronchoscope is removed, this technique can still provide jet ventilation until spontaneous respiration is restored in these patients.

3.1.1 Efficacy of manual jet ventilation using Manujet III for bronchoscopic airway foreign body removal in children

3.1.1.1 Patients and methods

Approval was obtained from the hospital's Human Research Committee prior to the study. The study was carried out from February of 2005 to June of 2009. A total of 360 children, ASA I or II, aged from 10 months to 12 years, weighing 8 - 35 kg, who required removal of an airway FB were enrolled in the study. All surgical manipulations were performed with Karl-Storz rigid bronchoscopes under general anesthesia. Informed consent was obtained from parents or legal guardians before the initiation of anesthetic and surgical procedure. Exclusion criteria included: (1) inability to obtain parental consent, (2) no foreign body found by bronchoscopy, and (3) absence of spontaneous breathing, cyanosis, or SpO2 <90% was detected prior to the operation. The presence of a supraglottic/glottic foreign body suggested by clinical symptoms and chest radiography findings or confirmed by laryngoscopy was also excluded from the study. The data were collected in the operating room and ward. Each outcome was observed under the same set of conditions and recorded at same time to avoid bias. Participants were blinded, observers were partially blinded, while surgeons and anesthetists were not blinded in the study.

3.1.1.2 Management of anesthesia and ventilation

Atropine (0.01 mg/kg) and methylprednisolone (2 mg/kg) was given intravenously to all patients before anesthetic induction. Patients were randomly divided into three groups (n = 120). In group S, anesthesia was induced with propofol (2 mg/kg) and ghydroxybutyrate sodium (70 mg/kg) and maintained by bolus administration of 1 - 2 mg/kg propofol as needed. The patient was allowed to breathe spontaneously at this level of anesthesia. Following successful insertion of a rigid bronchoscope, pure oxygen was delivered at a flow rate of 8 L/min by connecting the respiratory circuit to the side arm of the bronchoscope.

In Group P, anesthesia was induced with propofol (4 - 5 mg/kg), fentanyl (1 - 2 mg/kg) and succinylcholine (2 mg/kg) and maintained by bolus administration of 1 - 2 mg/kg propofol and 2 mg/kg succinylcholine as needed. The respiratory circuit was connected to the side arm of the bronchoscope and manual intermittent positive pressure ventilation (IPPV) was performed at the rate of 16 - 35 ventilations/min. A larger than normal tidal volume was delivered to offset the leakage of oxygen through the open eye piece of bronchoscope. The chest wall movement of the patients was closely observed to assure adequate ventilation.

In group J, patients received the same anesthetic protocol as in Group P. A small catheter was inserted transnasally into the trachea under the guidance of a laryngoscope and connected to the Manujet III device. Jet ventilation was manually controlled throughout the operation with the driving pressure of 0.6 - 1 bar in children aged less than 12 months or 1 - 2.5 bar in children aged more than 1 year (1 bar = 105 Pa) at a frequency of 20 - 35 ventilations/min. The effectiveness of ventilation was assessed by degree of chest excursion. After the FB removal, spontaneous respiration or assisted ventilation was maintained through a facemask in Groups S and P. In Group J, the jet catheter was kept in the trachea and jet ventilation was continued until spontaneous respiration resumed.

Prior to the start of the insertion of bronchoscope, 1% lidocaine aerosol was sprayed over the epiglottis using laryngoscopic guidance in all groups of patients.

3.1.1.3 Measurements

The condition for insertion of bronchoscope was regarded as satisfactory when the bronchoscope was inserted successfully on the first attempt with a clear view of the glottis and without patient's body movement or bucking. Hypoxemia was defined as a decrease in pulse oxygen saturation (SpO2) < 90% for >5 s.

Beside the baseline medical conditions and condition that required the procedure, the following information was recorded for each patient: successful insertion of bronchoscope on the first attempt, occurrence of hypoxemia during bronchoscopy and after withdrawing the bronchoscope, successful rate of FB removal, the duration of the operation, the time of emergence and recovery from anesthesia, and perioperative side effects including laryngospasm, arrhythmias, breath holding, and post-op restlessness. Patients were discharged from this study if no foreign body was found during the operation. If the presence of a foreign body was confirmed but could not be removed in the first attempt of bronchoscopy, a second attempt was made 3 - 5 days later, and a thoracotomy should be taken after two times of unsuccessful bronchoscopy. The ventilation mode and anesthetic technique for the second bronchoscopy were chosen based on the anesthetist's preference, and, in some cases, on the surgeon's preference. In those cases, only the first attempt was included in the study and was classified as unsuccessful foreign body removal. Whether the second attempt was successful or not, the patient was not included in the study. No thoracotomy was performed in the study.

3.1.1.4 Results

The data structure of each group was identical, and demographic and epidemiologic data were comparable among the three groups (Table 1). Table 2 presents the clinical and surgical data for the three groups. Compared with group S, groups P and J showed significantly higher success rates of bronchoscope insertion on the first attempt, lower rates of intra- and post-operative hypoxemia, lower rates of perioperative complications, shorter durations of operation, and faster recoveries and emergence from anesthesia ($P < 0.05$). The incidences of hypoxemiawere lower in Group J comparedwith that in Group P (2.5% versus 16.7%,$P < 0.05$). There were no significant differences among groups for the other data that were collected.

3.1.1.5 Discussion

In the current study, three types of ventilation methods were compared in patients undergoing rigid bronchoscopy for airway FB removal. We found that the patients with spontaneous breathing during the procedure had lower success rates for bronchoscope

	Group S	Group P	Group J
Sex (male/female)	81/39	74/46	83/37
Age (months)	17 (22–36)	17 (14–24)	20 (14–24)
Weight (kg)	14±3	13±4	14±4
Duration of foreign body in the airway (days)	3 (1–11)	3 (1–9)	3 (1–7)
Location of the foreign body (n)			
main	9	13	11
left	53	51	49
right	57	53	58
both	1	3	2

Table 1. Clinical characteristics of the patients (n = 120 per group). Parameters presented as mean±SD. Data structure of each group was identical; demographic and epidemiologic data were comparable among the three groups.

	Group S	Group P	Group J
Successful bronchoscope insertion (%)	70.8	97.5*	98.3*
Duration of operation (min)	29.1±6.2	16.7±2.1*	15.2±2.2*
Duration of emergence from anesthesia (min)	32.7±6.8	9.1±2.4*	9.2±2.0*
Percentage of cases with foreign body removal (%)	90.8	92.5	96.7
Intraoperative hypoxemia (%)	40.8	16.7*	2.5*†
Postoperative hypoxemia (%)	19.2	6.7*	4.2*
Body movement during operation (%)	73.3	17.5	10.8*
Perioperative side effects (%)	34.2	10.8*	9.2*
Laryngospasm(cases)	5	1	1
Arrhythmia(cases)	3	2	0
Breath holding(cases)	21	11	9
Restlessness(cases)	13	8	9
other(cases)	7	4	3

*P<0.05 versus Group S; †P<0.05 versus Group P.

Table 2. Clinical characteristics of surgery for the three groups (n = 120 per group). Parameters presented as mean±SD.

insertions, higher incidences of hypoxemia and perioperative adverse events and a longer operation times. We speculated that the cause for these findings was due to an inadequate depth of anesthesia in group S. Lighter anesthesia would make a patient's airway more sensitive and reactive to the presence of the bronchoscope, frequently leading to bronchospasm, breath-holding and bucking. Deeper anesthesia increases the risk of inhibiting respiration or causing shallow respiration. All of these factors may have contributed to the higher incidence of hypoxemia in group S. The duration of the operation was also significantly longer in group S because extra time was needed for frequent adjustment of the depth of anesthesia or management of complications. In contrast, the controlled ventilation techniques used in groups P and J provided a good anesthetic status for surgery, and the muscle relaxation caused by succinylcholine gave a further advantage for bronchoscope manipulation. Therefore, decreased rate of complications and reduced duration of operation were observed in both groups P and J.

Jet ventilation during rigid bronchoscopy was first introduced by Sanders. Since then, it has been modified and is now widely used in suspension laryngoscopy. The route used for jet ventilation can be classified as either intratracheal jet ventilation (ITJV) or supraglottic jet ventilation (SJV). Both have a low incidence of complications when compared with traditional jet ventilation. Neither ITJV nor SJV are widely advocated in pediatric airway FB removal. From a practical point of view, SJV is unlikely to be attached to a rigid bronchoscope because of the incompatibility of the instruments. ITJV can be performed through the lateral aperture of the rigid bronchoscope by propelling air through the lumen of the bronchoscope. In the case, however, that the bronchoscope must be inserted distally to the FB, ventilation through the bronchoscope becomes limited to the bronchus, which is actually obstructed by the FB. In this situation, jet ventilation via the bronchoscope will be much less efficient and hypoventilation may occur quickly. To circumvent this problem in this study, we used a modified catheter that was connected directly to Manujet III, and was placed transnasally into the trachea; therefore, the jet ventilation and the bronchoscopic procedures were performed separately. This design made continuous ventilation to the nonobstructed lung or both lungs possible because the tip of the catheter was placed in the trachea, and did not interfere with bronchoscopic operation. The advantage of this method is that it can provide continuous ventilation to the clear lung with a catheter separate from the bronchoscope. This was confirmed by results from the present study in which the incidence of hypoxemia was lower in Group J than in Group P. Another advantage of the MJV is that it can offer unhurried conditions for bronchoscope insertion while continuous ventilation takes place through the transnasal catheter. This method appears superior to the IPPV method, in which the delay in initiating artificial ventilation is likely to be too long to maintain adequate oxygen saturation if the bronchoscope is not inserted successfully on the first or second attempt.

The use of transtracheal manual jet ventilation has been suggested for emergent airway management in the "can't intubate, can't ventilate" scenario described in the "Failed Ventilation Guidelines" formulated by "The Difficult Airway Society" Manujet III is a device widely used in emergency departments, intensive care units, recovery rooms and operating rooms for patients needing emergency ventilation. We utilize this kind of device for bronchoscopic foreign body removal. The device sprays hyperbaric oxygen into the airway through the jet catheter, and at the same time, air around the jet oxygen flow is also driven into the airway because of the "Venturi" effect. The final tidal volume is composed of the jet oxygen flow and its surrounding air flow. The highest oxygen pressure designed for this device can reach to 3 bar (300kPa). The driving pressure of the jet flow can be regulated as needed. The recommended driving pressure is dependent on the age of the patient: 0.1 - 1 bar for infants, 1 - 2.5 bar for children and 2.5 - 3.5 bar for adults.

Barotrauma is the most severe complication associated with jet ventilation. Blockage of airway outflow and trauma on the tracheal mucosa are the two most common causes of barotraumas. In the current study, no cases of barotrauma were observed when Manujet III was used. However, Manujet III has the potential to aggravate an existing pneumothorax because of the high pressure of airflow; the patient should be closely monitored and the necessary preventive strategies should be applied. First, a smaller jet catheter should be used to avoid blocking the airway outflow and disturbing the surgical procedure. Second, the location and position of catheter should be checked frequently to prevent it from slipping deeper, and preventing air accumulation caused by severe bronchotracheal occlusion. Third, the jet of the Manujet should be manipulated by the Manujet operator in a pattern of slow jetting-quick release using a high frequency and a low driving pressure. Finally, successful jet ventilation is highly operatordependent and should be done by experienced attendant anesthesiologists or residents under the guidance of attendants.

Manual jet ventilation with Manujet III has become the standard technique in our hospital for FB removal by rigid bronchoscopy. There are several advantages in using this device: (1) it provides continuous ventilation during all steps of the procedure;(2) it avoids inadequate ventilationto aunilateral lungwhenthe bronchoscope is inserted distal to the FB;(3) it shortens the duration of operation and emergence from anesthesia; (4) spontaneous respiration is possible because of the minimal stimulation by a small transnasal catheter and a manually controlled ventilation mode adaptable to patients' status of respiration; and (5) it minimizes the post-operative hypoxemia by decreasing bucking, coughing, or laryngospasm induced by oral secretions accumulated under the glottis if ventilated through mask during the emergence from anesthesia. In cases with a supraglottic/glottic foreign body, manual jet ventilation is not suggested, while in cases with bilateral bronchus obstruction, jet ventilation should be cautiously usedwhile keeping the catheter in themain tracheal airway. Although it is impossible to detect the end tidal CO_2 levels in an open airway during rigid bronchoscopy, CO_2 retention has not been a problem according to our previous study using jet ventilation with a frequency of 20 - 60 ventilations/min in suspension laryngoscopy.

In conclusion, manual jet ventilation using Manujet III is a safe and effective technique for airway FB removal by rigid bronchoscopy in children. It offers more favorable outcomes when compared with spontaneous respiration. Attention should be paid to carefully observe the chest excursion of the patients for the assessment of the efficiency of jet ventilation and to check the location of the catheter to avoid barotrauma caused by bronchotracheal occlusion.

3.1.2 MJV using Manujet III to removal long retained airway FB

Delayed diagnosis in AFB aspiration in children leads to prolonged foreign body retention in the brochus, causing pathological changes in the lungs, such as pneumonia, bronchitis, emphysema, breathing difficulties, asthma, choking, etc. The longer the foreign body retention, the more the respiratory problems and aggravated pathological changes, which have increased the risk of foreign body removal surgery, particularly the incidence of intraoperative hypoxia

3.1.2.1 Materials and method

We reviewed the records of all children who underwent the removal of airway foreign bodies(FBs) using rigid bronchoscopy in our Eye and ENT hospital between June 2004 and

September 2008. The patients whose time from FBs aspiration to retrieval exceed 30 days were admitted into our study. The subjects who underwent MJV using Manujet III constituted for Group m, and those who underwent ventilation through lateral aperture of rigid bronchoscopy were Group n, and the narcotic drugs must be identical in Group m and Group n. To analyze the distribution of patients and complications before operation, to analyze the incidence of hypoxemia during and after the operation, to analyze the rate of success of FB removal, to analyze the duration of operation and emergence from anesthesia and the other perioperative side effects.

3.1.2.2 Results

From June 2004 to September 2008, there were 1263 patients who were subjected to FB removal. Among them, 67 children (5.30%) accorded to our study qualification, age ranging from 9 months to 131 months (median 25 months), weight ranging 9~33kg (median 13kg), ASA I~III,The duration of FB aspiration was 30days to 370 days (median 87days). 46 children (68.66%) with no FB history, in others 21 (31.34%) cases with positive clinical history(but not chest film findings, or not early symptoms or negative bronchoscopy findings). There was no signification difference between Group m and Group n about the distribution of patients and complications before operation, The incidence of hypoxemia during operation was lower in Group m than in Group n (P<0.05), and the duration of operation and emergence from anesthesia were shorter in Group m than in Group n (P<0.05). There was no significant difference in other compared factors (P>0.05) (see Table 3,4,5).

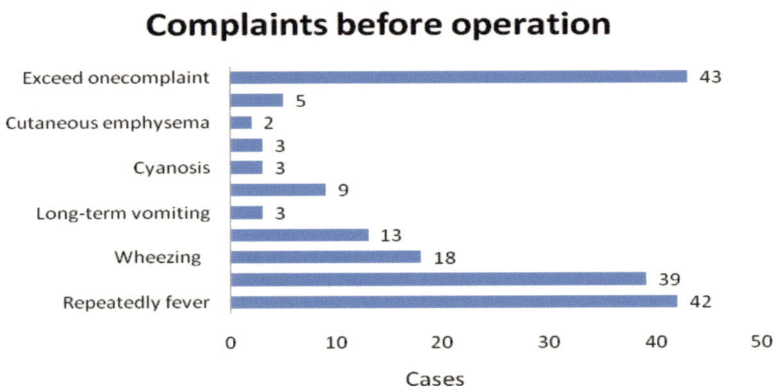

Fig. 3. Complaints before operation

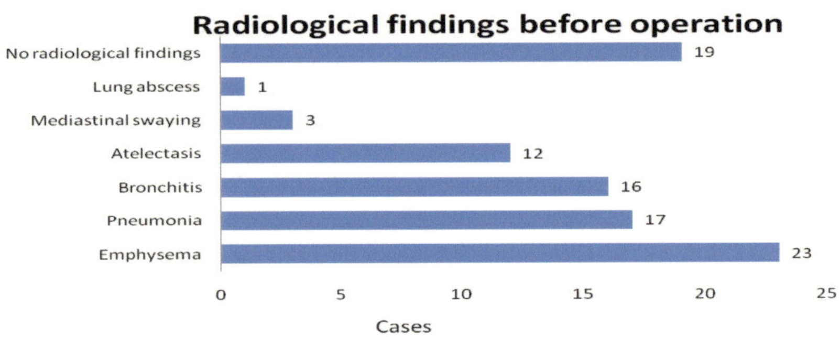

Fig. 4. Radiological findings before operation

	Number(cases)	percentage
Exceed 30 days	67	
From rural	56	83.58%
From urban	11	16.42%
No FB history	46	68.66%
FB history	21	31.34%
Organic FB	57	85.07%
Left	36	53.73%
Right	31	46.27%

Table 3. Distribution of patients

	Number(cases)	Percentage
Complaints		
Repeatedly fever	42	62.69%
Chronic cough	39	58.21%
wheezing	18	26.87%
appetite depress	13	19.40%
long-term vomiting	3	4.48%
dyspnea	9	13.43%
cyanosis	3	4.48%
vomica	3	4.48%
cutaneous emphysema	2	2.99%
no complaint	5	7.46%
exceed onecomplaint	43	64.18%
Radiological findings		
emphysema	23	34.33%
pneumonia	17	25.37%
bronchitis	16	23.88
atelectasis	12	17.91%
mediastinal swaying	3	4.48%
lung abscess	1	1.49%
No radiological findings	19	28.36%

Table 4. Complaints and radiological findings before operation

Compared items	Group m (cases and percentage)	Group n (cases and percentage)
patients studied (cases)	40(59.70%)	27(40.30%)
hypoxia during perform	7(17.5%)●	11(40.74%)●P=0.035 χ=4.431
hypoxia postoperation	5(12.5%)	4(14.81%) P=0.785 χ=0.074
Time of perform(minutes)	21.3±3.7◆	37.2±6.3◆ P=0.031 χ=5.016
Time of analepsia (minutes)	16.2±4.1■	19.1±4.3■ P=0.043 χ=3.426
extracted FB(cases)	39(97.5%)	27 (100%) P=0.145 χ=2.219
respiratory tract obstruction postoperation(cases)	3(7.5%)	3(11.11%) P=0.612 χ=0.258
recover from chronic respiration symptoms(cases)	33(82.5%)	22(81.48%) P=0.915 χ=0.011
remain respiration symptoms(cases)	7(17.5%)	5(18.52%) P=0.915 χ=0.011

●、◆、■ ($P<0.05$)

Table 5. Comparison between Group m and Group n

3.1.2.3 Discussion

Airway foreign bodies often occur in 8 months to 3 years old children. However, in many children, there was no clear history of FB or lacked of self-reported or parent-witnessed events. As a result, diagnosis of FBA was often delayed. In addition, medical imaging sensitivity and specificity in the diagnosis of airway FB was low. If lack of obvious early respired symptoms, often led to prolonged FB retention. Although fiberoptic bronchoscopy approach is a highly successful diagnosis approach, in our country, many doctors lack of AFB consciousness, and they seldom give a suggestion of taking fiberoptic bronchoscopy. In our study, organic FBs accounted for 85.07%. The most important feature of organic FBs (such as plant seeds) was that they contain unsaturated fatty acids, which may release arachidonic acid and plant protein. These molecules trigger a inflammatory response that involves the release of inflammatory chemokines, and other substances, causing inflammation of tracheal mucosa, resulting in mucosal swelling and congestion, bronchitis, pneumonia, wheezing, airway obstruction, etc. In addition, the plant seeds are rich with in protein and sugar, with affinity to water, thus the longer the retention time, the softer and more swollen the mucous membrane, exacerbating bronchial obstruction. Consequently, pulmonary secretions can not be discharged in time, increasing the risk of lung infections and "asthma syndrome". Lan F.T found that lung extracellular matrix remodeling, and triggered a series of lung pathological changes in the long FB retained children.

FB removal in the children with complicated lung pathological changes is a high risk procedure. The risks were ventilate disorder and hypoxemia with the most severe life-threatening, and the most commonest risk being a high incidence of intraoperative hypoxia. So the appropriate ventilation mode was important. We had tried a variety ways of anesthesia ventilation, every method had themselves advantages and disadvantages. In the manual jet ventilation method by Manujet III, a small catheter was inserted transnasally into the trachea and connected to the Manujet III device, that take up airway as little as possible, and provide more space for hard-placed laryngoscopy. Manual jet ventilation can give adequate ventilation and less carbon dioxide retention. In our this retrospective study, manual jet ventilation using Manujet III significantly reduced the occurrence of hypoxia and shorten the operation time. Why was Manujet III manual jet ventilation more adequate? Probably because the jet tube was in main airway, ventilated through bilateral lung, when rigid bronchoscopy into the side of the bronchial airway, the other side of the pulmonary could be ventilated; the ventilated method through lateral aperture of rigid bronchoscopy, when rigid bronchoscopy into the side of the bronchial airway, the other side of the pulmonary could't be ventilated well, If rigid bronchoscopy into the "disease lung" side, that became "disease lung" ventilation and "healthy lung" no ventilation, so the ventilation is inadequate. Manujet III manual jet ventilation in children with complete muscle relaxation can be fixed, good ventilation and good operating vision, can creating favorable conditions for removal of foreign body, reduce operation time.

But Manujet III manual jet ventilation is a positive pressure ventilation, need to pay attention to the outlet of gas and muscle relaxation, the pressure should be appropriate (the baby was 0 ~ 1bar, children 1 ~ 2.5bar, adult 2.5 ~ 3.5bar), the chest wall motion should be closely observed to estimate the efficacy of ventilation. Therefore, we recommend the users were to be well trained before used Manujet III. Furthermore, characteristics of the air flow dynamics of manual jet ventilation using Manujet III was not clear, the potential risks need further study.

This retrospective study confirmed that MJV using Manujet III in FB removal can offer sufficient ventilation and shorten operation time and fasten analepsia, and prove the advantages in FB removal surgery in the children with a long retained airway foreign body.

Manual jet ventilation using Manujet III has many, it should be recommended, but for the possible adverse events, the operator should be well trained in advance.

3.2 Main complications relevant to MJV

3.2.1 Pneumothorax

A Pneumothorax is the most serious complication associated with MJV. Reports of the occurrence of this complication vary in the literature. A retrospective review , which covered 942 laryngeal jet ventilation cases (via suspension laryngoscope) collected for as long as 10 years, revealed that pneumothoraces were reported in 4 patients. It is thought that two factors accounted for the pneumothoraces; these were airway damage and high airway pressures. Leemann, et al reported one case involving a combined pneumothorax and subcutaneous emphysema that was caused by airway mucosal damage after laser surgery. In a discussion of this case presented by Sosis, it was regarded that once the pneumothorax and subcutaneous emphysema were observed in the first surgery, jet ventilation should not have been used in the second surgery, because the highly pressurized air flow could pass through the injured mucosal into the pleural and subcutaneous tissues and resulted in the pneumothorax and subcutaneous emphysema. Airway pressure has always been one of the most conspicuous causes of mucosal injury seen in clinical practice. But according to the opinion provided by Bourgain, et al., the occurrence of complications such as pneumothoraces could not be reduced even when pressure-controlled jet ventilation device was used. It is also regarded that the degree of airway pressure after initiation of jet ventilation depends on not only the rate of aspirating gas stream and diameter of the catheter but also the size of the environment arround the aspirating gas stream, such as, diameter of the airway, cross sectional area of the trachea and the distance from distal end of the catheter to glottis vera. When driving pressure is fixed, the obstruction of airway outflow is the main reason for increased airway pressure and occurrence of pneumothoraces. In upper airway surgeries, possible reasons for airway outflow obstruction include, but are not limited to, severe laryngotracheal stenosis, upper airway blocked by a neoplasm, aggravated airway mucosal edema caused by the operation procedures, and a totally blocked airway possibly due to the surgical procudure or position of surgical devices. Baer pointed out that the monitoring of airway pressure curve has prevented the occurrence of pressure relevant damages, such as pneumothoraces, from happening since this practice was in use for nearly 20 years. Rezaie-Majd also speculated that the most important measure in preventing pressure related damages was to ensure there was no outflow obstruction. The advantage in using the Manujet is that the ventilation device has a pressure-controlling design that can keep gas pressure within the prescribed safety ranges. The ventilation frequency can be adjusted manually by operators. Therefore, this ventilation technique, adopted during surgery, facilitates the cooperation between anesthesiologists and surgeons, and ensures good oxygen supply as well as an unobstructed airway outflow to patients throughout operations. In our hospital, more than 2000 airway foreign body removals were finished under the ventilation model of MJV since 2007, 7 cases of pneumothorax occurred. There was no evidence that could indicate MJV was associated with higher rate of pneumatothoraces than any other ventilation models. So, we consider that MJV can play a safe part in the airway foreign body removal when correctly used.

3.2.2 Hypoxemia

Although most of the literatures indicate that jet ventilation can provide adequate oxygen supply, hypoxemia is still the most commonly observed complication. Most of the upper airway surgeries were taken in an open airway under suspension laryngoscope or rigid bronchoscope, and jet-propelled entrainment of atmosphere into the airway causes an atmospheric inhaled gas that occupies 25–60% of the tidal volume, attributing to a fraction of inspired oxygen of 32–42% .

3.2.3 Carbon dioxide retention

Carbon dioxide retention is another complication associated with jet ventilation, especially when the operation is prolonged. This complication is more commonly observed during HFJV and may be attributed to low tidal volume and inhalation of the expiratory gas. In low frequency MJV, the incidence of carbon dioxide retention is low, the elimination of carbon dioxide was mainly influenced by the compliance of thorax.

4. Experiences for the application of MJV using Manujet III device for FB removal

4.1 Driving pressure level, frequency and inspiration/expiration ratio

In jet ventilation, gas flow volume is proportional to driving pressure. Therefore, with an increase in driving pressure, tidal volume will increase linearly and $PaCO_2$ will decrease.

However, if tidal volume is to be increased by raising the driving pressure, the barotrauma risk will be increased as a result of high airway pressure. With the increase in frequency, there is a corresponding decrease in tidal volume; the contraflow effect of intrapulmonary gas also becomes weak, and the eliminating rate of carbon dioxide decreases proportionally. The ideal ratio of inspiration to whole respiration period is 20–30%. According to our clinical experience, when performing Manu-jet, the driving pressure should be set less than 15 psi in infants, and between 15–35 psi in children (usually less than 25 psi), and 35–59 psi in adults with a frequency of 15-30 times/minute in children and 12–20 times/minute in adults.

4.2 Maintaining adequate depth of anesthesia and degree of muscle relaxation

When the depth of anesthesia is not adequate or the degree of muscle relaxation is not enough, the glottis vera will close due to the contraction of laryngeal muscles and gas expiration will be inhibited; this creates turbulent air flow which is indicated by a sound of whistle. Therefore, to avoid barotraumas, MJV has to be stopped immediately when a whistle is heard until adequate anesthesia and muscle relaxation are attained.

4.3 Attending chest visualization and auscultation

During ventilation, it is very necessary to closely observe the chest excursions and listen to the sound of gas flow passing in and out of airway. By doing this, airway obstruction can be found immediately if it occurs. The surgical manipulation in the airway may dislodge the jet catheter, so it is important to frequently check the location of the catheter by lung auscultation.

5. Conclusions

Manual jet ventilation using Manujet III is a safe and effective technique for airway FB removal by rigid bronchoscopy in children. It offers more favorable outcomes compared with spontaneous respiration. But attention should be paid to closely observe the chest excursion of the patients for the assessment of the efficiency of jet ventilation and to check the location of the catheter to avoid barotrauma caused by bronchotracheal occlusion.

However, the time of MJV with Manujet III wasn't long, its mechanism of airflow dynamics isn't clear enough. the advanced research will focus on the mechanism which can make us use Manujet better.

6. Acknowledgment

The authors acknowledge Dr. Wu, an anesthesiologist in Cincinnati Children's Medical Center, USA. for the helps in English language; Dr. TianYu Zhang, a rhinolaryngologist in Eye and ENT hospital, China, for the co-operation in foreign body removal; Dr. Dan Chen, an anesthesiologist in Eye and ENT hospital, China, for recording clinical documents; others are YaoZhen, YeMing, et al.

7. References

Baer GA. (2000). No need for claims: facts rule performance of jet ventilation. *Anesth Analg*,Vol.91,No.4, （October 2000）, pp.1040-1041, ISSN 0003-2999

Bourgain J.; Desruennes E. & Fischler M.(2001).Transtracheal high frequency jet ventilation for endoscopic airway surgery: a multicenter study. *Br J Anaesth,*Vol.87,(August, 2001),pp.870–5, ISSN 0007-0912

Brown R. ; Greenberg R. & Wagner E.(2001). Efficacy of propofol to prevent bronchoconstriction. *Anesthesiology,*Vol. 94,(May 2001),pp. 851–855, ISSN 0003-3022

Chen L.; Zhang X. & Li S.;et al.(2009). The risk factors for hypoxemia in children younger than 5 years old undergoing rigid bronchoscopy for foreign body removal. *Anesth Analg,*Vol.109,No.4,(October 2009),pp.1079-1084, ISSN 0003-2999

Chih-Yung C.; Kin-Sun W. & Shen-Hao L.;et al.(2005). Factors Predicting Early Diagnosis of Foreign Body Aspiration in Children. *Pediatric Emergency Care,* Vol.21, No. 3, (March 2005), pp.161-164, ISSN: 0749-5161

D'Haese J. ; Camu F. & Noppen M.(1996). Total intravenous anesthesia and high-frequency jet ventilation during transthoracic endoscopic sympathectomy for treatment of essential hyperhidrosis palmaris: A new approach. *J Cardiothorac Vasc Anesth,*Vol. 10,No.6, (October 1996), pp.767-771, ISSN 1053-0770

Divisi, D.; Tommaso, S. & Garramone, M.(2007).Foreign bodies aspirated in children: role of bronchoscopy. *Thorac. Cardiovasc. Surg.,* Vol.55, No.4,(June 2007), pp. 249-252, ISSN 0022-5223

Farrell PT. (2004).Rigid bronchoscopy for foreign body removal: anaesthesia and ventilation. *Pediatr Anesth,*Vol.14, (January 2004),pp.84–9, ISSN 1155-5645

Gree G. ; Bauman N. & Smith R.(2000). Pathogenesis and treatment of juvenile onset recurrent respiratory papillomatosis. *Otolaryngol Clin North Am,*Vol. 33,No.1,pp. 187–207, ISSN 0030-6665

Ihra G. & Aloy A. (2000).On the use of Venturi's principle to describe entrainment during jet-ventilation. *J Clin Anesth,* Vol. 12,No.5, (Aug. 2000),pp.417-419, ISSN 0952-8180

Ihra G.; Hieber C. & Schabernig C.;et al. (1999). Supralaryngeal tubeless combined high-frequency jet ventilation for laser surgery of the larynx and trachea. *Br J Anaesth,* Vol. 83,no.6,(June 1999),pp.940-942, ISSN 0007-0912

Jaquet Y. ; Monnier P. & Van Melle G. ; et al. (2006).Complications of different ventilation strategies in endoscopic laryngeal surgery: a 10-year review. *Anesthesiology,*Vol. 104,No.1,(January 2006),pp. 52–59,ISSN 0003-3022

Karakoc F.; Cakir E. & Ersu R.;et.al. (2007). Late diagnosis of foreign body aspiration in children with chronic respiratory symptoms. *Int.J Pediatric Oto,*Vol. 71,No.2, (February 2007),pp. 241-246, ISSN 0165-5876

Karen B. & Ronald S.(2009). Pediatric airway foreign body retrieval: surgical and anesthetic perspectives. *Pediatric Anesthesia,* Vol. 19, No.(Suppl. 1),(July 2009),pp.109–117, ISSN:1155-5645

Kugelman R.; Shaoul M. & Goldsher I. (2006). Persistent cough and failure to thrive: a presentation of foreign body aspiration in a child with asthma. *Pediatrics,* Vol.117,No.5,(May 2006),pp.1057-1060, ISSN 00314005

Leemann B.; Heidegger T. & Grossenbacher R.; et al.(2004). A severe complication after laser-induced damage to a transtracheal catheter during endoscopic laryngeal surgery. *Anesth Analg,*Vol. 98,No.6,(June 2004),pp.1807-1808, ISSN 0003-2999

Lev S.; Salim M. & Yosef R.; et al. (2010). Foreign body aspiration in children: the effects of delayed diagnosis. *Am J Otolaryngol,*Vol.31, No.5, (September-October 2010),pp.320-4, ISSN: 0196-0709

Li S.; Liu Y. & Tan F.(2010). Efficacy of manual jet ventilation using Manujet III for bronchoscopic airway foreign body removal in children. *Int J Pediatr Otorhinolaryngol,*Vol. 74,No.12,(December 2010),pp.1401-1404, ISSN 0165-5876

Mallick M.; Khan A. & Al-Bassam A. (2005). Late presentation of tracheobronchial foreign body aspiration in children. J. Trop. *Pediatr,*Vol.51,No.3, (June 2005), pp. 145-148, ISSN 0142-6338

Metrangolo S.; Monetti C. & Meneghini L. (1999).Eight years' experience with foreign-body aspiration in children: what is really important for a timely diagnosis. *J Pediatr Surg,* Vol.34,No.8, (August 1999), pp.1229–31, ISSN 0939-7248

Mu L.; He P. & Sun D.(1991). The causes and complications of late diagnosis of foreign body aspiration in children. Arch Otolaryngol. *Head Neck Surg,* Vol.117,No.8, (August 1991),pp. 876-879, ISSN 0886-4470

Nouraei S. ; Giussani D. & Howard D. ; et al.(2008). Physiological comparison of spontaneous and positive-pressure ventilation in laryngotracheal stenosis. *Br J Anaesth,*Vol. 101,No.3,(June 2008),pp. 419–423, ISSN 0007-0912

Paola Z.; Amulya K. & Saxena. (2009).Management Strategies in Foreign-Body Aspiration. *Indian J Pediatr,*Vol. 76,No.2,(February 2009),pp. 157-161, *ISSN*: 0019-5456

Patel R.(1999). Percutaneous transtracheal jet ventilation. A safe, quick and temporary way to provide oxygenation and ventilation when conventional methods are unsuccessful. *Chest,* Vol. 116,No.6, (December 1999), pp.1689-1694, ISSN 0012-3692

Peng S.; Xia S. & Zhong L.;et al.(1997). Clinical research on the normal pressure and frequency jet ventilation during suspension laryngoscopy. *Chi J Anesth,*Vol.17,No.7,pp.407-410

Perrin G.; Colt H. & Martin C.;et al.(1992).Safety of interventional rigid bronchoscopy using intravenous anaesthesia and spontaneous assisted ventilation, a prospective study. *Chest* ,Vol.102,No.5, (November 1992), pp.1526–30, ISSN 0012-3692

Perry RH. Ejector performance. In: Perry RH, Chilton CH, eds. *Chemical Engineer's Handbook.* New York, NY: McGraw-Hill, 1973:29-32, ISBN/ISSN 0070494797

Rezaie-Majd A.; Bigenzahn W. & Denk D.;et al. (2006).Superimposed high-frequency jet ventilation (SHFJV) for endoscopic laryngotracheal surgery in more than 1500 patients. *Br J Anaesth,*Vol.96,No.5,(March 2006), pp.650–9, ISSN 0007-0912

Richards SD, Kaushik V, Rothera MP et al.(2005). A tubeless anaesthetic technique for paediatric laryngeal laser surgery. *Int J Pediatr Otorhinolaryngol,*Vol.69,No.4,(April 2005),pp. 513–516, ISSN:0165-5876

Sameh I., Usama A., Wael A. (2005). Inhaled foreign bodies: management according to early or late presentation. *European Journal of Cardio-thoracic Surgery,* Vol. 28,No.3, (September 2005),pp.369–374,ISSN 1010-7940

Shikowitz M.; Abramson A. & Liberatore L.(1991). Endolaryngeal jet ventilation: a 10- year review. *Laryngoscope,* Vol.101,No.5,(May 1991),pp.455-461, ISSN 0023-852X

Sırmalı M.; Türüt , H. & Kısacık E. et al.(2005). The Relationship between Time of Admittance and Complications in Paediatric Tracheobronchial Foreign Body Aspiration. *Acta chir belg,*Vol.105,pp. 631-634, ISSN:0001-5458

Soodan A.; Pawar D. & Subramanium R. (2004).Anaesthesia for removal of inhaled foreign bodies in children. *Pediatr Anaesth,*Vol.14,No.11,(November 2004),pp.947–52 ,ISSN 1155-5645

Sosis M.(2004). Should CO2 laser jet ventilation be abandoned? *Anesth Analg,*Vol. 99,No.6,(December 2004),pp.1882, ISSN 0003-2999

Spoerel W.; Narayanan P. & Singh N. (1971). Transtracheal ventilation. *Br J Anesth,*Vol. 43,No.10,pp.932-939, ISSN 0007-0912

Spoerel W. & Greenway R.(1973). Technique of ventilation during endolaryngeal surgery under general anaesthesia. *Can Anaesth Soc J,*Vol. 20,No.3,pp.369-377, ISSN 0008-2856

Su-Mi S.; Woo S. & Jung E. et,al.(2008). CT in Children With Suspected Residual Foreign Body in Airway After Bronchos opy. *AJR,* vol.192,(September 2008.),pp.1744 - 1751,ISSN 0361-803X

The Difficult Airway Society. Failed ventilation guidelines. 18.12.2010, Available from *http://www.das.uk.com/guidelines/cvci.html*

Theroux M. ; Grodecki V. & Reilly J. ; et al.(1998). Juvenile laryngeal papillomatosis: scary anaesthesia. *Paediatr Anaesth,*Vol. 8,No.4,(July 1998),pp. 357-361, ISSN 1155-5645

Tremblay L. & Slutsky A.(2000). Continuous gas flow and high frequency ventilation. In: Shoemaker WC, ed. Textbook of Critical Care, 4th edn. Philadelphi, *PA: W.B. Saunders Company,* pp.1297-1298, ISSN 0279-5442

Vourc'h G.; Fischler M. & Michon F.;et al.(1983). Manual jet ventilation v. high frequency jet ventilation during laser resection of tracheo-bronchial stenosis. *Br J Anaesth,* Vol. 55,No.10, (October 1983), pp.973-975, ISSN 0007-0912

Weisberger E. & Emhardt J.(1996). Apneic anesthesia with intermittent ventilation for microsurgery of the upper airway. *Laryngoscope,*Vol. 106,No.9 , (September 1996),pp. 1099–1102, ISSN 0023-852X

Yadav, S.; Singh, J. & Aggarwal, N.;et,al. (2007). Airway foreign bodies in children: experience of 132 cases. *Singapore Med. J.,* Vol.48, No.9, (September 2007),pp. 850-853, ISSN 0037-5675

12

Utility of Pediatric Flexible Bronchoscopy in the Diagnosis and Treatment of Congenital Airway Malformations in Children

Yong Yin, Shuhua Yuan, Wenwei Zhong and Yu Ding
Department of Respiratory, Shanghai Children's Medical Center
Affiliated to Shanghai Jiaotong University School of Medicine, Shanghai
China

1. Introduction

Bronchoscopy is an indispensable tool in the clinical evaluation and management of pediatric airway and lung disease. Common indications for pediatric bronchoscopy are varied and extend over a spectrum of congenital, infectious, structural conditions and diagnostic applications . Indications for flexible bronchoscopy in children include the evaluation of stridor, persistent or recurrent wheezing, chronic cough, hemoptysis, atelectasis, suspected airway foreign body, suspected airway anomaly, tracheoesophageal fistula, vascular ring and pneumonia/lower respiratory tract infection. Of note, congenital airway malformations are of specific clinical concern in children with the potential to present as an acute emergency. Airway malformations can cause recurrent wheezing, respiratory distress with, repeated pneumonia by poor drainage of lung segments or aspiration, and life-threatening airway obstruction. Flexible bronchoscopy plays an important role in the diagnosis, evaluation and management of such congenital lung malformations.

The major advantages of flexible bronchoscopy as compared to rigid bronchoscopy, include smaller external diameter of the new pediatric flexible scopes, the ability to change direction (flex and extend within the airway), fine illumination with fibreroptic technology and airway dynamics evaluation. Bronchoscopy is a minimally invasive and superior technique for directly visualizing and evaluating airway anatomy and mucosa compared with chest radiography, high resolution CT scan and bronchogram. Advances in technology leads to more and more sophisticated interventions and therapeutic options in the field of adult bronchoscopy including airway stenting, balloon dilatation, cryotherapy and endobronchial laser therapy. As the development of experience and expertise in the field of pediatric flexible bronchoscopy in clinic, we hope that the versatility of the flexible bronchoscopy can extend the range of diagnostic and therapeutic interventions in children.

2. Choice of pediatric flexible bronchoscope for neonates and children

The pediatric bronchoscopist should be experienced with expertise in maneuvering the bronchoscope deftly and safely in the pediatric airway. The bronchoscopist should also have a thorough understanding of bronchoscope structure, functions, and reprocessing protocols and adherence to strict infection control precaution both during the procedure, reprocessing and storage of the equipment. This is essential as fiberoptic bronchoscopes are fragile instruments that need careful handling at each step. The pediatric bronchoscopist should also work closely with the anesthesiologist in deciding and developing an appropriate sedation protocol according to the age, underlying medical condition and respiratory status of each child.

Airway size can be largely determined by the age of the patient and the appropriate sized bronchoscope chosen accordingly. Table 1 depicts the different sizes of bronchoscope that can be selected according to the age of the patient.

Particularly in neonates, infants and young children, the smallest sized bronchoscope available should be used, in order to reduce obstruction of the airway lumen by the bronchoscope during the procedure (which would impair ventilation) and to minimize local mucosal trauma.

The flexible bronchoscope with a 3.6 mm external diameter is useful for infants and young children; the bronchoscope with a 4.8mm external diameter can be used in older children. Both bronchoscopes posses a working/suction channel of 1.2 mm diameter sufficient for suctioning and obtaining a diagnostic bronchoalveolar lavage. The smaller bronchoscope with a 2.8 mm external channel is useful to evaluate neonates and small infants in whom congenital airway malformations and abnormal airway anatomy is suspected. The neonatal bronchoscope with 2.2mm external diameter without a suction channel, and can be used for visualization of the airway in neonates, particularly low birth weight infants, and those intubated with endotracheal tubes of 3.0 diameter or less. The quality of images obtained and visualization increases with the increase in diameter (and hence the number of fiberoptic cables) of the flexible bronchoscope.

O.D. mm	Pt/wt (age)	Suction Channel mm	Biopsy	Brush	Picture Clarity	Tool durability	Pass through tube No.	Extra features
2.2	>700g	No	No	-	Fair	Very delicate	>3	Limited use in very small airway
2.8	>1.5kg	1.2	Small	+	Good	Delicate	>4	Useful as has suction channel
3.6	>3kg	1.2	Small	+	Very good	Good	>5	In major use
4.0	>10 kg	2.0	Good	+	Very good	Very good	>5.5	Working channel good for laser and for biopsy

Table 1. Types flexible bronchoscopes in children and characteristic features.

3. Sedation and anesthesia for bronchoscopy in children

Appropriate sedation is important for a well-tolerated bronchoscopic procedure particularly for pediatric patients. Pre-procedure assessment of the child is essential in order to evaluate safety and tolerability of bronchoscopy in addition to anticipating potential difficulties and procedure and anesthesia related complications. Individual pre-anesthetic assessment should include a comprehensive evaluation of baseline respiratory status and underlying medical conditions. Flexible bronchoscopy can be performed using either conscious sedation or general anesthesia .Various protocols for anesthesia may be used during flexible bronchoscopy in pediatric patients entailing administration of either intravenous drug combination (e.g. midazolam, meperidine, propofol, ketamine, remifentanyl), or inhalational agents (premixed nitrous oxide, sevoflurane). Regardless of the choice of sedation, and it is essential to ensure adequate delivery of oxygen (either by nasal prongs, face mask, laryngeal mask airway or endotracheal intubation). Ideally, allowing the patient to maintain spontaneous ventilation will provide valuable information on airway dynamics which is an advantage as compared to deep anesthesia and paralysis with controlled ventilation as used during rigid bronchoscopy. The most frequent complication of sedation during flexible bronchoscopy is hypoxaemia, either alone or in association with larygospasm and/or bronchospasm. Hypoxemia should be monitored for continuously before, during and after the procedure; and can be secondary to partial or total airway obstruction by the bronchoscope and/or central respiratory depression due to sedation. Pre-operative identification of high-risk patients, administration of appropriate anesthesia individually tailored for each patient and close monitoring are essential for minimizing potential complications and successful completion of the procedure.

4. Applications in the diagnosis of congenital airway malformations

Flexible bronchoscopy enables internal visualization of a child's airways starting from the external nares, via the pharynx, larynx, trachea and large central airways down to the bronchi limited only by the relative size of the child's airways and the external diameter of the bronchoscope. Flexible bronchoscopy in a lightly sedated child who is breathing spontaneously, allows assessment of airway dynamics (not provided by rigid bronchoscopy which requires deep sedation and paralysis) which is critical in diagnosing certain airway abnormalities (Table 2). A detailed inspection of dynamics and movements of the glottis, vocal cords and the trachea is invaluable in the systematically evaluating pediatric airway conditions, such as airway collapse caused by tracheomalacia or external compression. Furthermore, bronchoscopy allows direct examination of the internal surface of the airways, their diameter, and characteristics of the tracheal and bronchial mucosa, and respiratory tract secretions.

Laryngomalacia	Tracheal Cartilaginous Sleeve
Vocal Cord Paralysis	Complete Tracheal Rings
Posterior Laryngeal Cleft	Tracheal Diverticulum
Laryngeal web	Tracheal Bronchus
Subglottic Stenosis	Tracheomalacia and Bronchomalacia
Subglottic Hemangioma	Tracheoesophogeal Fistula
Subglottic Cyst	Bronchial Atresia/Agenesis
Tracheal Stenosis	Bronchial Stenosis
Tracheal Web	External Compression by a Vascular Ring

Table 2. Common airway anomalies that can be visualized during bronchoscope

4.1 Laryngomalacia

Larygomalacia is a usually benign, self-limited disorder; it is the most common congenital laryngeal anomaly (50-75%) and the most common cause of stridor in infants (approx.60%) [1].The term 'laryngomalacia' suggests that the cartilage of the larynx is abnormally soft, but there is no definitive evidence supporting this hypothesis; studies have reported dominance of submucosal edema and lymphatic dilation in the histopathology of tissue excised during supraglottoplasty for the treatment of severe laryngomalacia [2]. Thus, whether laryngomalacia is primarily an anatomical abnormality or whether it is due to delayed neuromuscular development remains under debate. Laryngomalacia is frequently associated with gastro-esophageal reflux, and infants with laryngomalacia may have episodes of micro-aspiration as well [3-5]. The natural history of laryngomalacia is characterized by an onset of inspiratory stridor usually within the first 4-6 weeks of life; the infant's voice and cry are normal. The stridor varies considerably with posture and airflow, is loudest with increased turbulence in airflow such as with crying, agitation and increased respiratory efforts with feeding. The stridor is also louder and appears worse during intercurrent respiratory tract infections. Some patients will have increasing symptoms during the first few months of life but thereafter stridor tends to resolve with time during the latter half of infancy into the second year of life as the supportive tissues mature and the diameter of the airway increases with somatic growth. In some instances, depending on the severity and structural anatomy, stridor may persist beyond the first year of life or even up to several years. Surgical treatment (i.e. supraglottoplasty) may be indicated in severe cases with prolapse of the supraglottic structures into the laryngeal inlet, feeding difficulties with failure to thrive and respiratory distress.

Flexible bronchoscopy demonstrates supraglottic collapse, i.e.prolapse of the epiglottic and/or the aryepiglottic folds and/or arytenodis during inspiration into the glottis (Fig.1).The state of consciousness and respiratory efforts of the patient may be critical in the examination of the dynamics of the larynx and laryngeal structures during spontaneous breathing; some children may be stridulous only when crying, others only when they are asleep. Topical anesthesia can potentially exaggerate the findings associated with laryngomalacia; thus, the larynx should be examined before applying topical anesthesia [6].

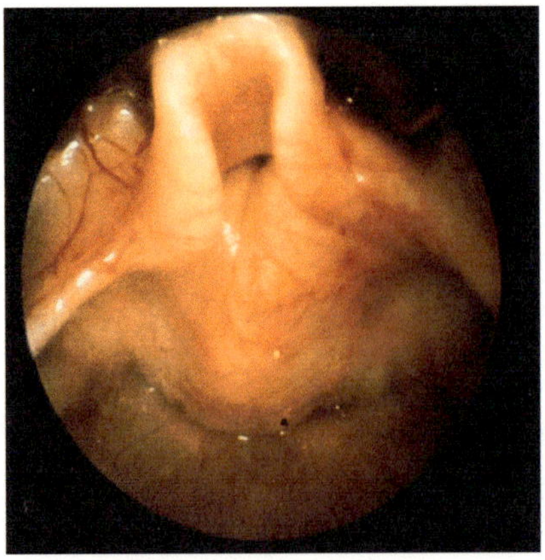

Fig. 1. The epiglottis and the aryepiglottic folds prolapse during inspiration into the glottis.

4.2 Vocal cord paralysis

In the pediatric population, vocal cord paralysis is the second most common congenital laryngeal anomaly (Fig.2). Central nervous system aetiologies of congenital disorders resulting in bilateral vocal cord paralysis include myelomeningocele, Arnold-Chiari malformation, hypoxic ischemic encephalopathy, cerebral hemorrhage and hydrocephalus. Other causes are traumatic and idiopathic factors which can cause vocal cord paralysis[7,8]. Most frequent causes of unilateral vocal cord paralysis are linked to cardiovascular surgery for correction of heart defects that may cause injury to the recurrent laryngeal nerve and esophageal surgery for esophageal atresia with tracheo-oesophageal fistula[9].

Bilateral vocal cord paralysis is characterized by a high-pitched inspiratory stridor along with a normal or near normal cry with the vocal cords assuming a midline or paramedian position. Unilateral vocal cord paralysis is characterized by a mild, position-dependent inspiratory stridor with a hoarse, breathy cry and potential risk for feeding difficulties and aspiration [10].

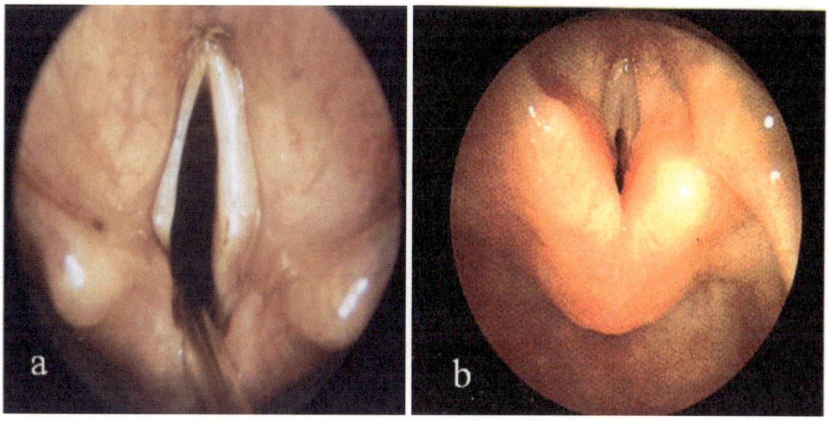

Fig. 2. (a)Left vocal cord paralysis (b) Bilateral vocal cord paralysis

4.3 Posterior laryngeal cleft

Posterior laryngeal clefts are rare congenital anomalies characterized by a failure of fusion of the posterior cricoid lamina that creates an abnormal communication between the larynx and hypopharynx (Fig.3). The anatomic severity of the cleft can range from the absence of interarytenoid muscle above the superior margin of the cricoid cartilage to the absence of the tracheoesophageal septum. Clinical symptoms include combined feeding-respiratory difficulties, such as coughing, choking and cyanotic attacks during feeding, aspiration, recurrent pneumonia, atelectasis, and even death. Other anomalies like cleft lip and palate and congenital cardiovascular anomalies may accompany the laryngeal cleft.

A high index of suspicion is required and bronchoscopy and microlaryngoscopy are needed to make a definitive diagnosis. Posterior laryngeal clefts can be either treated conservatively with medical management to prevent gastroesophageal reflux and aspiration, or surgical repair by endoscopy[11].Early medical management may prevent complications, surgery is needed when conservative measures fail. Depending on the severity of the comorbidities and the respiratory condition, some patients with mild symptoms don't need special treatments, while severe patients may require feeding through a nasogastric tube.

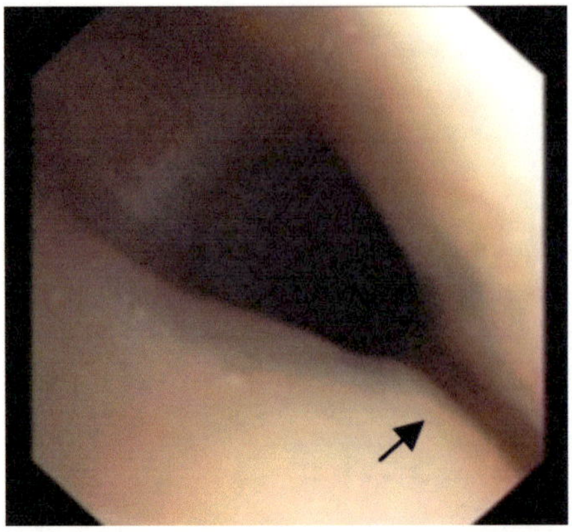

Fig. 3. Laryngeal cleft extending inferiorly to - but not through - the cricoid cartilage;

4.4 Laryngeal web

A congenital laryngeal web is a malformation in which abnormal tissue forms between two structures within the larynx. All patients present with some degree of dysphonia, ranging from mild hoarseness to aphonia. Airway obstructive symptoms increase with the extent of the web compromising or occluding the airway, with the most severe cases warranting a tracheotomy to secure the airway[12]. Anterior glottic webs less than 2- to 3-mm thickness are often asymptomatic and do not require treatment. Larger webs can cause symptoms which range from dysphonia and decreased exercise tolerance to severe airway obstruction[13-14].

Laryngoscopy is used to assess precisely the subglottic extension of the web and the size of the residual airway lumen. Webs of the glottis are classified as anterior, posterior, or complete; and may be located at the glottic, supraglottic or infraglottic level. Most commonly found are webs in the anterior portion of the glottis[15].

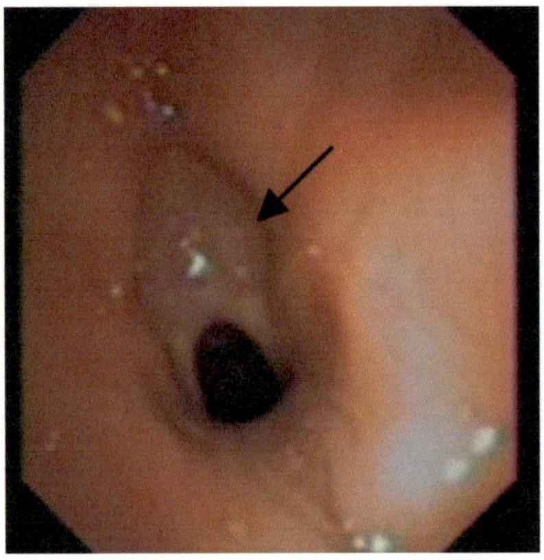

Fig. 4. Anterior Laryngeal web

4.5 Subglottic stenosis

Subglottic stenosis is narrowing of the subglottic airway, which is housed in the cricoid cartilage. It is the third most common congenital anomaly of the larynx [16] after laryngomalacia and vocal cord paralysis. The subglottic airway is the narrowest area of the airway because it is a enclosed by the complete cartilaginous ring of the cricoid, unlike the trachea, which has a posterior membranous section, and the larynx, which has a posterior muscular section. Subglottic stenosis is characterized by recurrent episodes of croup or prolonged croup with a barking cough. Acquired subglottic stenosis is related to a variety of causes, including prolonged endotracheal intubation[17], gastroesophageal reflux, infection, autoimmune disorders, and iatrogenic disorders. The Myer-Cotton grading system for subglottic stenosis (SGS) is widely used in the pediatric community [18]. It classifies SGS into four grades of luminal obstruction (Fig.5).

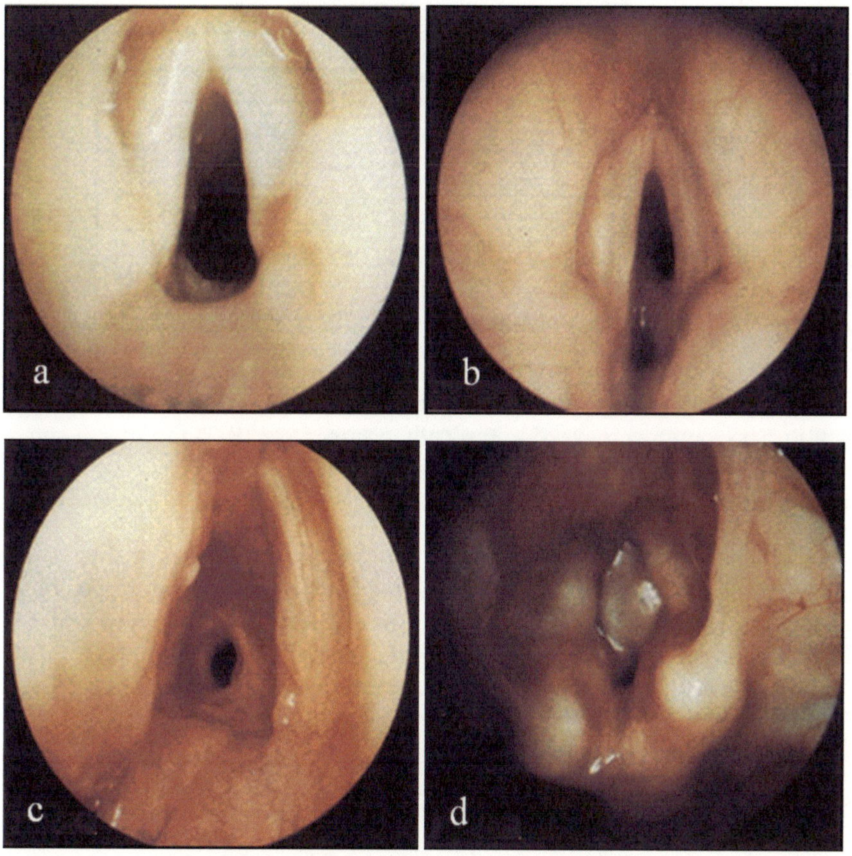

Fig. 5. The Myer-Cotton grading system for subglottic stenosis. (a)Grade 1: ≤50% obstruction. (b)Grade 2:51-70% obstruction. (c)Grade 3:71-99% obstruction. (d)Grade 4: no detectable lumen.

4.6 Subglottic hemangioma

Congenital subglottic hemangioma is the most common neoplasm of the airway in children (Fig.6). It is a benign tumor associated with hyperplasia of the endothelial cells, mast cells, pericytes, fibroblasts and macrophages. In the absence of treatment, it's potentially life-threatening during the proliferative phase (occurring below the age of 6-12 months) causing airway obstruction which necessitates medical or surgical intervention [19].

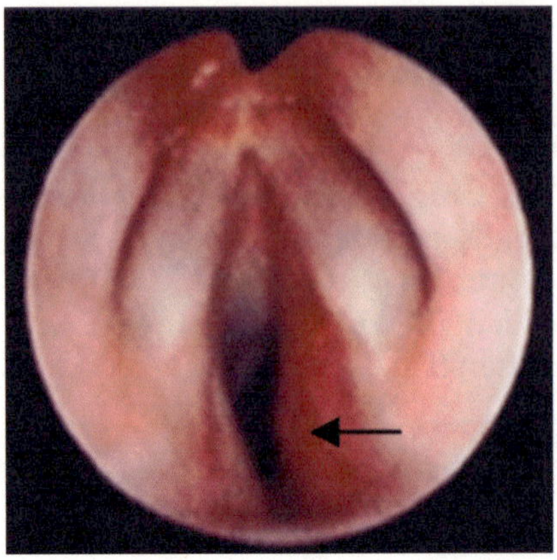

Fig. 6. Right-sided subglottic haemangioma

During the first weeks of life, the infant may be asymptomatic. Usually, symptoms of inspiratory stridor followed by biphasic stridor with barking cough and slight hoarseness start at around the age of 2-4 months. Symptoms of respiratory distress with suprasternal and chest retractions, feeding difficulties and failure to thrive depend on the severity of the airway obstruction. If symptoms worsen, then early intervention is indicated.

This may consist of a tracheotomy, general or local treatment with steroids, interferon, propranolol or vincristine therapy, LASER treatment, or open surgery with laryngo-tracheal reconstruction. Spontaneous regression typically occurs after 18-24 months of age [20].

4.7 Tracheal web

Congenital tracheal web is a rare congenital anomaly. It consists of a thin layer of tissue draped across the tracheal lumen. The web is not complete, and the degree of ventilatory symptoms that may occur is directly related to the size of the remaining functional tracheal lumen. Symptoms consist of stridor, dyspnea and respiratory failure resulting in death in severe cases. Tracheal web may often be misdiagnosed as refractory asthma as symptoms may include recurrent respiratory infections, dyspnea or wheezing. Postintubation tracheal

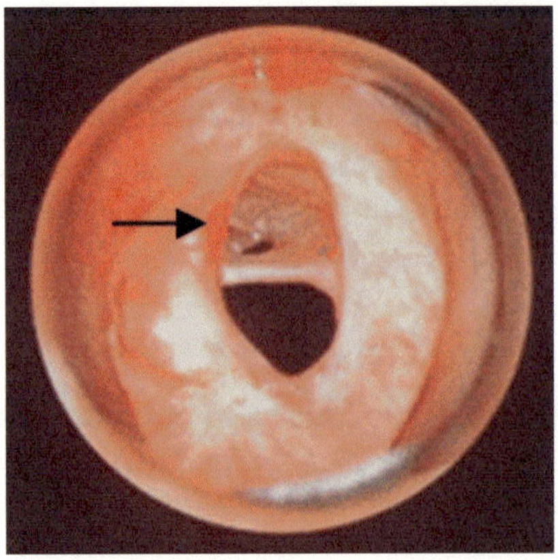

Fig. 7. Tracheal stenosis caused by a tracheal web

web may result as a complication of airway mucosal injury following endotracheal intubation. Although some patients may remain asymptomatic until detected incidentally, most present with symptoms of acute airway obstruction.

Treatment consists of rupturing the web. The first case was reported by Miller et al.[21] in 1978, as an 8-year-old girl presenting with a six year history of frequent colds, wheezing, and dyspnea in whom the tracheal web was successfully excised after failure of bronchoscopic dilation. In 2004, Alan et al. [22] removed a 9-year-old girl's web by endoscopic argon laser treatment.

4.8 Complete tracheal rings

Congenital complete tracheal rings are a rare anomaly, reported by Scheid et al. in 1938 at the first time. They usually present in the first year of life with respiratory distress[23], and often associated with vascular slings[24], or other malformations such as tracheoesophageal fistula and esophageal atresia. In complete tracheal rings, the normally C-shaped cartilaginous tracheal rings are fused posteriorly replacing the membranous posterior part of the trachea, becoming O shaped(Fig.8). As a consequence, the trachea is often narrower than normal. The complete rings may be localized to the region where the sling passes around the trachea, or may extend to a certain length of the trachea, creating a long-segment tracheal stenosis, causing recurrent wheezing, breathing difficulties, cyanosis, and is potentially life-threatening.

It is very important to observe and examine the contours of tracheal cartilages during the passage of the bronchoscope through the trachea during diagnostic bronchoscopy, which is considered as the gold standard. CT scan may be used to aid the diagnosis and assess the degree of involvement, a single tracheal ring or short or long segment involvement. Definitive treatment is surgical with primary resection of a single ring or short segment with end-to end anastomosis; longer length involvement will require tracheal reconstructive surgery. In cases of associated pulmonary vascular sling anomaly, reimplantation of the anomalous left pulmonary artery is performed. Laser division of complete tracheal rings has

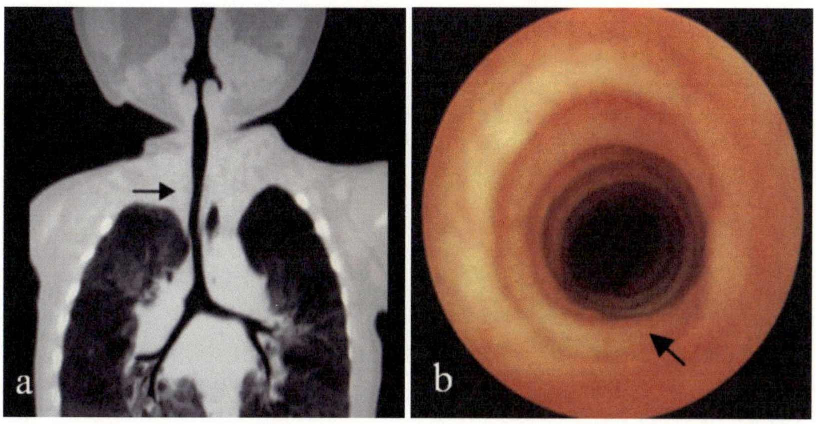

Fig. 8. (a) Coronal projection of the CT scan showing the associated long-segment tracheal stenosis with severe distal deviation and obstruction (Pulmonary artery sling). (b) Complete cartilaginous tracheal rings, the posterior membranous component of the trachea is absent.

only been described in a small number of cases and may provide an alternative approach in patients who are not able to undergo an open procedure or in an emergency situation [25].

4.9 Tracheal diverticulum

Tracheal diverticulum was firstly described by Rokintansky in 1938[26]. It is a rarely encountered entity. The frequency of the tracheal diverticulum found in some autopsy series has been estimated to be about 1% [27], and in children older than 10 yr it is reported as 0.3% [28]. The tracheal diverticulum is usually located approximately 4-5 cm below vocal cords or just above the carina. It projects posteriorly where the cartilage rings are deficient and usually lies towards the right where there is no esophagus supporting the paratracheal tissue (Fig.9). Tracheal diverticulum may be congenital or acquired. Congenital diverticulum is not normally detected in infancy unless it is suggested by recurrent episodes of tracheobronchial infection or in association with other congenital malformations[29-30]. The acquired form is thought to be due to prolonged increase in intraluminal pressures as occurs with a chronic cough. Although usually asymptomatic, the tracheal diverticulum may accumulate respiratory secretions that become infected and lead to cough or tracheobronchitis.

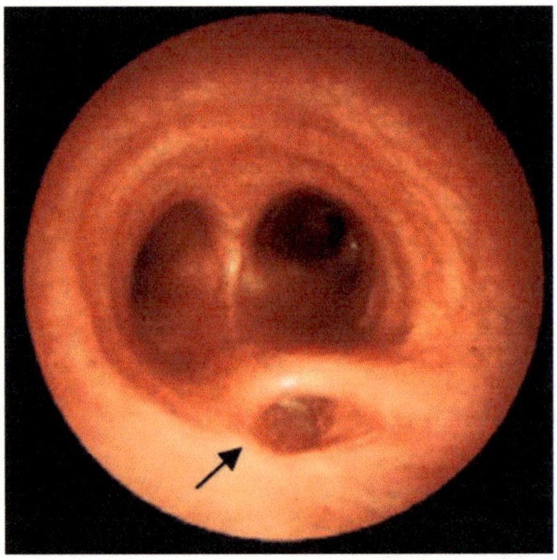

Fig. 9. Tracheal diverticulum in the membranous posterior part of the trachea above the carina.

4.10 Tracheal bronchus

A tracheal bronchus originates from the right lateral wall of the trachea above the level of the main carina and courses to the right (Fig. 10). It was firstly described by Sandifort in 1785. The frequency of the tracheal bronchus is approximately from 0.1% to 3%. In most cases, the tracheal bronchus supplies the apical segment of the right upper lobe. In such case, there is usually an additional orifice proximal to the bifurcation of the trachea, and the usually positioned right upper lobe bronchus has only 2 visible segmental branches (instead of three). Less frequently, the tracheal bronchus is associated with other anomalies, such as stenosis of the right main stem bronchus or it may supply additional, dysplastic pulmonary tissue. Patients in whom the tracheal bronchus is undetected, may undergo atelectasis of the right upper lobe when undergoing endotracheal intubation as the endotracheal tube will

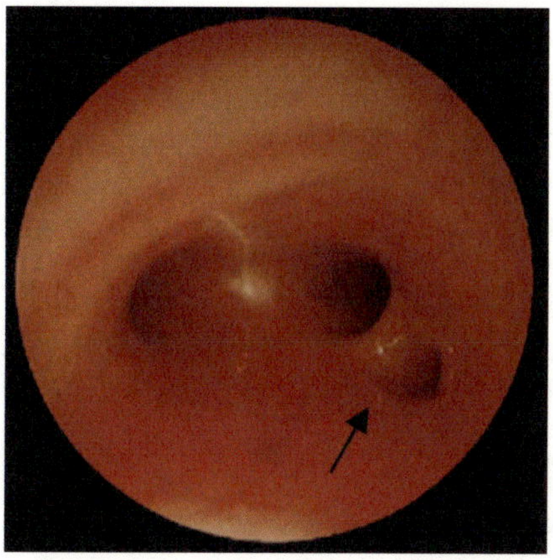

Fig. 10. A tracheal bronchus originates from the right lateral wall of the trachea above the level of the main carina and courses to the right.

obstruct the orifice. In a series of 35 patients with tracheal bronchus, 28 originated from the right wall and 7 from the left wall of the trachea as reported by Ghaye[31]. Other research by Bertrand suggests that the frequency of the tracheal bronchus in children with Down syndrome is up to 20.8%[32].

4.11 Tracheomalacia and bronchomalacia

Tracheobronchomalacia can be divided into two different types: congenital (or primary) and secondary tracheobronchomalacia [33].The cause of congenital tracheobronchomalacia is abnormal cartilaginous ring formation with small, malformed or excessively pliable rings and sometimes absent or defective cartilage affecting the trachea partially or completely. Secondary tracheobronchomalacia may occur due to airway compression by vascular structures, tumor, enlarged lymph nodes, thymus, and even excessive fat. Complicated cardiac abnormalities associated with tracheobronchomalacia may result in a higher mortality.

Congenital tracheobronchomalacia is usually caused by abnormal cartilage formation of the trachea and bronchi during the embryonic period. Several changes in cartilage can be found on histopathologic examination, including reduced volume, thinned depth, piecemeal shape of cartilage and even its absence. Acquired tracheobronchomalacia may occur in patients with tracheal cannulation as with prolonged endotracheal intubation, tracheotomy, abnormal left pulmonary artery or vascular ring or sling anomalies, space occupying lesion that compress the airway (for example, goiter), following tracheoesophageal fistula repair , cardiac dilatation and post lung transplantation [34-38]. Secondary tracheobronchomalacia may be related to recurrent bronchitis and infections causing chronic inflammation of airway mucosa. In tracheomalacia, the trachea and bronchi lose their normal horseshoe-shape and this leads to the narrowness in airway and limitation of airflow, turbulent or eddied flow and wheezing.

Bronchoscopy has been considered the gold standard in diagnosis of tracheobronchomalacia with direct visualization of dynamic airway collapse with respiration.(Fig.11,Fig.12). Pulsation may be noted at the site of vascular compression as well. These bronchoscopic findings help differentiate tracheomalacia from tracheostenosis in which there is a fixed and narrowed airway lumen.

Congenital (primary) tracheobronchomalacia is not uncommon, with an incidence of 1/2100 in some estimates[39].Most patients will often outgrow their symptoms at the age of 1-2 years with growth and development. Secondary tracheobronchomalacia occuring in association with cardiac and vascular abnormalities, in which the trachea and bronchi are extrinsically compressed by the enlarged heart chambers or anomalous vascular structures. Most children with tracheobronchomalacia may only need conservative treatment to manage respiratory infections, timely anti-infective agents, physical therapy for clearance of airway secretions and good nutrition for lung and body growth. Continuous positive airway pressure (CPAP) or mechanical ventilator support through a tracheostomy tube may be required in children with severe tracheobronchomalacia.. In some cases, surgical intervention with aortopexy or airway stents may be indicated.

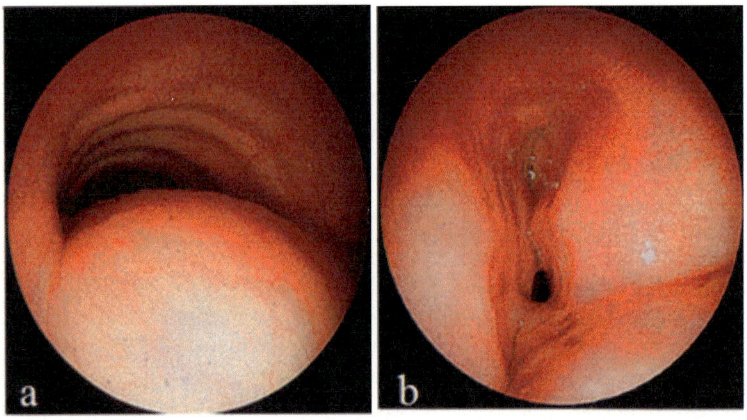

Fig. 11. Two characteristic features of tracheobronchomalacia on bronchoscopy. (a) Dynamic collapse of at least 50% of the airway lumen diameter, during expiration, cough or spontaneous breathing.(b) A ratio of cartilage to membranous wall area of < 3:1

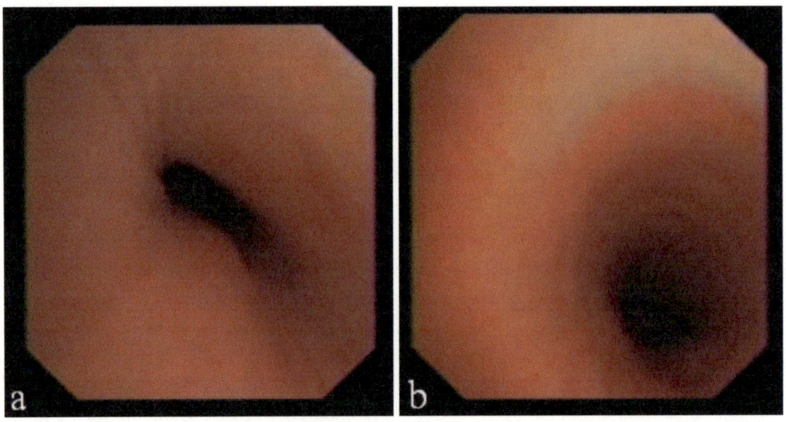

Fig. 12. Dynamic changes of trachea during respiratory period under bronchoscopy. (a) Airway collapse during expiration. (b) Airway dilation during inspiration.

4.12 Tracheo-esophogeal fistula

Congenital tracheo-esophogeal fistula (TEF) with esophageal atresia occurs with an incidence of approximately 1 in 3500 live births. TEF is potentially lifethreatening in the neonatal period requiring surgical correction. Gibson reported the first case of esophageal atresia with TEF in 1697. Since the report by Laddand and Levin in successful multistage correction of 2 cases of TEF patients in 1939; and technological and clinical advances in neonatal management there has been significant reduction in mortality due to TEF . Surgical correction is well established and survival rates of over 90% can be expected[40]. Survival has been reported to be lower in infants with TEF weighing less than 1500g and with associated cardiac abnormalities.

Tracheoesophageal fistula results from failure of the primitive gut to separate and recanalize during early embryonic development resulting in an abnormal fistulous connection between the trachea and esophagus[41]. Five types of TEF with esophageal atresia are described: Type 1:,esophageal atresia, in which both the proximal (upper) and distal (lower) segments of the esophagus end in blind pouches. Neither segment is connected to the trachea; Type 2: Esophageal atresia with tracheoesophageal fistula in which the proximal (upper) segment of the esophagus forms a fistula (TEF) to the trachea. The distal (lower) segment of the esophagus ends in a blind pouch; Type 3: Esophageal atresia with tracheoesophageal fistula, in which the proximal (upper) segment of the esophagus ends in a blind pouch and the distal (lower) segment of the esophagus is attached to the trachea (TEF). Type 4: Esophageal atresia with tracheoesophageal fistula, in which both segments (proximal and distal) of the esophagus are attached to the trachea. Type 5: Tracheoesophageal fistula in which there is no esophageal atresia. An H-type fistula is present between the esophagus and the trachea. The most common type of TEF is type 3, with an incidence around 85%-93%(Fig.14). Type 5 (H type TEF) which is not associated with esophageal atresia potentially display the mildest symptoms, and occur at an incidence of around 4%. Secondary TEF usually results from injury to the esophagus as occurs with swallowing of corrosive agents, erosion by mediastinal granuloma or tumors or accidental perforation during tracheo-esophageal

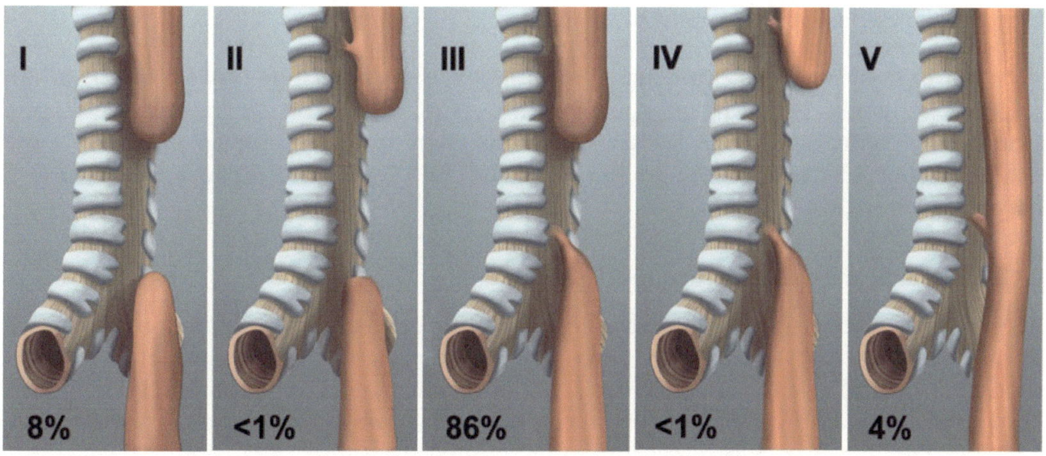

Fig. 13. Types of tracheo-oesophageal fistula and esophageal atresia malformations: The type III with a blind proximal esophageal pouch and a distal TE fistula is by far the most common (Reproduced from Holinger [42]. With permission)

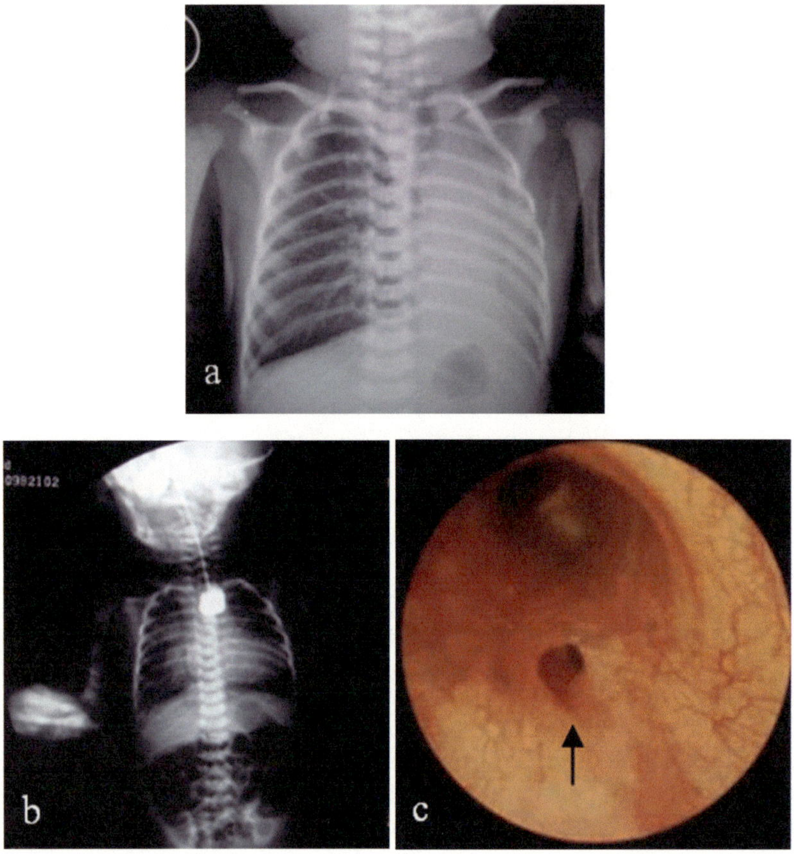

Fig. 14. (a) Chest radiograph shows a gastric tube coiled in blind esophageal pouch (b) Chest radiograph shows round or pocket-like blind esophageal pouch after meglumine diatrizoate injection via gastric tube. (c) Bronchoscopy demonstrates fistulous opening at the posterior aspect of the trachea just 1cm above the carina.

surgery. Complications of primary TEF surgical repair include development of an anastomotic fistula, recurrent laryngeal nerve paralysis, vocal cord paralysis, esophageal stenosis and recurrence of TEF. Recurrent TEF can result from compromise of blood supply and circulation of the area around the original fistula leading to tissue breakdown and fistula recurrence.

4.13 Tracheobronchial absence and agenesis

Agenesis of the trachea is a rare congenital malformation with an incidence below 1 in 50000. The entire trachea is usually absent and air reaches the bronchi through a fistulous connection with the esophagus; the lungs are normally formed. About half the infants are born premature, and a male predominance has been reported. It was first described by Payne in 1900 when he was dissection an infant died from disease[43].Those patient didn't cry when was born, and with progressive severe dyspnea, cyanosis and even dead. It is usually combination with other severe malformation and can barely survive under current technique.

Floyd classified tracheal agenesis into 3 types of malformation according to the anatomical location [44] (Fig.15). In Type I, accounting for approximately 20% of the malformations, there is atresia of part of the trachea with a normal but short distal trachea, normal bronchi and a tracheo-esophageal fistula (TEF). Sixty percent of the reported cases are of Type II, where there is complete tracheal atresia, the bronchi communicate at the carina (as the TEF) with normal distal bifurcation and bronchi (Fig.15-17). Type III, accounting for 20% of cases, comprises no trachea or carinal development and both mainstem bronchi arise directly from the esophagus.

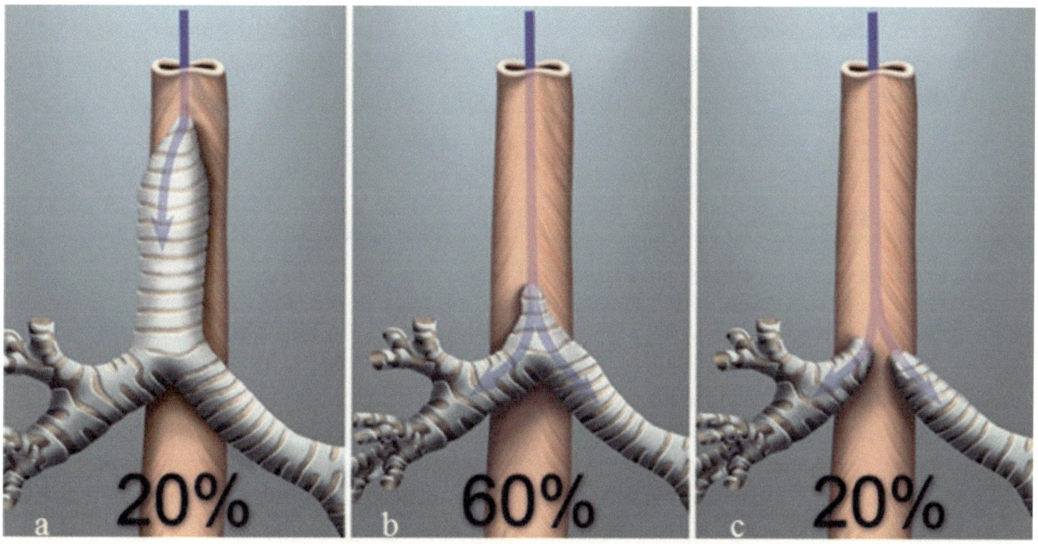

Fig. 15. Illustration of agenesis of trachea. (Reproduced from Monnier[45]. With permission)

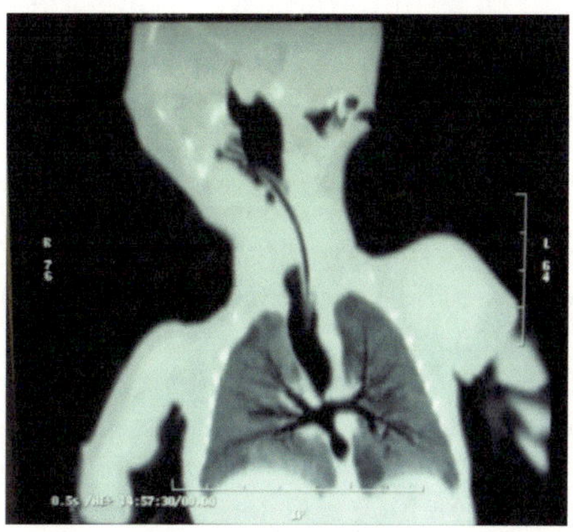

Fig. 16. CT airway reconstruction in coronal view: show left and right main bronchi arising directly from the mid-esophagus. No trachea is present, actually, the endotracheal tube goes though the esophagus.

Hiyama et al. described their surgical experience with 2 neonates; one of which had complex cardiac malformations, and died of cardiac failure 1 week after birth. The second with tracheal agenesis with a proximal TEF was managed successfully with multiple surgical

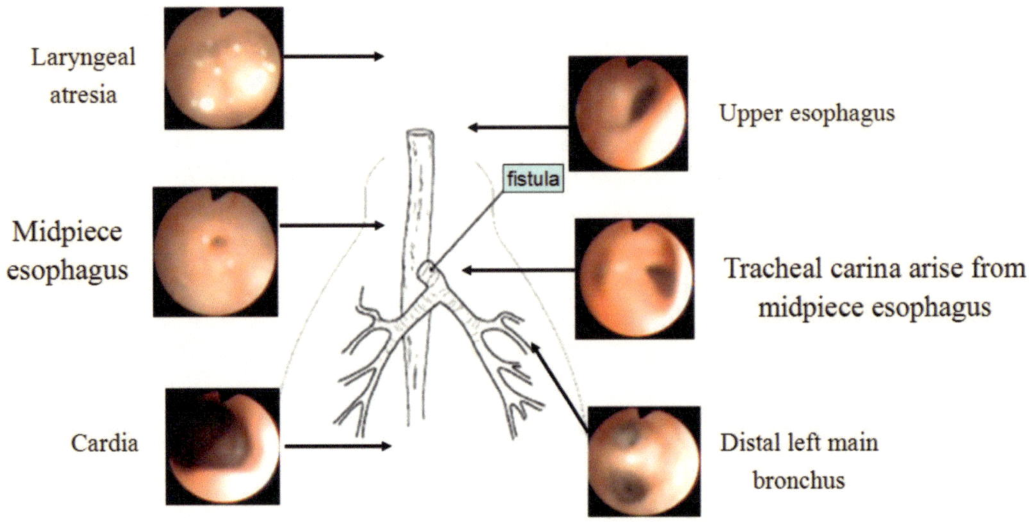

Fig. 17. Bronchoscopic findings in tracheal agenesis

procedures, including tracheotomy, with a long T-tube to maintain airway patency beyond the proximal TEF and esophageal reconstruction with a colonic interposition graft.[46]. It is essential to suspect this malformation and diagnose at birth, maintain airway patency with initial palliative surgerical procedures which are lifesaving until reconstructive surgery can be performed for successful outcomes. We hypothesize that tracheal transplantation could be a promising therapy in the future; with advances in tissue engineering, there is potential for the prognosis of this disease to be largely improved.

5. The therapeutic benefit of bronchoscopy in children with congenital airway malformation

5.1 Assisting identification and localization of the tracheoesophageal fistulae prior to and during surgery

It is necessarily important but also understandably technically difficult to locate the distal communicating ends of the tracheoesophageal fistula precisely prior to surgical correction of H-type TE fistulae. Precise dissection is required during the surgical procedure to avoid injury of surrounding and adjacent tissue. This is particularly true for patients who require secondary surgical correction; as it is a surgical challenge as there significant post-operative adhesions may have formed. Flexible bronchoscopy assists in locating the fistula precisely using transillumination of the airway by the inserted bronchoscope. This technique can shorten surgical time spent in searching and locating the communicating ends of the TE fistula. Blanco-Rodriguez et al reported their experience with 3 neonates utilizing preoperative catheterization of H-type tracheoesophageal fistula with either a rigid bronchoscope or a nasolaryngoscope. to facilitate identification, plan the surgical approach, and to reduce operating times and the extent of surgery. [47]. Several surgeons recommend locating the TE fistula by insertion of a catheter into the visualized orifice during bronchoscopy, however, with little success because of migration of catheter during operation. Garcia et al used bronchoscopy and oesophagoscopy perfomed simultaneously to establish a guide wire loop between the tracheoesophageal fistulae in 6 cases of isolated tracheoesophageal fistula (Fig.18) Their success in locating and separating the TE fistula without recurrence in all cases, was the basis for their suggestion that this method be used in H-type TEF[48] .

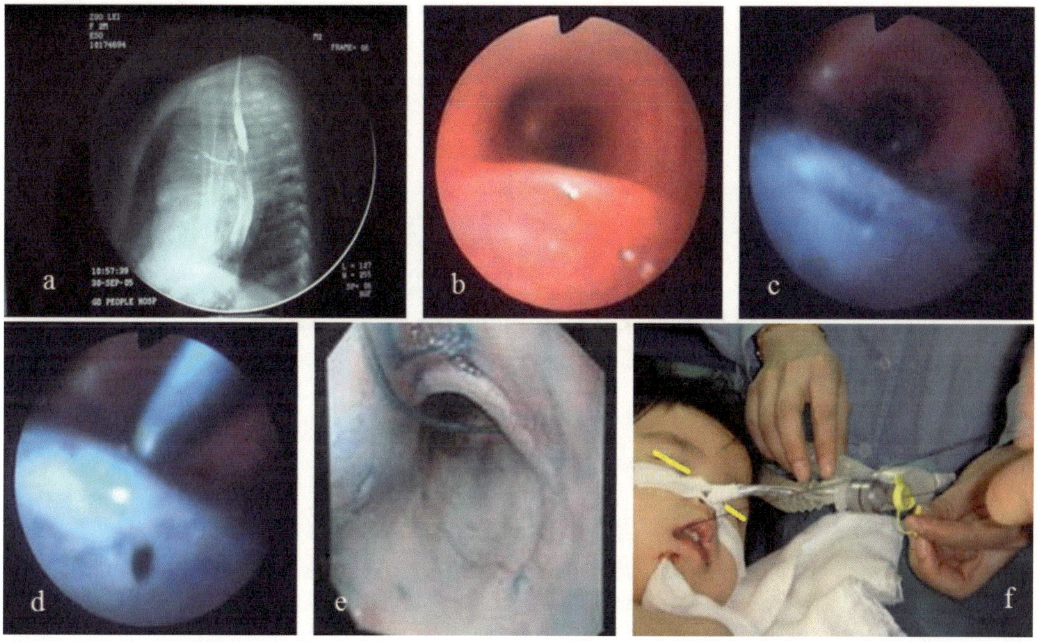

Fig. 18. (a) Shows contrast media passing through abnormal fistulous connection in the mid-esophagus during injection of meglumine diatrizoate via gastric tube. (b) Shows fistula located at the posterior tracheal wall visualized during bronchoscopy. (c) Shows color staining of the tracheal fistula after injection of methylene blue via gastroscopy. (d) Shows insertion of a guide wire towards the esophagus via bronchoscopy. (e) Shows the guide wire entering the esophagus. (f) Shows the guide wire loop between trachea and esophagus.

5.2 Laser treatment in laryngomalacia

With super-pulse or ultra-pulse technology, the CO2 laser is more precise than microscissors in resecting the desired amount of tissue without causing much bleeding. Further, depending on each individual child and clinical situation, the CO2 laser allows for additional vaporisation of tissue to achieve a tailored resection (Fig.19). If appropriate CO2 laser parameters are used, then a char-free resection with less than 50μ (four to five cells) depth of coagulation necrosis is achieved . This technique offers more versatility and precision than a microscissors resection.

Holinger et al [49] performed supraglottoplasty using CO2 laser which provided 6~9W of power with approximately 0.5mm diameter spot. The CO2 laser can relieve upper airway obstruction caused by laryngomalacia with less bleeding and higher accuracy. McClurg FL [50] summarized indications for supraglottoplasty using CO2 laser in 1994 to include the following: collapse of the glottis during inspiration, arrest of development, obstructive apnea, cor pulmonale, severe reflux and asphyxia in awake patients. Andrew et al reported

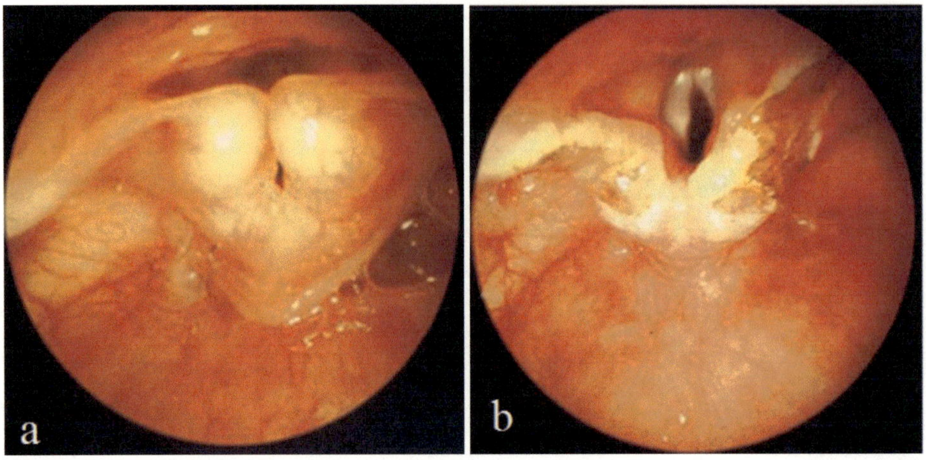

Fig. 19. (a) Inward collapse of the aryepiglottic folds. (b) CO2 laser resection of the excessive mucosa with preservation of the pharyngo-epiglottic folds.

on 76 cases of laryngomalacia over a 10 year period; CO2 laser supraglottoplasty resulted in a resolution of symptoms in 80% of the cases.

5.3 Stent insertion for tracheobronchomalacia

Tracheobronchomalacia, results in airflow limitation due to dynamic airway collapse and can be either a primary developmental abnormality of cartilage, or secondary to external compression (such as abnormal vasculature, cysts or tumor). Theoretically, insertion of an airway stent can maintain airway lumen and diameter, preventing collapse and thereby improving symptoms (Fig.1). Tracheobronchomalacia occurs fairly commonly in patients with congenital cardiovascular abnormalities with an incidence of 20-58%. Mortality may be high in patients with severe tracheobronchomalacia [51]. Bronchomalacia usually occurs in the left mainstem bronchus because of its proximity to the left atrium and left pulmonary artery, abnormal enlargement of which and pulsatility could compress the left main bronchus leading to bronchomalacia.

There are two methods to place airway stents, one surgical and the other non surgical. Fayon[51] treated 14 patients with left bronchomalacia using silicone stents with success in 6 patients (43%) ; one patient died of stent obstruction .With the development of newer types of stents and delivery devices, non surgical insertion and deployment is utilized, most often using special stent delivery device to place the stent precisely at the required location under bronchoscopic visualization.

However, it must be noted that in the pediatric age group, airway stents are infrequently used given the potential complications and limitations including formation of granulation tissue, potential for stent migration and penetration of adjacent structures. Other problems include technically difficult removal of the stent, potential for stent obstruction and death, stent fracture, the need for a larger stent placement or need to dilate the stent as the child grows and the airway diameter increases with growth and development. Currently, stents are used only in limited situations in children and when conventional therapy has failed.

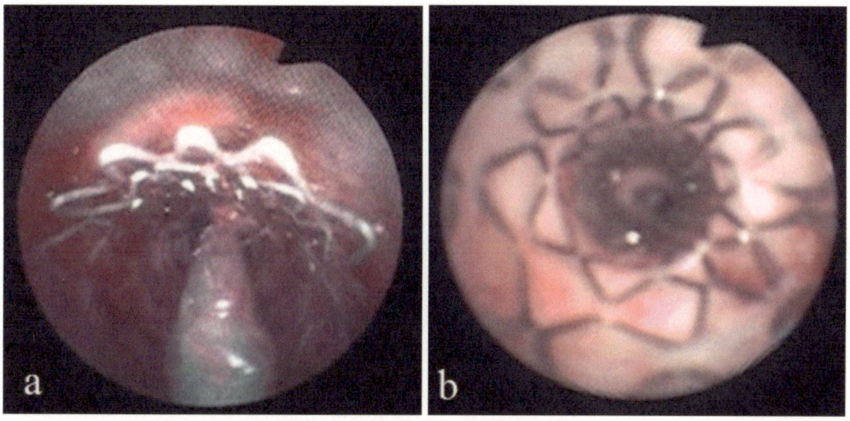

Fig. 20. (a) Expanding of a metal stent in airway carried by delivery device. (b) Full reopening of the collapsed airway with the expansion of the placed stent.

5.4 Balloon dilation for airway stenosis

The mechanism of balloon dilation of the airway relies on expanding the narrowed airway by creating longitudinal splits in the airway mucosa and tissues when the placed balloon is inflated by a pressure syringe device. The longitudinal splits around narrowed tracheal wall will be eventually filled with healing and fibrous tissue enlarging the narrowed airway (Fig.21). Balloon catheters that impart radially directed forces and can be precisely placed under bronchoscopic visualization and guidance are gradually inflated and utilized.

Cohen [52]reported a case of a 28 month old patient with congenital tracheobronchial stenosis who encountered restenosis after surgical tracheobronchoplasty which manifested as progressive dyspnea. The patient was anesthetized and tracheal and bilateral bronchial balloon dilatation was performed under fluoroscopic visualization. Andre et al[53] described balloon tracheoplasty cases in children over a 15 year period; 37 patients underwent 158 procedures for airway balloon dilation performed under bronchoscopic visualization ; with 90% of short-term efficacy and 54% long-term efficacy.

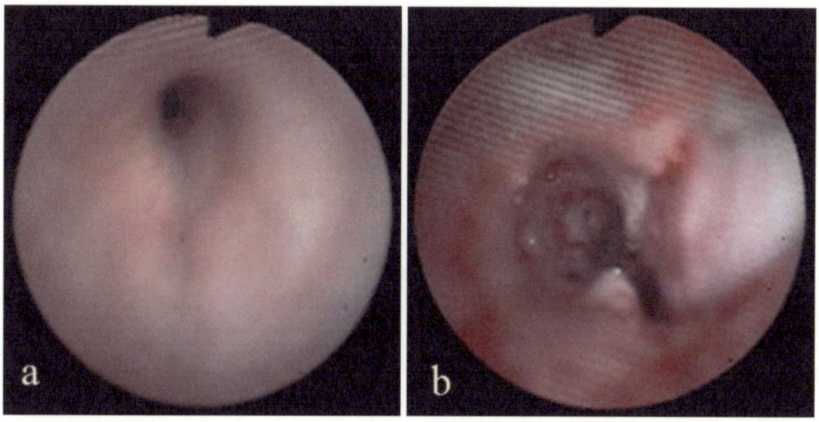

Fig. 21. (a) Narrowed mid part of trachea. (b) Narrowed tracheal segment that has been enlarged after balloon dilatation.

6. Future trends

During the past 30 years, flexible bronchoscopy has become an indispensible and useful tool in the diagnosis and management of pediatric respiratory disease. The use of the flexible bronchoscope provides significant insight into the pathogenesis of clinical pulmonary symptoms and assistance to the therapy and surgical interventions in children.

7. References

[1] Holinger LD, Congential laryngeal anomalies; in Holinger LD, Lusk RP, Greene CG(eds): Pediatric Larynogology and Bronchoesophagology. Philadelphia, Lippincott-Raven, 1997; 137-164.

[2] Chandra RK, Gerber ME, Holinger LD. Histological insight into the pathogenesis of severe laryngomalacia. Int Pediatr Otorhinolaryngol, 2001; 61:31-38.

[3] Bibi H, Khvlis E, Shoseyov D, et al. The prevalence of gastroesophageal reflux in children with tracheomalacia and larynogomalacia. Chest, 2001; 119:409-413.

[4] Midulla F, Guidi R, Tancredi G, et al. Microaspiration in infants with larynogomalacia. Laryngoscope, 2004; 114:1592-1596.

[5] Dickson JM, Richter GT, Meinzen-Derr J, et al. Secondary airway lesions in infants with laryngomalacia. Ann Otol Rhinol Laryngol, 2009; 118:37-43.

[6] Nielson DW, Ku PL, Egger M. Topical lidocaine exaggerates laryngomalacia during fllexible bronchoscope. Am Respir Crit Care Med, 2000; 161:147-151.

[7] Miyamoto, R.C., Parikh, S.R., Gellad, W., et al. Bilateral congenital vocal cord paralysis: a 16-year institutional review. Otolaryngol. Head Neck Surg, 2005; 133:241-245.

[8] Daya, H., Hosni, A., Bejar-Solar, I., et al. Pediatric vocal fold paralysis: a long-term retrospective study. Arch. Otolaryngol. Head Neck Surg, 2000; 126:21-25.

[9] Oestreicher-Kedem, Y., DeRowe, A., Nagar, H., et al. Vocal fold paralysis in infants with tracheoesophageal fistula. Ann.Otol. Rhinol. Laryngol, 2008; 117:896-901.

[10] Smith, M.E. Vocal fold paralysis in children. In: Sulica, L., Blitzer, A. (eds.) Vocal Fold Paralysis, Springer, Berlin/Heidelberg, 2006; 225-235.

[11] Sivi Bakthavachalam, James W Schroeder Jr, Lauren D Holinger. Diagnosis and Management of Type I Posterior Laryngeal, The Annals of Otology, Rhinology & Laryngology, 2010; 119:239-10.

[12] S.R. Cohen, J.W. Thompson, Ventral cleft of the larynx: a rare congenital laryngeal defect, Ann. Otol. Rhinol. Laryngol, 1990; 99:281-285.

[13] B.W. Rotenberg and R.G. Berkowitz, Delayed failure of open repair of an anterior glottic web in the neonatal time period, Int J Pediatr Otorhinolaryngol Extra, 2006; 1(3):204-206.

[14] J. Edwards, N. Tanna and S.A. Bielamowicz, Endoscopic lysis of anterior glottic webs and silicon keel placement, Ann Otol Rhinol Laryngol, 2007; 116:211-216.

[15] S. Men, A.O. Ikiz, I. Topcu, H. Cakmakci and C. Ecevit, CT and virtual endoscopy findings in congenital laryngeal web, Int J Pediatr Otorhinolaryngol, 2006; 70:1125-1127.

[16] Narcy, P., Bobin, S., Contencin, P., et al. Laryngeal anomalies in newborn infants. A propos of 687 cases. Ann. Otolaryngol. Chir. Cervicofac, 1984; 101:363-373.

[17] M. L. G. Duynstee, R. R. de Krijger, Ph. Monnier, et al. Subglottic stenosis after endolaryngeal intubation in infants and children: result of wound healing processes, International Journal of Pediatric Otorhinolaryngology, 2002; 62(1):1-9.

[18] C.M. Myer, D.M. O'Connor, R.T. Cotton, Proposed grading system for subglottic stenosis based on endotracheal tube sizes, Ann. Otol. Rhinol. Laryngol, 1994; 103:319-323.

[19] Catherine Blancheta, Richard Nicollasb, Michèle Bigorrec, et al. Management of Hemangiomas and Other Vascular Tumors. Clinics in Plastic Surgery, 2011; 38:45-63.

[20] Catherine Blancheta, Richard Nicollasb, Michèle Bigorrec, et al. Management of infantile subglottic hemangioma: Acebutolol or propranolol? Clinics in Plastic Surgery, 2011; 38:45-63.

[21] Miller BJ, Morrison MD. Congenital tracheal web - a case report. J Otolaryngol, 1978; 7:218-222.

[22] Alan C. Legasto, Jack O. Haller, Robert J. Giusti. Tracheal web. Pediatr Radiol, 2004; 34: 256-258.

[23] L.D. Hollinger, Congenital abnormalities of the larynx. In: R.E. Bchrman and R.M. Kliegman, Editors, Nelson Textbook of Pediatrics (17th ed.), Elsevier Science, Philidelphia, 2004:. 1409-1413.

[24] M.I. Ali, C.D. Brunson, J.F. Mayhew, Failed intubation secondary to complete tracheal rings: a case report and literature review, Pediatr. Anaesth, 2005; 15:890-892.

[25] W.A. Clement, N.K. Geddes, C. Best, Endoscopic carbon dioxide laser division of congenital complete tracheal rings: a new operative technique, Ann. Thorac. Surg, 2005; 76:687-689.

[26] Frenkiel S, Assimes IK, Rosales JK. Congenital tracheal diverticulum. A case report. Ann Otol Rhinol Laryngol, 1980; 89:406-408.

[27] MacKinnon D .Tracheal diverticula. J Pathol Bacteriol, 1953; 65:513-517.

[28] Caversaccio MD, Becker M, Zbaren P .Tracheal diverticulum presenting with recurrent laryngeal nerve paralysis. Ann Otol Rhinol Laryngol , 1998; 107:362-364.

[29] Hernandez JM, Pe´rez L, Batista JJ, et al. Intratracheal diverticulum. J Bronchol, 2005; 12:104-105.

[30] Restrepo S, Villamil MA, Rojas IC, et al. Association of two respiratory congenital anomalies: tracheal diverticulum and cystic adenomatoid malformation of the lung. Pediatr Radiol, 2004; 34:263-266.

[31] Ghaye B, Szapiro D, Fanchamps J-M, et al. Congenital bronchial abnormalities revisited. Radiographics, 2001; 21(1):105–119.

[32] Bertrand P, Navarro H, Caussade S, et al. Airway anomalies in children with Down syndrome: endoscopic findings. Pediatr Pulmonol, 2003 Aug; 36(2):137-41.

[33] Carden K, Boiselle PM, Waltz D, et al. Tracheomalacia and tracheobronchomalacia in children and adults: an in-depth review of a common disorder. Chest, 2005; 127:984-1005.

[34] Mair EA, Parsons DS. Pediatric tracheobronchomalacia and major airway collapse. Ann Otol Rhinol Laryngol, 1992; 101:300-309.

[35] Blair GK, Cohen R, Filler RM. Treatment of tracheomalacia: eight years' experience. J Pediatr Surg, 1986; 21:781-785.

[36] Andrews TM, Myers CMI, Gray SP. Abnormalities of the bony thorax causing tracheobronchial compression. Int J Pediatr Otorhinolaryngol, 1990; 19:139-144.

[37] Jacobs IN, Wetmore RF, Tom LW, et al. Tracheobronchomalacia in children. Arch Otolaryngol Head Neck Surg, 1994; 120:154-158.

[38] Shaha AR, Alfonso AE, Jaffe BM. Operative treatment of substernal goiters. Head Neck Surg, 1989; 11:325-330.

[39] Boogaard R, Huijsmans SH, Pijnenburg MWH, et al. Tracheomalacia and bronchomalacia in children: Incidence and patients characteristics. Chest, 2005; 128:3391-3397.

[40] Houben CH, Curry JI. Current status of prenatal diagnosis, operative management and outcome of esophageal atresia/tracheo-esophageal fistula. Prenatal Diagnosis, 2008; 28(7):667-675.

[41] Kluth D, Fiegel H. The Embryology of the Foregut. Semin Pediatr Surg, 2003; 12:3-9.

[42] Holinger, L.D., Green, C.G., Benjamin, B., et al. Tracheobronchial tree. Pediatric Laryngology and Bronchoesophagology, 1997; 187–214.

[43] Das, B.B., Nagaraj, A., Rao, A.H., et al. Tracheal agenesis: report of three cases and review of the literature. Am. J. Perinatol, 2002; 19:395-400.

[44] Floyd, J., Campbell Jr., D.C., Dominy, D.E.. Agenesis of the trachea. Am. Rev. Respir. Dis, 1962; 86: 557-560.

[45] Monnier Philippe (Ed.), Congenital Tracheal Anomalies. Pediatric Airway Surgery: Management of Laryngotracheal Stenosis in Infants and Children, 2011; 157-179.

[46] Hiyama, E., Yokoyama, T., Ichikawa, T., et al. Surgical management of tracheal agenesis. J. Thorac. Cardiovasc. Surg, 1994; 108: 830-833.

[47] G. Blanco-Rodríguez, J. Penchyna-Grub, A. Trujillo-Ponce, et al. Preoperative Catheterization of H-Type Tracheoesophageal Fistula to Facilitate its Localization and Surgical Correction. Eur J Pediatr Surg, 2006; 16:14-17.

[48] N.M. Garcia, J.W. Thompson, D.B. Shaul. Definitive Localisation of Isolated Tracheoesophageal Fistula Using Bronchoscopy and Esophagoscopy for Guide Wire Placement. Pediatric Surgery, 1998; 33:1645-1647.

[49] Holinger LD, Konior RJ. Surgical management of severe laryngomalacia. Laryngoscope, 1989; 99(2):136-42.

[50] McClurg FL, Evans DA. Laser laryngoplasty for laryngomalacia. Laryngoscope, 1994; 104:247-52.

[51] Fayon M, Donato L, de Blic J. French experience of silicone tracheobronchial stenting in children. Pediatr Pulmonol, 2005; 39(1): 21-27.

[52] Cohen MD, Weber TR, Rao CC. Balloon dilatation of tracheal and bronchial stenosis. AJR Am J Roentgenol, 1984; 142(3):477-8.

[53] Andre Hebra, David D.Powell, Charles D. Smith, et al. Balloon traceoplasty in children: results of a 15-year experience. Journal of Pediatric Surgery, 1991; 26(8):957-961.